Substance Abuse Treatment: Addressing the Specific Needs of Women

A Treatment Improvement Protocol

TIP
51

U.S. DEPARTMENT OF HEALTH AND HUMAN SERVICES
Substance Abuse and Mental Health Services Administration

1 Choke Cherry Road
Rockville, MD 20857

Acknowledgments

This publication was prepared under contract numbers 270-99-7072 and 270-04-7049 by the Knowledge Application Program (KAP) with the Substance Abuse and Mental Health Services Administration (SAMHSA), U.S. Department of Health and Human Services (HHS). Christina Currier served as the Government Project Officer.

Electronic Access and Printed Copies

This publication may be ordered from or downloaded from SAMHSA's Publications Ordering Web page at http://store.samhsa.gov. Or, please call SAMHSA at 1-877-SAMHSA-7 (1-877-726-4727) (English and Español).

Recommended Citation

Center for Substance Abuse Treatment. *Substance Abuse Treatment: Addressing the Specific Needs of Women*. Treatment Improvement Protocol (TIP) Series, No. 51. HHS Publication No. (SMA) 15-4426. Rockville, MD: Center for Substance Abuse Treatment, 2009.

Originating Office

Quality Improvement and Workforce Development Branch, Division of Services Improvement, Center for Substance Abuse Treatment, Substance Abuse and Mental Health Services Administration, 1 Choke Cherry Road, Rockville, MD 20857.

HHS Publication No. (SMA) 15-4426

Printed 2009
Revised 2010, 2012, 2013, 2014, and 2015

Contents

Figures

Advice to the Clinician and Administrator Boxes

What Is a TIP?

Treatment Improvement Protocols (TIPs) are developed by the Center for Substance Abuse Treatment (CSAT), part of the Substance Abuse and Mental Health Services Administration (SAMHSA) within the U.S. Department of Health and Human Services (HHS). Each TIP involves the development of topic-specific best-practice guidelines for the prevention and treatment of substance use and mental disorders. TIPs draw on the experience and knowledge of clinical, research, and administrative experts of various forms of treatment and prevention. TIPs are distributed to facilities and individuals across the country. Published TIPs can be accessed via the Internet at http://store.samhsa.gov.

Although each consensus-based TIP strives to include an evidence base for the practices it recommends, SAMHSA recognizes that behavioral health is continually evolving, and research frequently lags behind the innovations pioneered in the field. A major goal of each TIP is to convey "front-line" information quickly but responsibly. If research supports a particular approach, citations are provided. When no citation is provided, the information is based on the collective clinical knowledge and experience of the consensus panel.

Consensus Panel

Note: The information given indicates each participant's affiliation as of 2008, when the panel was convened, and may no longer reflect the individual's current affiliation.

Chair

Norma B. Finkelstein, Ph.D., M.S.W.
Executive Director
Institute for Health & Recovery
Cambridge, Massachusetts

Co-Chair

Juana Mora, Ph.D.
Professor
Northridge Chicano/a Studies Department
California State University, Northridge
Northridge, California

Workgroup Leaders

Karen Allen, Ph.D., R.N., FAAN
Professor/Chair
Department of Nursing
Andrews University
Berrien Springs, Michigan

Hortensia Amaro, Ph.D.
Distinguished Professor
Center on Health and Social Science Research
    Director
Institute on Urban Health Research
Northeastern University
Boston, Massachusetts

Stephanie S. Covington, Ph.D., LCSW
Co-Director
Center for Gender and Justice
Institute for Relational Development
La Jolla, California

Francine Feinberg, Psy.D., CISCW
Executive Director
Meta House
Whitefish Bay, Wisconsin

Beth Glover Reed, Ph.D.
Associate Professor
Social Work and Women's Studies
School of Social Work
University of Michigan
Ann Arbor, Michigan

Brenda L. Underhill, M.S., CAC
President
Underhill and Associates
El Cerrito, California

Panelists

Belinda Biscoe, Ph.D.
Assistant Vice President for Public and
    Community Services
Director, Region VII Comprehensive Assistance
    Center
Director, Education, Training, Evaluation,
    Assessment and Measurement Department
    (E-TEAM)
University of Oklahoma
Norman, Oklahoma

Vivian B. Brown, Ph.D.
Founder, Board Member Emeritus
PROTOTYPES
Culver City, California

Margaret A. Cramer, Ph.D.
Clinical Psychologist/Instructor
Massachusetts General Hospital
Boston, Massachusetts

Gloria Grijalva-Gonzales
Certified Sr. Substance Abuse Case Manager/
    Counselor
Allies Project
San Joaquin County
Stockton, California

Tonda L. Hughes, Ph.D., R.N.
Professor
Department of Health Systems Science
University of Illinois at Chicago
Chicago, Illinois

Marty A. Jessup, Ph.D., R.N., M.S.
Associate Adjunct Professor
Department of Family Health Care Nursing
Institute for Health and Aging
University of California, San Francisco
San Francisco, California

Karol A. Kaltenbach, Ph.D.
Clinical Associate Professor of Pediatrics,
    Psychiatry and Human Behavior
Director, Maternal Addiction Treatment
    Education and Research
Department of Pediatrics
Jefferson Medical College
Thomas Jefferson University
Philadelphia, Pennsylvania

Robin A. LaDue, Ph.D.
Clinical Psychologist
Department of Psychiatry and
Behavioral Sciences
University of Washington
Renton, Washington

LaVerne R. Saunders, B.S.N., R.N., M.S.
Founder/Partner
Dorrington & Saunders and Associates
Framingham, Massachusetts

Starleen Scott-Robbins, M.S.W., LCSW
Women's Treatment Coordinator
Best Practice Consultant
Developmental Disabilities and Substance Abuse
    Services
Division of Mental Health
North Carolina Department of Health and
    Human Services
Raleigh, North Carolina

Sally J. Stevens, Ph.D.
Executive Director
Southwest Institute for Research on Women
University of Arizona
Tucson, Arizona

Sharon Wilsnack, Ph.D.
Professor
Department of Clinical Neuroscience
Medical School for the Public
School of Medicine & Health Sciences
University of North Dakota
Grand Forks, North Dakota

Rita Zimmer, M.P.H.
Founder
Women in Need, Inc.
New York, New York

Editorial Board

Note: The information given indicates each participant's affiliation during the time the board was convened and may no longer reflect the individual's current affiliation.

KAP Expert Panel and Federal Government Participants

Note: The information given indicates each participant's affiliation during the time the panel was convened and may no longer reflect the individual's current affiliation.

Barry S. Brown, Ph.D.
Adjunct Professor
University of North Carolina at Wilmington
Carolina Beach, North Carolina

Jacqueline Butler, M.S.W., LISW, LPCC, CCDC III, CJS
Professor of Clinical Psychiatry
College of Medicine
University of Cincinnati
Cincinnati, Ohio

Deion Cash
Executive Director
Community Treatment and Correction
    Center, Inc.
Canton, Ohio

Debra A. Claymore, M.Ed.Adm.
Owner/Chief Executive Officer
WC Consulting, LLC
Loveland, Colorado

Carlo C. DiClemente, Ph.D.
Chair
Department of Psychology
University of Maryland Baltimore County
Baltimore, Maryland

Catherine E. Dube, Ed.D.
Independent Consultant
Brown University
Providence, Rhode Island

Jerry P. Flanzer, D.S.W., LCSW, CAC
Chief, Services
Division of Clinical and Services Research
National Institute on Drug Abuse
Bethesda, Maryland

Michael Galer, D.B.A.
Chairman of the Graduate School of Business
University of Phoenix - Greater Boston Campus
Braintree, Massachusetts

Renata J. Henry, M.Ed.
Director
Division of Alcoholism, Drug Abuse,
and Mental Health
Delaware Department of Health and Social
    Services
New Castle, Delaware

Joel Hochberg, M.A.
President
Asher & Partners
Los Angeles, California

Jack Hollis, Ph.D.
Associate Director
Center for Health Research
Kaiser Permanente
Portland, Oregon

Mary Beth Johnson, M.S.W.
Director
Addiction Technology Transfer Center
University of Missouri—Kansas City
Kansas City, Missouri

Eduardo Lopez, B.S.
Executive Producer
EVS Communications
Washington, DC

Holly A. Massett, Ph.D.
Academy for Educational Development
Washington, DC

Diane Miller
Chief
Scientific Communications Branch
National Institute on Alcohol Abuse
    and Alcoholism
Bethesda, Maryland

Harry B. Montoya, M.A.
President/Chief Executive Officer
Hands Across Cultures
Espanola, New Mexico

Richard K. Ries, M.D.
Director/Professor
Outpatient Mental Health Services
Dual Disorder Programs
Seattle, Washington

Gloria M. Rodriguez, D.S.W.
Research Scientist
Division of Addiction Services
NJ Department of Health and Senior Services
Trenton, New Jersey

Everett Rogers, Ph.D.
Center for Communications Programs
Johns Hopkins University
Baltimore, Maryland

Jean R. Slutsky, P.A., M.S.P.H.
Senior Health Policy Analyst
Agency for Healthcare Research & Quality
Rockville, Maryland

Nedra Klein Weinreich, M.S.
President
Weinreich Communications
Canoga Park, California

Clarissa Wittenberg
Director
Office of Communications and Public Liaison
National Institute of Mental Health
Kensington, Maryland

Consulting Members:

Paul Purnell, M.A.
Social Solutions, L.L.C.
Potomac, Maryland

Scott Ratzan, M.D., M.P.A., M.A.
Academy for Educational Development
Washington, DC

Thomas W. Valente, Ph.D.
Director, Master of Public Health Program
Department of Preventive Medicine
School of Medicine
University of Southern California
Alhambra, California

Patricia A. Wright, Ed.D.
Independent Consultant
Baltimore, Maryland

Foreword

The Substance Abuse and Mental Health Services Administration (SAMHSA) is the agency within the U.S. Department of Health and Human Services that leads public health efforts to advance the behavioral health of the nation. SAMHSA's mission is to reduce the impact of substance abuse and mental illness on America's communities.

The Treatment Improvement Protocol (TIP) series fulfills SAMHSA's mission to improve prevention and treatment of substance use and mental disorders by providing best practices guidance to clinicians, program administrators, and payers. TIPs are the result of careful consideration of all relevant clinical and health services research findings, demonstration experience, and implementation requirements. A panel of non-Federal clinical researchers, clinicians, program administrators, and patient advocates debates and discusses their particular area of expertise until they reach a consensus on best practices. Field reviewers then review and critique this panel's work.

The talent, dedication, and hard work that TIPs panelists and reviewers bring to this highly participatory process have helped bridge the gap between the promise of research and the needs of practicing clinicians and administrators to serve, in the most scientifically sound and effective ways, people in need of behavioral health services. We are grateful to all who have joined with us to contribute to advances in the behavioral health field.

Pamela S. Hyde, J.D.
Administrator
Substance Abuse and Mental Health Services Administration

Daryl W. Kade
Acting Director
Center for Substance Abuse Treatment
Substance Abuse and Mental Health Services Administration

Executive Summary

Clinicians and program administrators are increasingly aware of the important differences between men and women with regard to the physical effects of substance use and the specific issues related to substance use disorders. They are also recognizing that these differences have an impact on treatment—that gender does make a difference. When women's specific needs are addressed from the outset, improved treatment engagement, retention, and outcomes are the result.

This TIP endorses a biopsychosociocultural framework based on clinical practice and research centered on women. By placing emphasis on the importance of context, many topics examine the role of factors that influence women's substance use from initiation of use to engagement of continuing care treatment services, i.e., relationships, gender socialization, and culture. The knowledge and models presented here are grounded in women's experiences, built on women's strengths, and based on best, promising, or research-based practices. The primary goal of this TIP is to assist substance abuse treatment providers in offering effective, up-to-date treatment to adult women with substance use disorders.

The TIP is organized into eight chapters. The following section summarizes the content of each chapter to present an overview of this publication.

Creating the Context

The consensus panel for this TIP proposes that substance abuse treatment for women be approached from a perspective that encompasses the contexts of women's lives. These contexts include a woman's social and economic environment; her relationships with family, extended family, and support systems; and the impact of gender and culture. As a framework to explore women's substance use disorders, treatment needs, and treatment approaches, this TIP adopted two systemic models: Bronfenbrenner's ecological model and CSAT's *Comprehensive Substance Abuse Treatment Model for Women and Their Children*. Both models endorse the relevance and influence of multisystems and their bidirectional influence upon women's lives.

What makes gender an important clinical issue in substance abuse treatment? Are there gender differences in the development and pattern of substance use disorders? Do these differences warrant specific treatment approaches? To date, there is considerable evidence denoting that gender differences do exist, and these differences begin with early risk factors for substance use and extend throughout the course of treatment and recovery. Grounded in research, this TIP begins with unique biopsychosocial and developmental issues of women that create or intensify gender differences across the continuum of care. Knowledge of these unique factors is essential for treatment providers to fully understand the contexts of women's lives and their needs.

Based on the premise and knowledge that women are biopsychosocially unique in ways that are relevant to substance use, substance use disorders, and substance abuse treatment, this consensus panel endorses core principles for gender responsive treatment for women, such as—

- Acknowledging the importance as well as the role of the socioeconomic issues and differences among women.
- Promoting cultural competence specific to women.
- Recognizing the role as well as the significance of relationships in women's lives.
- Addressing women's unique health concerns.
- Endorsing a developmental perspective.
- Attending to the relevance and influence of various caregiver roles that women often assume throughout the course of their lives.
- Recognizing that ascribed roles and gender expectations across cultures affect societal attitudes toward women who abuse substances.
- Adopting a trauma-informed perspective.
- Using a strengths-based model for women's treatment.
- Incorporating an integrated and multidisciplinary approach to women's treatment.
- Maintaining a gender responsive treatment environment across settings.

- Supporting the development of gender competency specific to women's issues.

Patterns of Use: From Initiation to Treatment

Numerous factors influence the reasons for initiation of substance use among women, and a number of these factors are more prevalent among women than men. Women often report that stress, negative affect, and relationships precipitate initial use. In fact, women are often introduced to substance use by a significant relationship such as boyfriend, family member, or close friend. Though genetics also may be a significant risk factor for women, more research supports familial influence—a combination of genetic and environment effects. Less is known about familial influence of illicit drugs, but parental alcohol use increases the prevalence of alcohol use disorders among women by at least 50 percent. Family of origin characteristics play a role too. Exposure to chaotic, argumentative, and violent households, or being expected to take on adult responsibilities as a child, are other factors associated with initiation and prevalence of substance use disorders among the female population.

Women are significantly influenced by relationships, relationship status, and the effects of a partner's substance abuse. Women dependent on substances are more likely to have partners who have substance use disorders. At times, women perceive shared drug use with their partner as a means of connection or of maintaining the relationship. Often, rituals surrounding drug use are initiated by a male partner, and women bear more risk in contracting HIV/AIDS and hepatitis by sharing needles or having sexual relationships with men who inject drugs. Relationship status similarly influences use and potential development of substance use disorders. Marriage appears protective, whereas separated, never married, or divorced women are at greater risk for use and the development of substance use disorders. Relationship influence does not stop at the point of treatment entry; relationships also significantly influence treatment engagement, retention, and outcome among women.

Other risk factors associated with initiation of use and the prevalence of substance use disorders include sensation-seeking, symptoms of depression and anxiety, posttraumatic stress and eating disorders, and difficulty in regulating affect. Women with a history of trauma, including interpersonal and childhood sexual abuse, are highly represented in substance abuse samples. In addition, sociocultural issues play a significant role across the continuum beginning with enhanced risk for substance use. Degree of acculturation, experiences of discrimination, and socioeconomic status are prominent risk factors from the outset but continue to influence women's substance use, health status, treatment access, and help-seeking behavior.

Among women, six patterns of substance use clearly emerge from empirical data. First, the gender gap is narrowing for substance use across ethnicities, particularly among young women. Second, women are more likely to be introduced to and initiate substance use through significant relationships, while marital status appears to play a protective role. Third, women accelerate to injecting drugs at a faster rate than men, and rituals and high-risk behaviors surrounding drug injection are directly influenced by significant relationships. Fourth, women's earlier patterns of use (including age of initiation, amount, and frequency) are positively associated with higher risks for dependency. Next, women are more likely to temporarily alter their pattern of use in response to caregiver responsibilities. And last, women progress faster from initiation of use to the development of substance-related adverse consequences.

Substance use is not as prevalent among women as it is among men, but women are as likely as men to develop substance use disorders after initiation. Women who are pregnant are likely to reduce or remain abstinent during pregnancy; however, continued use is associated with a wide range of issues and effects—from less prenatal care to potential irreparable harm to the child from fetal exposure. Among those entering treatment, women are more likely to report drug use as the main reason for admission.

Physiological Effects of Alcohol, Drugs, and Tobacco on Women

Women develop substance use disorders in less time than men. Some factors that either influence or compound the physiological effects of drugs and alcohol include ethnicity, health disparity, socioeconomic status, developmental issues, aging, and co-occurring conditions. Although research on the physiological effects of alcohol and illicit drugs on women is limited and often inconclusive, significant differences have been found in the way women and men metabolize alcohol. Women have more complications and more severe problems from alcohol use than do men, and these complications and problems develop more rapidly. This phenomenon is known as "telescoping." Complications include liver disease and other organ damage; cardiac-related conditions such as hypertension; reproductive consequences; osteoporosis; cognitive and other neurological effects; breast and other cancers; and greater susceptibility and progression of infections and infectious diseases, including HIV/AIDS and hepatitis C virus (HCV).

Although many physiological effects of licit and illicit drugs have not been well studied, research has shown that abuse of substances such as stimulants, opioids, and some prescription (e.g., anxiolytics, narcotic analgesics) and over-the-counter (e.g., laxatives, diuretics, diet pills) drugs causes adverse effects on women's menstrual cycles and gastrointestinal, neuromuscular, and cardiac systems, among others. With regard to nicotine use, women who smoke increase their risk of lung cancer. Currently, cancer is the second leading cause of death among women, with mortality rates higher for lung cancer than breast cancer. Other physiological consequences of tobacco use include, but are not limited to, increased risks for peptic ulcers, Crohn's disease, estrogen deficiencies, strokes, and atherosclerosis. Women who smoke are more likely to have chronic obstructive pulmonary disease and coronary heart disease.

Women who use alcohol, drugs, or tobacco while pregnant or nursing expose their fetuses or infants to these substances as well. The most thoroughly examined effect of alcohol on birth outcomes is fetal alcohol syndrome, which involves growth retardation, central nervous system and neurodevelopmental abnormalities, and craniofacial abnormalities. Alcohol and drug use by pregnant women is associated with many complications, including spontaneous abortion, prematurity, low birth weight, premature separation of the placenta from the uterine wall, neonatal abstinence syndrome, and fetal abnormalities. Likewise, women who are pregnant and use tobacco are more likely to deliver premature and low birth weight infants.

Screening and Assessment

Understanding the extent and nature of a woman's substance use disorder and its interaction with other areas of her life is essential for accurate diagnosis and successful treatment. This understanding can be acquired through screening and assessment. Screening is typically a brief process for identifying whether certain conditions may exist and usually involves a limited set of questions to establish whether a more thorough evaluation and referral(s) are needed. Sociocultural factors—ethnicity, culture, acculturation level, language, and socioeconomic status—are particularly relevant in screening and assessment selection, in determining the appropriateness of the instruments, and in interpreting the subsequent results. Sociocultural and socioeconomic characteristics of the client can affect testing expectations and behavior of both the counselor and client during the screening and assessment process; e.g., the client's distrust and subsequent reluctance in the testing process or the counselor's expectation that a woman with lower socioeconomic status will have a positive screening for alcohol or drug use.

For women, general alcohol and drug screening that determines current or at-risk status for drug and alcohol use during pregnancy is essential. However, healthcare professionals sometimes overlook the necessity of drug and alcohol screening for older, Asian, and/ or middle- and upper-class women who are pregnant. Screening is more likely based on preconceived beliefs concerning greater prevalence of substance abuse among women from diverse ethnic groups. Counselors and intake personnel may also alter their behavior when working with diverse populations, such as eye contact, body language, and communication styles, that ultimately affect clients' responses and trust in the screening process.

Other screenings involve the determination of co-occurring risks, conditions, or disorders, including general mental disorders, mood and anxiety disorders, risk of harm to self or others, history of childhood trauma and interpersonal violence, and eating disorders. Considering women's likely involvement with health care providers, screening for substance use and abuse should be a standard practice. Yet, the implementation of screening, regardless of setting, is only as good as the protocol in providing feedback, referral, and follow-up. Screening is not an intervention. What makes the difference is how a woman's positive endorsement of screening questions leads to feedback, referral, further assessment, and intervention, if warranted.

The difference between screening and assessment is that assessment examines several domains in a client's life in detail so that diagnoses can be made for substance use disorders and possible co-occurring mental disorders. Assessment is an ongoing process in which the counselor forms an increasingly clearer picture of the client's issues, how they can best be addressed, and how the client is changing over time. An assessment interview, such as a structured psychosocial interview, an unstructured psychosocial and cultural history, and/or the Addiction Severity Index, needs sufficient time to complete. The degree to which it is possible or advisable to probe in depth in different areas of functioning depends on the individual issues, the needs of the woman, the complexity of her issues, and the level of rapport between the client and clinician. Equally important, assessment processes should explore coping styles, strengths, and available support systems. An assessment process would not be complete without a health assessment and medical examination.

In sum, screening and assessment for women must be approached from a perspective that allows for and affirms cultural relevance and strengths. Whenever possible, instruments that have norms established for specific population groups should be used. Counselors' sensitivity to the clients' cultural values and beliefs, language, acculturation level, literacy level, and emotional ability to respond facilitates the assessment process and helps women engage in treatment.

Treatment Engagement, Placement, and Planning

Women face many obstacles and challenges in engaging in treatment services: lack of collaboration among social service systems, limited options for women who are pregnant, lack of culturally congruent programming, few resources for women with children, fear of loss of child custody, and the stigma of substance abuse. On one hand, intake personnel and counselors can help women tackle and overcome personal barriers to treatment (such as issues of motivation and shame); yet, on the other hand, programming and administrative policies must address obstacles surrounding program structure, interagency coordination, and service delivery to improve treatment engagement. In recent years, more effective engagement strategies have been implemented. Outreach services, pretreatment intervention groups, and comprehensive and coordinated case management can effectively address the numerous barriers and the array of complex problems that women often express in their role as caregivers.

Treatment placement decisions are based not only on the woman's individual needs and the severity of her substance use disorder but also on the treatment options available in the community, her financial circumstances, and available healthcare coverage. To determine treatment placement, the American Society of Addiction Medicine's Patient Placement Criteria, Second Edition Revised (ASAM's PPC-

2R), are used widely, and the levels determined by these criteria are useful to standardize treatment placement. To date, empirical literature supporting specific placement criteria for women is limited. The treatment levels suggested by the consensus panel and supported by ASAM criteria include pretreatment or early intervention; detoxification; outpatient treatment; intensive outpatient treatment (IOT); residential and inpatient treatment; and medically managed, intensive inpatient treatment. Specific placement criteria must also account for pregnancy, child placement, and children services. Treatment services for women must extend beyond standard care to address specific needs for women, pregnant women, and women with children such as medical services, health promotion, life skills, family- and child-related treatment services, comprehensive and coordinated case management, and mental health services.

When clients participate fully in decisions related to treatment, they are more likely to understand the process and develop realistic expectations of treatment. Active involvement of clients in all aspects of treatment planning and placement significantly contributes to both recovery and empowerment and is essential to the development of meaningful, effective services for women.

Substance Abuse Among Specific Population Groups and Settings

Women who are of different racial and ethnic groups, different sexual orientations, in the criminal justice system, living in rural areas, older, and who speak languages other than English are among the population groups that may experience unique challenges that affect their substance use or abuse and its treatment.

The risk for substance abuse and its consequences and optimal processes for treatment and recovery differ by gender, race, ethnicity, sexual orientation, and other factors. The complex interplay of culture and health—as well as the influence of differing attitudes toward, definitions of, and beliefs about health and substance use among cultural groups—affects the psychosocial development of women and their alcohol, drug, and tobacco use and abuse. Women's risks for substance abuse are understood best in the social and historical context in which the influences of gender, race and ethnicity, education, economic status, age, geographic location, sexual orientation, and other factors converge. Understanding group differences across segments of the population of women is critical to designing and implementing effective substance abuse treatment programs for women.

Training helps staff members recognize the individual and group strengths and resiliency factors that can assist women from diverse identity groups in recovery. These include beliefs regarding health care and substance abuse; the value the individual or identity group places on family and spirituality; the effects of group history on current behaviors; how women are socialized in a particular culture; and the flexibility of gender norms, communication styles, rituals, the status of women, the stigma the group or individual faces, and attitudes toward self-disclosure and help-seeking behavior.

Substance Abuse Treatment for Women

Gender does not appear to predict retention in substance abuse treatment. Women are as likely as men to stay in treatment once treatment is initiated. Factors that encourage a woman to stay in treatment include supportive therapy, a collaborative therapeutic alliance, onsite child care and children services, and other integrated and comprehensive treatment services. Sociodemographics also play a role in treatment retention. Studies suggest that support and participation of significant others, being older, and having at least a high school education are important factors that improve retention. Criminal justice system or child protective service involvement also is associated with longer lengths of treatment. Women are more likely to stay in treatment if they have had prior successful experiences in other life areas and possess confidence in the treatment process and outcome. Although pregnancy may motivate women in initiating treatment, studies suggest that pregnant women do not stay in treatment as long and that retention may be significantly affected by stage of pregnancy and the presence of co-occurring psychiatric disorders.

Limited research is available highlighting specific therapeutic approaches for women outside of trauma-informed services. In recent years, more attention has been given to effective women's treatment programming across systems with considerable emphasis on integrated care and the identification of specific treatment issues and needs for women. Gender specific factors that influence the treatment process and recovery evolve around the importance of relationships, the influence of family, the role of substance use in sexuality, the prevalence and history of trauma and violence, and common patterns of co-occurring disorders. Among women with substance use and co-occurring mental disorders, diagnoses of posttraumatic stress and other anxiety disorders, postpartum depression and other mood disorders, and eating disorders are more prevalent than among men who are in treatment for substance use disorders. Consequently, clinical strategies, treatment programming, and administrative treatment policies must address these issues to adequately treat women. Likewise, women often need clinical and treatment services tailored to effectively address pregnancy, child care, children services, and parenting skills.

Recovery Management and Administrative Considerations

Empirical data suggest that women are as likely as men to attend continuing care services. Transition from a more intensive level of care to less intensive services has proven to be challenging for all clients, but evidence suggests that women will continue with services if they stay within the same agency and/or effort is made to connect them to the new service provider prior to transition.

Gender does not consistently predict treatment outcome. For example, women have comparable abstinent rates with men and are as likely to complete treatment. Even so, women are more likely to have positive treatment outcomes in the following ways: less incarceration, higher rates of employment, and more established recovery-oriented social support systems. Women and men do not differ in relapse rates. It is more likely that individual characteristics hold the key in determining who may be a greater risk for relapse. However, there is a delineation of the types of risks and triggers that make women versus men more vulnerable to relapse, and women exhibit different emotional and behavioral responses during and after relapse. Women report more interpersonal problems and strong negative affect, including symptoms of depression, severe traumatic stress reactions to early childhood trauma, and low self-worth, as precipitants of relapse. They also display a lack of coping skills, greater difficulty in severing their connections with individuals who use, and a failure in establishing new recovery-oriented friends. Conversely, women who relapse are more likely to seek help and have shorter relapse episodes.

Other considerations in providing treatment to women involve programmatic and administrative issues. First, full participation of clients as partners in treatment is important, and both the program and client will benefit if they are involved in program development and serve in an advisory capacity. Programs will likely improve the quality of services and clients will benefit from an increase in self-efficacy, the attainment of specific skills, and a reduced stigma from substance abuse treatment. Gender-responsive treatment involves a safe and non-punitive atmosphere, where staff hold a hopeful and positive attitude toward women and show investment in learning about women's experiences, treatment needs, and appropriate interventions. Administrators need to invest in staff training and supervision and show a commitment to training beyond immediate services. Training should include other social and healthcare facilities and personnel within the community to enhance awareness, identify women with substance use disorders, and increase appropriate referrals. As research, programming, and clinical experience expand along gender lines in substance abuse treatment, clinicians and administrators alike will have considerable opportunities in adapting new standards of care for women.

1 Creating the Context

Overview

Women with substance use disorders have unique biopsychosocial needs that should be addressed if their treatment is to be successful. This TIP examines the current state of women's substance abuse treatment needs, approaches, and experience; highlights promising strategies and best practices for treatment counselors working with female clients; and explores evidence-based research and clinical issues that affect treatment for women. The primary goals of this TIP are to help substance abuse treatment counselors and administrators provide effective treatment for women and to assist clinicians in equipping their female clients with the tools they need to maintain recovery.

Following is an introduction to many of the themes and issues discussed in greater depth in later chapters. This chapter presents a guiding framework for treatment of women who have substance use disorders. It highlights the multiple contexts of women's lives and treatment issues, provides gender responsive principles of treatment, and presents the unique biopsychosocial needs that characterize the issues women face in treatment. The chapter concludes with a discussion on guidelines for readers and definitions of terms and concepts used in this TIP.

Creating the Context

According to the Substance Abuse and Mental Health Services Administration's (SAMHSA's) National Survey on Drug Use and Health (NSDUH), 6.2 percent of females ages 12 and older were classified with substance dependence or abuse in 2004, but only 0.9 percent of females received treatment in 2004 (SAMHSA 2005).

The medical, social, emotional, and financial consequences and costs of these disorders to women's families and society are enormous.

By and large, women with substance use disorders must find a way to support themselves and their children, often with little experience or education and few job skills. They frequently have to overcome feelings of guilt and shame for how they treated their children while abusing substances. When a woman becomes pregnant, her motivation to seek treatment may rise greatly. However, pregnancy itself can be a barrier to treatment because substance abuse treatment programs are not always able to admit pregnant women or to provide the services required, such as medically indicated bed rest, transportation to prenatal care, and nutritious meals (Jessup et al. 2003). Some women fear the negative consequences that will result if their substance abuse becomes known. In many States, pregnant and parenting women can be reported to child protective services, lose custody of their children, or be prosecuted for using drugs. On top of additional healthcare needs, substance use during pregnancy confers stigma and shame, which may create another challenge in treatment.

A high proportion of women with substance use disorders have histories of trauma, often perpetrated by persons they both knew and trusted. A woman might have experienced sexual or physical abuse or witnessed violence as a child. She may be experiencing domestic violence such as battering by a partner or rape as an adult (Finkelstein 1994; Young and Gardner 1997). These traumas contribute to the treatment needs for women.

The societal stigma toward women who abuse substances tends to be greater than that toward men, and this stigma can prevent women from seeking or admitting they need help. Women who use alcohol and illicit drugs often have great feelings of shame and guilt, have low levels of self-esteem and self-efficacy, and often are devalued or disliked by other women. These feelings make it difficult for women to seek help or feel that they deserve to be helped—creating yet more treatment needs that must be addressed. Gender role expectations in many

cultures result in further stigmatization of substance use; additional challenges face women who are of color, disabled, lesbians, older, and poor.

Over the last decade, women with substance use disorders have increasingly been the subject of scientific study. Studies have explored the effects of alcohol and illicit drugs on pregnancy in greater detail, best practices in substance abuse treatment for women, the impact of trauma and the need for trauma-informed services, and the importance of incorporating a gender responsive framework. More recently, research is burgeoning in the area of outcome variables, relapse prevention, women and child services, and specific treatment approaches. This TIP seeks to help the substance abuse treatment system lower barriers, improve treatment, and assist clinicians in providing their female clients with the tools needed to maintain recovery. Improved collaboration within the current system of health care and social services will result in more comprehensive and responsive care for women in recovery.

Sociocultural Context

The consensus panel for this TIP approached substance abuse treatment for women from a perspective that encompasses the multiple contexts of women's lives. This TIP provides a systemic framework for looking at women with substance use disorders, and uses Bronfenbrenner's ecological model (1989), where women are engaged in multisystems and relationships that maintain a bidirectional influence—the systems and relationships influence the woman with a substance use disorder and the woman, along with the impact of her substance use, influences her relationships and the systems that interact with her. Figure 1-1 depicts a woman as the center of a circle, surrounded by other concentric rings.

Each ring represents a different system with the closest adjacent ring representing her most immediate relationships—the microsystem. The following ring, the mesosystem, represents the interrelationships between her immediate relationships and systems; e.g. the interaction between her family and school, the potential influence or conflict between her substance using peer group and her family. Next, the exosystem represents larger systems that directly influence the woman but where the woman has no direct active role; e.g., county funding for treatment or State and Federal laws pertaining to sentencing or child protective services. The macrosystem is the largest system that involves cultural values and beliefs, gender socialization, political ideologies, etc. Each system is influenced by chronology, or life events. These events, either normative or non-normative individual events at specific developmental periods or historical events, can have significant impact and influence on further development, treatment needs and recovery, and ultimately interactions among all systems.

Using a systems approach is appropriate regardless of gender, yet it is a vital framework for understanding women's treatment needs and the impact of substance use on their relationships and caregiving roles. Consistent

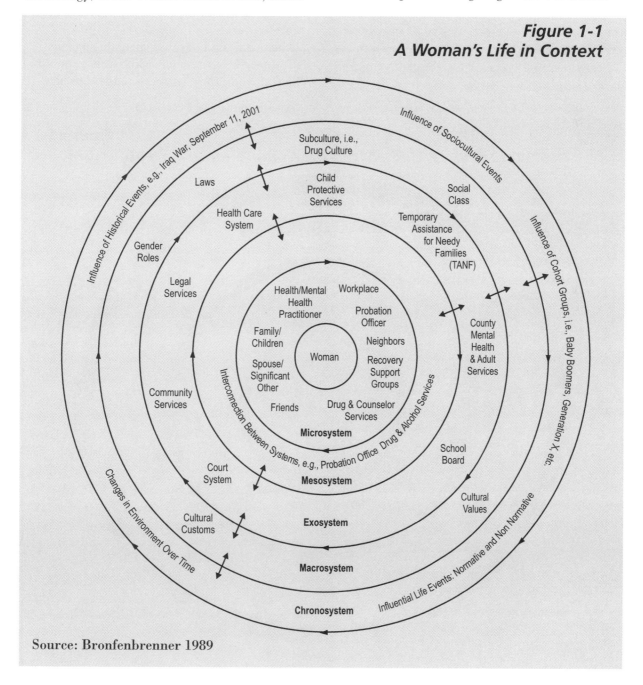

Figure 1-1
A Woman's Life in Context

Source: Bronfenbrenner 1989

with Bronfenbrenner's model, this TIP uses SAMHSA's Center for Substance Abuse Treatment's (CSAT's) *Comprehensive Substance Abuse Treatment Model for Women and Their Children* as the keystone in addressing women's treatment needs and services. Figure 1-2 highlights the four broad interrelated elements of CSAT's comprehensive model of care including clinical treatment services, clinical support services, community support services, and cultural competence. For more in-depth information about this model, refer to Appendix B. This model is an update of a model published in 1994 in *Practical Approaches in the Treatment of Women Who Abuse Alcohol and Other Drugs* (CSAT 1994a).

Gender Responsive Treatment Principles

The principles articulated by the consensus panel, which serve as the TIP's conceptual framework, are explained below. Each principle is derived from research that highlights the distinctive characteristics and biopsychosocial issues associated with women in general and specific to women with substance use disorders.

- **Acknowledge the importance and role of socioeconomic issues and differences among women.** Biological, cognitive–behavioral, and psychological dimensions of women's substance use and abuse should be framed in their socioeconomic contexts

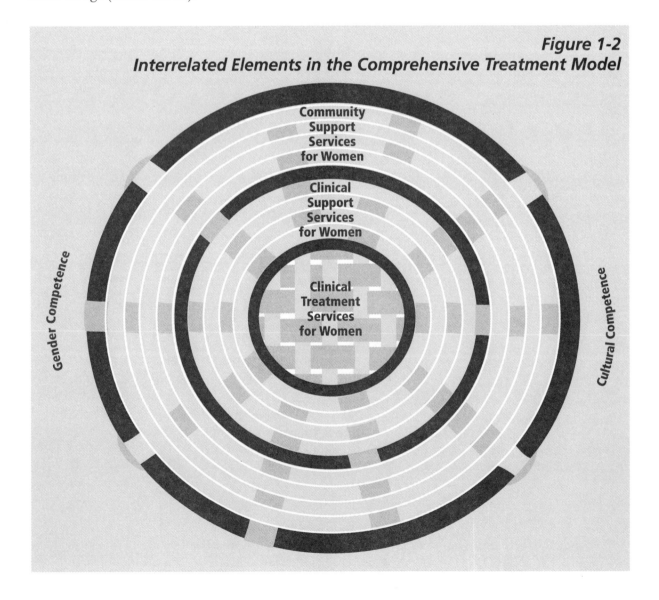

Figure 1-2
Interrelated Elements in the Comprehensive Treatment Model

Community Support Services for Women

Clinical Support Services for Women

Clinical Treatment Services for Women

Gender Competence

Cultural Competence

including, but not limited to, employment, educational status, transportation, housing, literacy levels, and income.

- **Promote cultural competence specific to women.** Treatment professionals and staff must understand the worldviews and experiences of women from different ethnic and cultural backgrounds, as well as the interaction among gender, culture, and substance use to provide effective substance abuse treatment. In addition, effective treatment will depend equally on attention and sensitivity to the vast diversity among the female population, including overlapping identities of race, class, sexual orientation, age, national origin, marital status, disability, and religion.

- **Recognize the role and significance of relationships in women's lives.** The relational model recognizes the centrality of relationships or connections in women's lives and the importance of those relationships with respect to alcohol, tobacco, and drug use. While substance use may initially play an integral role in making or maintaining connections in relationships, the relational approach views the development of substance use disorders as a "disconnection" and stresses the development and repair of connections to others, oneself, one's beliefs, and one's culture as critical for recovery. The relational model takes a family-focused perspective, using a broad definition of family as those individuals a woman views as her significant support system. In this model, a woman's children are included in her treatment, and prevention and treatment services must be provided directly to her children and family.

- **Address women's unique health concerns.** Women possess distinctive risk factors associated with onset of use, have greater propensity for health-related consequences from drug and alcohol consumption, exhibit higher risks for infectious diseases associated with drug use, and display greater frequency of various co-occurring disorders. Moreover, women who abuse substances are more likely to encounter problems associated with reproduction, including fetal effects from substance use during pregnancy, spontaneous abortion, infertility, and early onset of menopause. Substance abuse treatment needs to address women's unique health concerns throughout the course of treatment.

- **Endorse a developmental perspective.** In general, women experience unique life course issues. Specific to women who abuse substances, these life course issues, along with developmental milestones, impact their patterns of use, engagement in treatment, and recovery. Substance use and abuse affect women differently at different times in their lives. It is important to consider age-specific and other developmental concerns starting with the assessment process and continuing through continuing care and long-term recovery.

- **Attend to the relevance and influence of various caregiver roles that women often assume throughout the course of their lives.** Regardless of substance abuse, women are more likely to assume primary caregiving responsibilities for their children, grandchildren, parents, and other dependents. These roles may heavily influence a woman's willingness to seek help for substance abuse, and also may interfere with her ability to fully engage in the treatment process or to adhere to treatment recommendations.

- **Recognize that ascribed roles and gender expectations across cultures affect societal attitudes toward women who abuse substances.** Whether or not a woman neglects her roles as a caregiver, engages in alcohol or drug-induced sexual activity, continues to use despite pregnancy, or uses sex to secure her next supply of drugs or alcohol, women with substance use disorders are significantly stigmatized by societal attitudes and stereotypes of women who drink and use drugs. As a result, women may experience feelings of shame associated with their use and the consequences of their use.

- **Adopt a trauma-informed perspective.** Current and past violence, victimization, and abuse greatly affect many women who abuse alcohol and drugs. Substance abuse treatment approaches need to help women find safety, develop effective coping strategies, and recover from the effects of trauma and violence.

- **Utilize a strengths-based model for women's treatment.** A strengths-based approach builds on the woman's strengths and uses available resources to develop and enhance resiliency and recovery skills, deepen a sense of competency, and improve the quality of her life. These strengths may include personality traits, abilities, knowledge, cultural values, spirituality, and other assets; while resources may involve supportive relationships, environments, and professional support.

- **Incorporate an integrated and multidisciplinary approach to women's treatment.** Treatment needs to integrate current knowledge, research, theory, experience, and treatment models from diverse disciplines critical to understanding women and substance abuse treatment. In addition to incorporating and blending information from the mental health, women's health, and social and behavioral sciences fields, treatment providers must network and collaborate with other agencies to provide comprehensive case management and treatment planning to address the complexity of biopsychosocial and cultural issues that women may exhibit throughout treatment.

- **Maintain a gender-responsive treatment environment across settings.** Effective treatment for women begins with a collaborative environment that is nurturing, supportive, and empowering. Women with substance use disorders are more likely to remain in a treatment setting that feels familiar and safe, includes their children, utilizes proactive case management, and fosters the development of supportive relationships across the continuum of care.

- **Support the development of gender-competency specific to women's issues.** Administrative commitment and vigilance is needed to ensure that staff members are provided gender-specific training and supervision to promote the development of gender competency for women.

Women's Biopsychosocial Uniqueness

There is notable evidence to suggest that gender does make a difference. Whether examining risk factors to relapse potential, biological aspects to psychological issues, or treatment engagement to attrition rates, empirical evidence suggests that gender differences do exist in substance use disorders. For women, unique biopsychosocial and developmental issues create or intensify these differences, which require specific treatment needs across the continuum of care of substance use disorders.

This TIP is based on the premise that women are biopsychosocially unique in ways relevant to substance use, substance use disorders, and the treatment of these disorders. Specifically, this TIP takes the following position: There are biopsychosocial factors that may affect a significant proportion of women across the continuum of substance abuse services. The knowledge of these factors will likely assist the substance abuse counselor in better understanding and responding to the treatment needs of female clients.

Not only do women face numerous obstacles to entering and remaining in treatment, they also have specific needs while in treatment. Some obstacles stem from the frequently low economic status of women, the likelihood that they are custodial parents, the greater incidence of trauma and violence in female clients, and the societal stigma of substance abuse.

Additional treatment needs stem from a greater incidence of co-occurring mental disorders among female clients, and the growing realization that women respond better to treatment approaches that are supportive rather than confrontational and that promote relationships and positive connections among other clients in recovery and treatment providers.

Supported by research, this section highlights the biopsychosocial uniqueness of women and the impact that these characteristics may have on the onset of use, the development and progression of substance abuse and dependence, and the treatment of substance use disorders. The unique biopsychosocial characteristics are divided into three segments: biological and psychological, social, and developmental. This section does not focus on specific populations or on biopsychosocial, cultural, or developmental issues that are common in both men and women.

Biological and Psychological

Differences between women and men in genetics, physiology, anatomy, and sociocultural expectations and experiences lay the foundation—that women have unique health concerns related to substance use disorders as well as elevated risk for certain co-occurring physical and mental issues or disorders. This segment highlights and outlines the unique physiological and psychological issues that need attention across the continuum of care.

1. Women have different physical responses to substances.

Women have different physical responses to substances and typically display a quicker progression from initial use to the development of health-related problems (Antai-Otong 2006; Mann et al. 2005). Women become intoxicated after drinking smaller quantities of alcohol than men. For women who drink, they are affected more by alcohol consumption due to higher blood alcohol concentrations, proportionately more body fat, and a lower volume of body water to dilute alcohol.

Women develop substance use disorders and health-related problems in less time than do men, and this effect is known as telescoping. While research has studied the differences in metabolism with alcohol intake, studies highlighting gender differences with illicit drugs is limited (Brady and Ashley 2005; Greenfield and O'Leary 2002; Sherman 2006). A few preliminary studies (Katz et al. 2004) have identified perceptual differences between men

and women asserting that women report more intense or positive effects; yet findings across studies are inconclusive. Chapter 3 of this TIP provides a review of physical responses to substance use, beginning with the factors that influence these reactions including, but not limited to, ethnicity, acculturation, and aging.

2. Women with substance use disorder have greater susceptibility to as well as earlier onset of serious medical problems and disorders.

In general, women develop alcohol-related physical health problems at lower doses and over shorter periods of time than do men. Less evidence is available on gender differences regarding the effects and health consequences of other illicit drug use, but women also appear to have higher rates of health problems resulting from other substances (Sherman 2006). From moderate to heavy use, drugs and alcohol consumption increase specific health risks and physical disorders among women.

Alcohol consumption significantly increases risk for breast and other cancers (Bagnardi et al. 2001; Key et al. 2006; Tiemersma et al. 2003), osteoporosis in premenopausal women (Sampson 2002), peripheral neuropathy, and cognitive impairments (Flannery et al. 2007; Sohrabji 2002). Overall, women develop cirrhosis and heart muscle and nerve damage with fewer years of heavy drinking in comparison to men. Likewise, illicit drug use is associated with greater risk for liver and kidney diseases, bacterial infections, and opportunistic diseases. Chapter 3 presents an overview of the physiological effects and consequences of alcohol and drug use, including nicotine, among women.

3. Women who abuse substances have specific health issues and medical needs related to gynecology.

Routine gynecological care is fundamental to the prevention or early detection of a variety of serious health problems among women with substance use disorders, including cervical, breast, and other cancers; HIV/AIDS; and other infectious diseases. Evidence supports the havoc substances play on reproductive processes, such as the role of heavy alcohol use on infertility and drug use on menstrual cycles (Lynch et al. 2002; Reynolds and Bada 2003; Tolstrup et al. 2003). Even though gynecological concerns are frequently one of the main health concerns identified by women in substance abuse treatment, many young and low-income women have never had a gynecological examination. Moreover, women over 40 with substance use disorders are less likely to have received a mammogram than other women of similar age (Carney and Jones 2006). Refer to chapter 3 for more information on gynecological consequences related to substance use disorders.

4. In treating women of childbearing age who have a substance use disorder, pregnancy is a significant concern.

Women who are abusing or are dependent on alcohol or other drugs may not realize they are pregnant. At times, women may mistakenly associate early signs of pregnancy as symptoms related to use or withdrawal from substances. Often, women who are pregnant and using alcohol and illicit drugs do not begin prenatal care until well into their pregnancies. Some of the most negative effects of substance use on the developing embryo can occur in the first weeks of pregnancy.

Adequate prenatal care often defines the difference between routine and high-risk pregnancy and between good and bad pregnancy outcomes. Timely initiation of prenatal care remains a problem nationwide, and it is overrepresented among women with substance use disorders. In part, the threat of legal consequences for using during pregnancy and limited substance abuse treatment facilities (only 14 percent) that offer special programs for pregnant women (SAMHSA 2007) are key obstacles to care.

Numerous medical concerns can result from substance use during pregnancy as well as from detoxification and the medications used to treat substance use disorders. Thus, identification, comprehensive case management, and integrated services are essential in addressing these significant threats. The following chapters provide information on negative consequences of alcohol and drug use during pregnancy (chapter 3), specific screening questions and tools (chapter 4), engagement strategies and programming for pregnant women (chapter 5), and retention and review of treatment issues and needs for pregnant women with substance use disorders, including co-occurring disorders (chapter 7).

5. Women who abuse substances are more likely than other women to have co-occurring disorders.

In general, women with substance use disorders are more likely to meet diagnostic criteria for mood disorders specific to depressive symptoms, agoraphobia with or without panic attacks, posttraumatic stress, and eating disorders (Hudson et al. 2007; Piran and Robinson 2006; Tolin and Foa 2006). For women, literature suggests that the onset of psychiatric disorders is apt to precede substance use disorders. For instance, women who experience depression are more prone to develop alcohol problems after their first depressive episode (Caldwell et al. 2002; Wang and Patten 2002). Chapter 2 of this TIP addresses risk factors for substance use disorders, including the role of other psychological disorders. Chapter 4 offers screening tools to help counselors identify the need for further assessment due to presenting psychological symptoms. Chapter 7 identifies treatment needs and strategies for the more prevalent psychological symptoms and disorders among women with substance use disorders, including trauma, posttraumatic stress and other anxiety disorders, and mood and eating disorders.

6. Women who have substance use disorders are more likely to have been physically or sexually traumatized and subjected to interpersonal violence.

A high proportion of women with substance use disorders have histories of trauma, often perpetrated by persons they both knew and trusted. These women may have experienced sexual or physical abuse, domestic violence, or witnessed violence as a child. Studies have consistently found that rates of sexual abuse in both childhood and adulthood are higher for women than for men, and that a lifetime history of sexual abuse ranges from 15 to 25 percent (Leserman 2005; Tjaden and Thoennes 1998). Similarly, prevalence of lifetime domestic violence among women in the United States ranges from 9 to 44 percent, depending on the employed definition of domestic violence in each study (for review, see Thompson et al. 2006; Wilt and Olson 1996). While race/ethnicity is not generally associated with interpersonal violence, lower socioeconomic status appears to be associated with greater prevalence.

Women who have been abused as children are more likely to report substance use disorders as adults (Kendler et al. 2000). In a large study of female twins (*n*=3,536), childhood sexual abuse was associated with a greater likelihood of lifetime alcohol use, having the first drink at an early age, and alcohol dependence (Sartor et al. 2007). Likewise, physical and sexual dating violence were found to be "significant independent predictors of substance use" in other research (Silverman et al. 2001). Among women seeking treatment for crack/cocaine abuse/dependence, a history of sexual trauma was associated with a greater number of health issues related to substance use, dependence on a greater number of substances, and a greater number of substance abuse treatment episodes (Young and Boyd 2000). In a study focused on the severity of childhood trauma among men and women who were dependent on cocaine, only a history of childhood trauma among women created a greater susceptibility to relapse and escalation in use after relapse (Hyman et al. 2008).

Numerous studies on interpersonal violence have found a similar reciprocal relationship between substance abuse and domestic violence (Kilpatrick et al. 1997; Swan et al. 2000; Tjaden and Thoennes 1998, 2000, 2006). Rates of partner abuse appear highest for women who use cocaine/crack (Swan et al. 2000) or methamphetamine (Cohen et al. 2003). However, women with substance use disorders and a history of physical abuse (from a known person,

not necessarily a partner) are more likely to enter substance abuse treatment than women with substance use disorders who don't have such a history (Walton-Moss and McCaul 2006).

Clinical issues related to childhood sexual and physical abuse, interpersonal violence, and trauma are addressed throughout this TIP. More specific information is covered in the following chapters:

Chapter 2 addresses risk factors (including interpersonal violence, sexual abuse, and other traumas) associated with the development of substance use disorders.

Chapter 4 provides general screening and assessment guidelines, including tools for sexual victimization, childhood abuse, and interpersonal violence.

Chapter 7 highlights the treatment needs and interventions for these specific populations.

For more comprehensive reviews of domestic violence and child abuse, refer to TIP 25 *Substance Abuse Treatment and Domestic Violence* (CSAT 1997*b*); TIP 36 *Substance Abuse Treatment for Persons with Child Abuse and Neglect Issues* (CSAT 2000*b*); and the planned TIP *Substance Abuse and Trauma* (CSAT in development *h*).

Social

1. **Significant relationships and family history play an integral role in the initiation, pattern of use, and continuation of substance abuse for women.**

From a sociocultural perspective, women (more than men) tend to define themselves in terms of their webs of social relationships and obligations. Relationships with others have special significance for many women. Hence, family history may have a more profound effect on initiation of use among women than men. Women with alcohol use disorders are also more likely than men to report having had alcohol dependent parents, other alcohol dependent relatives, and dysfunctional family patterns (Jennison and Johnson 2001; Nelson-Zlupko et al. 1995).

Women are more likely to be introduced to and initiate alcohol and drug use through significant relationships including boyfriends, spouses, partners, and family members. This influence does not stop with initiation; it extends to greater use and higher incidence of substance use disorders when they have partners who abuse substances (Klein et al. 2003). In comparison to men, women with substance use disorders are more likely to have intimate partners who also have substance use disorders (Brady and Ashley 2005; Lex 1991; Riehman et al. 2003; Wright et al. 2007). In this TIP, chapter 2 addresses initiation, risk factors, and patterns of substance use and substance use disorders among women across the lifespan.

2. **Significant relationships and other adult family members may substantially influence and impact women's behavior associated with treatment seeking, support for recovery, and relapse.**

Women may have less support from family/partners than do men for seeking treatment. Women with alcohol problems are more likely to be left by their partners at the time of entry into treatment (Lex 1991), and their partners are less likely to stay with them after completion of treatment. Unless they themselves are involved in treatment or recovery, partners with substance use disorders may be unsupportive of women's treatment seeking (Brady and Ashley 2005). Couples in which both partners have substance use disorders and in those in which only the woman has a substance use disorder are more likely to spend time separated after treatment than are couples where only the man has a substance use disorder (Fals-Stewart et al. 1999). At the same time, husbands who do not themselves have substance use disorders expect greater change from wives with substance use disorders in treatment than if the circumstances were reversed (Fals-Stewart et al. 1999).

At times, substance use and the rituals associated with use may be a significant ingredient and symbol of intimacy and closeness in relationships. This history and relational pattern may make recovery more challenging during and after treatment. Especially in the early phase of recovery, women may believe that their decision to not use is or will be perceived as a direct threat against their significant relationship or family. Hence, women are more likely to relapse due to interpersonal problems and conflicts, and relapse is more likely to occur in the presence of a significant other (McKay et al. 1996; Rubin et al. 1996; Sun 2007). To obtain more information on relational factors that influence women across the continuum from risk factors to relapse, see chapters 2, 5, 6, 7, and 8.

3. **For women, pregnancy, parenting, and childcare influence alcohol and drug consumption and increase the likelihood of entering and completing substance abuse treatment.**

For many women, including those with substance use disorders, use of alcohol, tobacco, and/or illicit drugs significantly decreases after becoming aware of their pregnancy (Tough et al. 2006). It is also not uncommon for women who abstained from alcohol, drugs, and tobacco during pregnancy to return to use after childbirth. So, the impact of pregnancy on patterns of consumption can present a double-edged sword in treatment planning. On the one hand, pregnancy may represent a "teachable moment" where motivation to protect the fetus can be expanded to help motivate the mother to make more permanent changes in her substance use behavior. On the other hand, progress toward recovery made by pregnant women may be transient if this progress is primarily in response to the pregnancy itself.

Women are much more likely than men to enter treatment because it affects child custody (Grella and Joshi 1999). If they are able to have their children in treatment, women are more likely to enter treatment, participate and stay in the program, and maintain abstinence (Brady and Ashley 2005; Lungren et al. 2003; Szuster et al. 1996). Likewise, women with children in treatment have better treatment outcomes in major life areas in comparison to women who are without their children in treatment (Stevens and Patton 1998). Women in recovery see the support of their children as an essential ingredient for their recovery (Tracy and

Martin 2007). Every chapter of this TIP covers issues pertaining to pregnancy, parenting, or child care, with specific attention to treatment modalities and treatment issues highlighted in chapters 5 and 7.

4. **Women are more likely to encounter obstacles across the continuum of care as a result of caregiver roles, gender expectations, and socioeconomic hardships.**

   • Women with substance use disorders have enhanced treatment needs related to pregnancy, care of children, and other caregiver roles. Familiarity with these gender-based experiences can contribute to effective treatment programming and successful treatment outcomes. To begin with, pregnancy itself can be an obstacle to treatment because substance abuse treatment programs are not always able to admit pregnant women or to provide the services required. Beyond pregnancy, women often assume many other caregiver roles, and these roles can significantly interfere with treatment engagement and regular attendance at treatment services. Brady and Ashley (2005) reported that women are more likely to encounter difficulties surrounding treatment attendance due to family responsibilities. Often family expectations regarding responsibilities involve care for other family members and the need to attend to their significant relationship.

   • Most women with substance use disorders have to contend with economic and social factors as well as individual and family issues to negotiate their recoveries successfully. Because women frequently earn less than men for doing the same job, they face more economic barriers to entering and staying in treatment than do men. Women are less likely than men to be able to pay out-of-pocket for treatment, have less access to private health insurance, are less likely to have savings or other financial resources to support themselves while in treatment, and often cannot afford a car to take them to treatment. According to NSDUH (SAMHSA 2003), 34 percent of women who reported they did receive substance use treatment indicated that they could not cover treatment costs due to inadequate or nonexistent health insurance. As important, women with co-occurring serious mental illness and substance use disorders were less likely to be employed full-time than women with only a substance use disorder (SAMHSA 2003). Many female clients need assistance with transportation; affordable, safe housing; and onsite child care and other services for their children. To obtain more specific information on obstacles pertinent to women in treatment, refer to chapter 5.

5. **Despite the unique challenges, women are more likely to engage in help-seeking behavior and in attending treatment after admission.**

Women are more likely to seek health and mental health services than are men. Studies have found that women with alcohol use disorders as well as drug use disorders marked with severity are either as likely as or more prone to initiate treatment than men (Moos et al. 2006; Weisner et al. 2001). Once women are admitted to substance abuse treatment, they are at least as likely as men to participate and stay in treatment. Help-seeking behavior among women with substance use disorders appears to remain consistent across time. In one study, Chatham et al. (1999) found that women, in comparison to men, were more likely to seek further help for both psychological issues and drug use 1 year postdischarge from a methadone maintenance program. Another study found that women were also more apt to seek help after a relapse (McKay et al. 1996). Refer to chapter 5 of this TIP for treatment engagement strategies that help reinforce help-seeking behavior.

6. Women report more interpersonal stressful life events.

Overall, women report more interpersonal related stress in relation to negative affect whereas men report more legal and work-related stressful life events (Kendler et al. 2001). This difference is likely a reflection of gender role expectations and socialization, and is evident among men and women in substance abuse treatment. Specifically, women entering treatment report a greater level of family and social problems as measured by the Addiction Severity Index (Green et al. 2002; Weiss et al. 1997). During the week prior to relapse and on the initial day of relapse, women report interpersonal problems and negative affect as key stressors (McKay et al. 1996). For more information regarding interpersonal risk factors of use, relational treatment needs, and relapse risk factors associated with interpersonal stress among women, refer to chapters 2, 7, and 8, respectively.

7. Women often take different paths in accessing treatment for substance use disorders.

Women are more likely than men to seek out physical and mental health treatment, including substance abuse treatment. They are also more likely to make use of a variety of healthcare options including primary care and psychological counseling (Cherry and Woodwell 2002). Among women with substance use disorders, the most frequent source of referral to treatment was made by self-referral followed by the criminal justice system and other community referrals, including child protective services (Brady and Ashley 2005). Refer to chapter 2 of this TIP to review more information regarding treatment admission characteristics among women.

8. Women have unique client–counselor expectations and relational needs related to treatment.

Women's sociocultural role as caregivers predisposes them to define themselves in terms of social relationships and obligations. Through this lens, women are more likely to view relationship building as an essential treatment ingredient. If attention is given to establishing and maintaining relationships across the continuum of care, women are more likely to initiate, engage, and successfully complete treatment. Women have identified several counselor characteristics that they believe contribute to treatment success—a projection of acceptance and care, trust and warmth, a non-authoritarian attitude, and a sense of confidence in their abilities (Fiorentine and Anglin 1997; Sun 2006). Likewise, women are more likely to stay in treatment longer if they receive more intensive and individual care, are able to maintain their parenting role while in treatment, and either stay within the same treatment services or maintain a connection with treatment providers throughout the continuum of services, including continuing care. In this TIP, chapter 7 covers the main factors that influence retention; particular attention is given to women's treatment expectations surrounding environment, theoretical approach, therapeutic alliance, and counselor characteristics.

9. Women are uniquely stigmatized in relationship to substance abuse.

- Stigma is a significant barrier to treatment and recovery. Ascribed roles and gender expectations across cultures affect societal attitudes toward women with substance abuse. The societal stigma toward women who abuse substances tends to be greater than that toward men, which can prevent women from seeking or admitting they need help. According to NSDUH (SAMHSA 2003), women who reported not receiving or not perceiving a need for treatment attributed social stigma as the primary reason.

Women who use alcohol and illicit drugs often have great feelings of shame and guilt, have low levels of self-esteem and self-efficacy, and often are devalued by other women and men. These feelings make it difficult for women to seek help or feel that they deserve to be helped. Additionally, women may carry internalized feelings of guilt and shame concerning their failure in maternal roles (Ehrmin 2001). Some women fear negative consequences, including mandatory involvement with child protective services, loss of child custody, or other legal consequences, if their substance abuse becomes known. Gender role expectations in many cultures result in further stigmatization of substance use, and additional challenges face women who are of color, disabled, older, lesbians, and poor. For additional information on gender socialization and the role of stigma associated with substance abuse across specific populations, review chapter 6. For additional discussion and material on stigmatization, review risk factors in chapter 2 and sociocultural obstacles in chapter 5.

Developmental

1. Women have unique life-course issues and events.

Over the past two decades, the substance abuse field has increasingly recognized the importance of developmental issues over the entire lifespan (Klitzner 1992; White 2006). Changes in physiology, emotional and social development, and cognitive capacity as well as changes in social roles and expectations have all been associated with substance abuse and its treatment. Many of these life course issues are different or more salient for women than for men. The following segment covers the main developmental milestones for women, and additional information is interwoven throughout this TIP.

Identity and gender expectations—the younger years: During adolescence and young adulthood, young women are likely to face greater gender-based sociocultural expectations (Gilligan et al. 1990). Consistent with this notion is the finding that girls and young women may be more susceptible to substance use-related social influences than are boys (Dick et al. 2007). Substance use may play an essential role in exploring new experiences while forming identity, but it is as likely that substance use helps provide relief when identity formation and the negotiation of new gender role expectations becomes confusing or difficult (Arnett 2005).

Educational, employment, and career issues: In a recent summary of women's career development, Fitzgerald and Harmon (2001; p. 226) concluded that "life is, in many ways, less gendered than it was in the 1970s"; however, "there are still ways in which life and its opportunities are partially controlled by gender stereotypes" and roles. Several writers have argued that "women's work lives are more complex than men's" (Fitzgerald et al. 1995; p. 76). For example, the need to balance career endeavors—education, training, and employment—with caregiver responsibilities is a major developmental task that more often than not is unique to women.

While younger women are more likely and able to invest in earlier career development than the women of 50 years ago (Arnett 2005), they still do not characteristically encounter the same career opportunities, and for many women, early career aspirations may be placed on hold or pared down until years later due to pregnancy and childcare responsibilities. Disparity in employment opportunities, income, healthcare insurance, and/or childcare support presents unique challenges for all women, but significantly impacts women with substance use disorders and women seeking substance abuse treatment. Overall, women with substance use disorders have more pronounced employment barriers than men with substance use disorders and women without substance use problems, including women who are recipients of the Temporary Assistance to Needy Families program (TANF; McCoy et al. 2007; Meara 2006).

Pregnancy, parenting, and childcare issues: This developmental milestone and the issues involving substance use disorders and treatment are covered in the above social section, item 3.

Menopause: Menopause is a complex biopsychosocial transition for women. Rather than an event, menopause is a process that unfolds over many years as estrogen levels decrease. These decreases, in turn, may lead to a variety of physical and psychological symptoms, the onset of which may precede the cessation of fertility by as much as a decade (Stewart 2005). For some women, cessation of fertility occasions a re-examination of social roles, which may lead to depression or anxiety in some and a new sense of freedom in others. Studies evaluating the impact of hormonal changes on alcohol and drug metabolism and the consequences of substance use on the development of menopause are limited. Yet, preliminary studies reflect potential effects even though research remains mixed and methodological issues are evident. Most noteworthy, substance abuse and dependence may exacerbate postmenopausal risks for coronary heart disease, osteoporosis, and breast cancer in this population (Register et al. 2003).

Caring for parents and partners: Many more people than ever before are having to cope with caring for elderly parents in addition to the usual demands of work and family. The typical pattern is that sons offer financial assistance, and daughters and daughters-in-law provide the time-consuming, hands-on care. More than 60 percent of caregivers are female (National Alliance for Caregiving and American Association of Retired Persons [AARP] 2004). An estimated 80 percent of informal care for elders is imparted on family caregivers (International Longevity Center 2006), and these caretaking responsibilities can last 10 years or more.

Women may be caught between the responsibilities of providing care to their parents or parents-in-law while simultaneously taking care of their own dependent children. Time and energy spent caring for elderly parents often come at the expense of other family or occupational roles as well as self-care. Although unpaid family leave is now available to many workers, the demands of caring for an elderly parent force some women to make hard choices. They either have to reduce or stop work or have to find professional and institutional care. Some have had to switch to part-time work, pass up promotions, or quit their jobs altogether. This decision can lead to greater risk for living in poverty in the later years due to terminating

or decreasing hours of employment to care for aging parents (Wakabayashi and Donato 2006). For women with substance use disorders, the emotional, physical, and financial stressors are likely to exacerbate substance use. Moreover, unique obstacles exist for women with substance use disorders—balancing the need to care for their parents and the need for their own substance abuse treatment.

Longer life than male partners: Women are more likely than men to outlive their partners. According to the Centers for Disease Control and Prevention, the general life expectancy for women and men is 80.4 and 75.2 years, respectively. Data from the Census Bureau indicate that almost one-half of American women over the age of 65 are widowed (Fields and Casper 2001). A recent cross-sectional and longitudinal study of more than 70,000 American women ages 50–79 (Wilcox et al. 2003) found that widowed women were significantly more physically impaired than married women on a variety of measures, including general health and physical functioning, obesity, hypertension, and pain. Widowed women were also significantly lower in overall mental health and social functioning and significantly higher in depressed mood.

The later years: Various sources of data suggest that alcohol problems are ordinary events among the elderly, and estimates of the prevalence of heavy drinking or alcohol abuse range from 2 to 20 percent for this population (Benshoff and Harrawood 2003). There is also some suggestion that the baby-boom generation is more likely than earlier generations to have been exposed to drug and alcohol use and may drink or consume drugs at greater rates after age 65. The literature on the etiology of elder substance use disorders is limited, but spousal loss is one commonly cited factor (Benshoff and Harrawood 2003).

Creating the Context

Organization of this TIP

Scope

This TIP discusses treatment for women from diverse cultures, ethnicities, and sexual orientations; women living in urban and rural areas; women who are pregnant, parenting, or without children; and women of all ages, socioeconomic classes, and histories. Although alcohol and drug effects on fetuses and neonates are mentioned, the details and implications for fetuses and neonates are not discussed in detail. Female adolescents are not addressed in this TIP. Whereas some adolescents' needs may parallel those of women, their developmental stage requires specialized treatment. Information on treating adolescents can be found in TIP 32 *Treatment of Adolescents with Substance Use Disorders* (CSAT 1999*d*). Substance abuse treatment issues specific to male clients are addressed in the planned TIP *Substance Abuse Treatment and Men's Issues* (CSAT in development *f*).

Whenever possible, TIPs include empirical findings in support of practices they recommend. However, the field of substance abuse treatment is evolving and research can lag behind the innovations being pioneered in the field. Treatment recommendations included in this TIP are based on both consensus panelists' clinical experience and scientific literature. When the research supports a particular approach, citations are provided.

Audience

The primary audience for this TIP is substance abuse treatment clinicians and counselors who work with women. Secondary audiences include administrators, educators, researchers, policymakers for substance abuse treatment and related services, consumers, and other healthcare and social service personnel who work with women with substance use disorders.

Approach: Gender Responsive Treatment

This TIP draws on the systemic framework of Bronfenbrenner's ecological theory and CSAT's *Comprehensive Substance Abuse Treatment Model for Women and Children* (see Appendix B). It is based on clinical practice and research centered on women. It is not derived primarily by comparing women with men. The knowledge, models, and strategies presented are grounded in women's experiences and their unique biopsychosocial and cultural needs. The basic elements and principles of gender-responsive treatment are presented throughout this TIP, with suggestions and resources on how to implement such a system of care. Also presented are approaches to treating substance use disorders among women; these employ model treatment programs, evidence-based and best practices, and other research on women's issues along with knowledge from related fields.

Guidelines for Readers

The consensus panel recognizes the realities of substance abuse treatment sometimes precludes implementing the wide array of services and programs recommended in this volume. Nevertheless, by presenting a variety of techniques for addressing the specific treatment needs of women, the panel hopes to increase sensitivity to these needs and options for improving treatment. A special feature throughout the TIP, "Advice to the Clinician," imparts the TIP's most direct and accessible guidance for the counselor. Readers with basic backgrounds (such as addiction counselors or other practitioners) can study the Advice to the Clinician boxes for the most immediate practical guidance. Brief "Note(s) to the Clinician" and "Note(s) to the Clinician and Administrator" are offered to highlight specific issues in treatment services. The TIP also includes "Clinical Activity" inserts that provide counselors examples of practical individual or group activities that support specific treatment issues for women.

Terminology

African American: The term is used to identify women who live in the United States and whose ancestors at some point arrived from Africa. Although it blurs the distinction between women whose families came to this country from Caribbean nations and other countries and those who came directly from Africa, it is the term used by the U.S. Census Bureau and by SAMHSA and CSAT.

Co-occurring disorders: The term "co-occurring disorders" refers to a diagnosis of substance use disorder and one or more mental disorders.

Gender: This term is used not just as a biological category, but also as a social category meaning society or culture shapes the definition of gender and shapes the socialization of each woman. Gender affects how women live their lives, see their roles and their expectations of themselves and others, view and interpret the world, and handle the opportunities open to them and the constraints placed on them. People enact their gender in the world through transactions with others and are guided by social and cultural values and conceptions (West and Zimmerman 1987).

Gender responsive: "Being gender-responsive (or woman-centered) refers to the creation of an environment—through site selection, staff selection, program development, and program content and materials—that reflects an understanding of the realities of women's and girls' lives and that addresses and responds to their challenges and strengths" (Covington 2007, p. 1).

Hispanic/Latina: The use of the Spanish feminine term "Hispanic/Latina" indicates a woman of Hispanic heritage. The phrase "Hispanic/Latino" refers to men only or a group of men and women. The phrase "women of color" refers in this document to women of racial and cultural groups other than Caucasian, as well as women who consider themselves biracial or multiracial.

Substance abuse: The term "substance abuse" refers to both substance abuse and substance dependence (as defined by the *Diagnostic and Statistical Manual of Mental Disorders, Fourth Edition, Text Revision* [DSM-IV-TR] [American Psychiatric Association {APA} 2000a]) because substance abuse treatment professionals commonly use the term "substance abuse" to describe any excessive use of addictive substances. In this TIP, the term refers to the use of alcohol as well as other substances of abuse. Readers should attend to the context in which the term occurs to determine the possible range of meanings it covers; in most cases, however, the term refers to all varieties of substance use disorders described by DSM-IV-TR.

2 Patterns of Use: From Initiation to Treatment

Overview

This chapter addresses patterns of substance use, abuse, and dependence using a continuum beginning with initial risk factors and concluding with common attributes associated with women entering treatment for substance use disorders. Information pertaining to risk factors linked to initiation of use, abuse of alcohol and other drugs, and/or the development of substance dependence is explored. Also examined are the potential reasons for initiation of use, means of introduction, and other characteristics of drug and alcohol patterns of use among women. In addition, to shed light on common patterns, this chapter provides prevalence rates of substance use, abuse, and dependence, including specific populations of women and substances as well as psychosocial characteristics of women who enter treatment.

While this section provides a wealth of information on the unique psychosocial issues and patterns of use among women to aid in program development, the essential value for clinicians is recognizing that substance use disorders do not occur in a vacuum. By gathering information on the specific risk factors associated with initiation of use, people of introduction, and other individual characteristics, clinicians can identify clients' potential barriers to treatment engagement and retention along with high-risk relapse triggers. For example, women who identify that their initial use was influenced by a sexual relationship and that their present use involves a significant relationship will be more likely threatened by the potential loss of a relationship if they continue in treatment and recovery. In addition, the client may be greatly influenced by phone calls from boyfriends, spouses, or significant others that lead to premature termination of treatment. Thus, risk factors associated with either the initiation or continuation of use can assist clinicians in identifying specific problem areas, in anticipating intervention strategies for these specific risks, and in developing a compatible treatment plan and an individually tailored continuing care plan.

Initiation of Use Among Women

The reasons for initiation of substance use and the subsequent development of substance use disorders involve a network of factors among women (Maharj et al. 2005). No one biopsychosocial characteristic is solely responsible for substance initiation, abuse, or dependence. For women, initiation of substance use typically begins after an introduction of the substance by a significant relationship such as a boyfriend, partner, or spouse. Reasons for initiation of substance use vary among women; they frequently report that stress, negative affect, and relationships are very influential in first use. Depending on the physiological effects of the substance, some women report they initiate use due to a desire to lose weight or to have more energy; e.g., methamphetamine use (Brecht et al. 2004).

Women initiate substance use at an older age than do males. According to SAMHSA's Treatment Episode Data Set (TEDS; SAMHSA 2004), the average age of first use of drugs or alcohol for females is almost 20 years old. In reviewing gender differences in initiation of use between males and females, a key ingredient that appears paramount is the opportunity to use. While females currently have fewer restrictions than in the past, they generally encounter more parent-imposed restrictions and constraints on activities, greater parental monitoring, and higher expectations surrounding responsibilities in the home. These restrictions often limit drug and alcohol exposure and opportunity to use (van Etten and Anthony 2001). Yet, when women across ethnically diverse groups have the same opportunity as men, they are just as likely to initiate use. In recent years, women have had more opportunities and greater availability in accessing drugs and alcohol (van Etten et al. 1999).

Risk Factors Associated with Initiation of Substance Use and the Development of Substance Use Disorders Among Women

Why one woman uses a substance without becoming dependent while another progresses to abuse and dependence is not entirely clear. Substance use disorders have complex and interrelated causes. For women, some factors are associated only with initiation of use, while other factors are associated with progression from initial use to substance dependence; e.g., co-occurring disorders (Agrawal et al. 2005). Just as some factors increase the likelihood of women developing substance abuse problems, others decrease those chances. For example, having a partner can be a risk factor if that person abuses alcohol or drugs, but having a supportive, caring partner who does not use alcohol or drugs can be a protective factor. In this section, risk factors associated with initiation of use, ongoing alcohol and drug involvement, and alcohol and drug abuse and dependence are explored.

Familial Substance Abuse

Substance use disorders aggregate in families: relatives of people with substance use disorders are more likely to have a disorder. In all likelihood, both genetic and environmental factors play important and interconnected roles. Most research on familial aggregation has been done on alcohol use disorders and on male subjects. Reviews of several studies indicate that parental substance abuse can influence the development of substance use disorders in their children (Finkelstein et al. 1997; Heath et al. 1997). Jennison and Johnson (2001) cite a growing body of research on the risk for adult children of parents who abuse alcohol. The literature indicates that women are affected by familial substance abuse as much as men, with a prevalence of alcohol dependence from 10 to 50 times higher than women who do not have a parent who abuses substances.

Twin and adoption studies have established an important role for genetic influences in the etiology of alcohol use disorders in men. Some studies show that genetic factors appear to be important in women as well, making women similarly vulnerable to substance abuse from a genetic standpoint (Johnson and Leff 1999; Merikangas and Stevens 1998; Pickens et al. 1991). A study of 1,030 female twins found that alcohol use disorders were consistently higher in identical twins than in non-identical twins and suggested that women's genetic likelihood of developing an alcohol use disorder is in the range of 50 to 60 percent (Kendler et al. 1992). Kendler and Prescott (1998) found that among women, genetic risk factors have a moderate effect on the probability of ever using cannabis and a strong effect on the likelihood of heavy use, abuse, and, probably, dependence.

However, on the whole, the evidence for genetic influence on the development of alcohol use disorders in women is less consistent than for men. Interpretation of the literature is complicated by methodological issues, such as small sample sizes. Some research suggests that differences between men and women exist in the sets of genes that influence alcohol use disorder risk or perhaps in the interactions of genes contributing to alcohol use disorder risk with other genetic or cultural factors (Prescott 2002). A study of women who were adopted found that early-life family conflict and psychopathology in the adoptive family interacted with a biological background of alcohol use disorders. Among women with at least one biological parent with an alcohol use disorder, conflict or psychopathology in the adoptive family increased the probability of alcohol abuse or dependence (Cutrona et al. 1994).

A number of possible explanations could account for this genetic and behavioral parental impact (Heath et al. 1997; Johnson and Leff 1999). Parents who use alcohol and illicit drugs sometimes are unable to supervise their children

and protect them from physical or sexual abuse by other family members or strangers (Moncrieff and Farmer 1998). They more often are emotionally unavailable to nurture and help their children. According to Johnson and Leff's (1999) review of the literature, alcohol use by parents is both directly linked to alcohol use by children and indirectly linked to stress, less parental supervision, and greater emotional volatility. Jessup's (1997) review indicates that when parents have substance use disorders, it signals to a child that coping with problems by using alcohol and illicit drugs is acceptable behavior.

Family of Origin Characteristics

Across ethnic and cultural population groups, major risk factors for substance initiation and dependence among women include chaotic, argumentative, blame-oriented, and violent households. As a general tenet, women who grew up in families where they take on adult responsibilities as a child, including household duties, parenting of younger children, and emotional support of parents, are more likely to initiate drug and alcohol use. Women who are dependent on substances are more likely to have a history of over-responsibility with their family of origin (Nelson-Zlupko et al. 1995). While prevalence of alcohol dependence appears consistently higher among women who report parental alcohol abuse regardless of the number of adverse childhood experiences (Anda et al. 2002), these experiences, characterized by childhood abuse and various forms of dysfunctional households, significantly increase early initiation of use on or before the age of 14 (Dube et al. 2006).

Marital Status

Women (18 to 49 years of age) who are married have a lower rate of alcohol or illicit drug abuse or dependence than women of any other marital status (SAMHSA 2003). History of divorce is positively associated with illicit drug use, not drug dependence, among women (Agrawal et al. 2005). Approximately 11 percent of divorced or separated women and 16 percent of women who have never married (in age range of 18 to 49 years) abuse or are dependent on alcohol or an illicit drug compared to only 4 percent of married women (SAMHSA 2004).

Effect of Partner Substance Abuse

The "interaction, assistance, and encouragement of other people" are major factors in women's substance use and abuse (Finkelstein 1996, p. 30). One study found that to some degree partners influence each other's drinking patterns (Wilsnack et al.1998b). Men who drink alcohol more frequently than their partners influence them to drink more often, and women who drink lightly influence their partners to drink less (Wilsnack et al. 1998b).

Women dependent on illicit drugs are more likely than males dependent on illicit drugs to have partners who use illicit drugs (Lex 1995). Although alcohol and marijuana use often begins with peer pressure during adolescence, women are likely to be introduced to cocaine and heroin by men (Amaro and Hardy-Fanta 1995; Henderson et al. 1994). Some women continue using alcohol and illicit drugs to have an activity in common with their partners or to maintain the relationships. The man often supplies drugs, and the woman becomes dependent on him for drugs. Among women with partners who have alcohol-related problems, they are more likely to report mental health problems including mood, anxiety, and quality-of-life problems as well as substance use disorders (Dawson et al. 2007).

The dynamic of one partner being the supplier and the other using the drug to maintain the relationship is present also in some same-sex relationships. A few studies have examined the effects of partner substance abuse in lesbian relationships, especially the association between substance use and violence, but little is actually known (Hughes and Norris 1995; Schilit et al. 1990).

Women are at risk of contracting HIV/AIDS and hepatitis from sharing needles or having sexual relations with men who inject drugs or have sex with men. Some women may have unrealistic notions about intimacy, assume their partners are monogamous, or fear alienating their partners by demanding safe sex practices. Women with a history of abuse may have particular problems negotiating the use of these practices.

Although ending a bad relationship can lessen stress, it also causes psychological distress (Hope et al. 1999; Horwitz et al. 1996) and can increase alcohol use and related problems (Chilcoat and Breslau 1996; Neff and Mantz 1998; Power et al. 1999), especially among women (Fillmore et al. 1997; Horwitz et al. 1996). The situation is more complicated when a couple has a child and the woman may feel unable to leave the child's father for emotional or financial reasons (Amaro and Hardy-Fanta 1995).

Partners may prevent women from entering or staying in treatment (Tuten and Jones 2003). A study of male partners of women in treatment for crack/cocaine found that most of the men accepted their partners' drug use as long as the women managed to care for the home and children (Laudet et al. 1999). This study notes the difficulty of involving male partners in women's treatment. Despite the fact that nearly two-thirds of the men said they supported their partners in treatment, they found this support to be passive and inconsistent. Laudet and colleagues (1999) suggest a number of possible reasons for the male partners' detachment: the males' own alcohol and drug use, desire to maintain the status quo, different treatment goals, preoccupation with their own treatment, and fear of stigma.

Personality Measures

Novelty-seeking was positively associated more with initiation of illicit drug use than with

---

Protective Factor—Parental Warmth: If a woman comes from a family of origin that has high parental warmth, she is less likely to initiate use, abuse substances, or become dependent on alcohol or other substances (Agrawal et al. 2005)

Protective Factor—Partner Support: In their study of nearly 4,500 women, Jennison and Johnson (2001) found that a good marriage was protective against the development of alcohol abuse in women with a familial history of alcohol abuse. Partners can be the key motivators in successful interventions that bring a woman to treatment. Treatment readiness and willingness to accept help are higher in women whose partners have been in treatment (Riehman et al. 2000).

progression from use to abuse/dependence (Agrawal et al. 2005). Among women, sensation-seeking (risk-taking personality) has significant effects on substance use. One study (VanZile-Tamsen et al. 2006) that examined the impact of personality constructs on health risk behavior among women showed that sensation-seeking has large indirect effects on risky sexual behavior, affiliation with risky partners, and drinking and illicit drug use behavior, and that sensation-seeking is more strongly associated with substance use than with sexual risk behavior. Premorbid personality risk factors that lay the foundation for substance abuse (besides depressive features) include obsessiveness and anxiety, difficulty in regulating affect and behavior (such as temper tantrums and frequent tearfulness), and low self-worth and ego integration (Brook et al. 1998). According to Page (1993), a negative self-perception of physical attractiveness is associated with increased illicit drug use.

Sexual Orientation

Studies show higher rates of substance use and dependence in women who have sex with women compared with heterosexual women (Bickelhaupt 1995; Cochran et al. 2000; Diamant et al. 2000; UCLA Center for Health Policy Research 2005). Hughes and Wilsnack (1997) conclude that lesbians differ from heterosexual women in that they are less likely to abstain from alcohol, have higher rates of alcohol problems, and do not decrease alcohol intake as much with age. Conversely, Drabble and Underhill (2002) note that two studies found no significant differences in levels of drinking between lesbians and heterosexual women and that lesbians who did not drink were more likely to report being in recovery. Heffernan (1998) suggests these comparable rates of drinking among lesbian and heterosexual women are perhaps the result of a greater emphasis on sobriety in the lesbian community over the past decade.

Studies have reported greater prevalence of marijuana use in comparison to other illicit drugs among lesbians (Cochran et al. 2004). In a study reporting elevated rates of illicit drug use among lesbian and bisexual women, marijuana was the most prevalent (33 percent), followed by opioids other than heroin (15.1 percent), and tranquilizers (11.6 percent; Corliss et al. 2006). Lesbians who have moderate or high-risk levels of use, measured by patterns of drug use and severity, were also more likely to report depressive symptoms, and this pattern of depressive symptoms is reflected in Hispanic/Latina and Asian populations (Cochran et al. 2007). Among younger lesbians and bisexual women, they appear to be most likely to abuse prescription drugs (Kelly and Parson 2007). Empirical studies reveal that lesbians are more likely to smoke than heterosexual women (Hughes and Jacobson 2003).

Protective Factor—Religious and Spiritual Practices: Numerous studies (for review, see Matthews et al. 1998) highlight that higher levels of personal devotion, religious affiliation, and religious beliefs (defined as religiosity) reduce the risk for substance use and dependence. A female twin study found a negative association between religious beliefs and illicit drug use (Agrawal et al. 2005)—that religiosity is associated with a reduced risk for substance abuse. Consistent with other studies (Kendler et al. 1997; Kendler et al. 2003), this study suggests that religiosity is a protective factor in substance use and abuse, and that faith-based approaches may serve as a potential relapse prevention strategy.

Lesbians who have a history of child sexual abuse possess a heightened risk for lifetime alcohol abuse in comparison to lesbians without a similar abuse history (Hughes et al. 2007). Adolescent females and women who are either struggling with issues or prejudice surrounding sexual orientation also have greater risks in initiating and maintaining drug and alcohol use (McKirnan and Peterson 1992). More information on treating lesbian clients is available in *A Provider's Introduction to Substance Abuse Treatment for Lesbian, Gay, Bisexual, and Transgender Individuals* (CSAT 2001b).

History of Interpersonal Violence, Childhood Sexual Abuse, and Other Traumas

A history of traumatic events including, but not limited to, sexual and physical assaults, childhood sexual and physical abuse, and domestic violence, are significantly associated with initiation of substance use and the development of substance use disorders among women (Agrawal et al. 2005; Brady and Ashley 2005; Hawke et al. 2000; Pettinati et al. 2000). One review found a lifetime history of trauma in 55 to 99 percent of women who abused substances, compared with rates of 36 to 51 percent in the general population (Najavits et al. 1997). Although not every woman who has a history of trauma develops posttraumatic stress disorder (PTSD), it is important to note that traumatic experiences are associated with substance use and subsequent substance use disorders. Several interpretations have been offered to explain why substance abuse often accompanies trauma. Studies (Grayson and Noelen-Hoeksema 2005; Jarvis et al.1998; Schuck and Wisdom 2001; Testa et al. 2003; Ullman et al. 2005) suggest that some survivors of sexual and/or physical abuse may use substances to self-medicate their depression or the anxiety that results from the abuse. Some survivors who use primarily cocaine and amphetamines may be trying to increase their vigilance against further victimization. Others with low self-esteem may use alcohol to increase their sociability. Conversely, substance use disorders increase a woman's vulnerability to additional trauma, decrease her ability to

Note to Clinicians

For those women who are more likely to seek out novel events and thrive on risk-taking behavior or those women who are accustomed to living in high stress or in crisis, one of the challenges in maintaining recovery is learning to engage in day-to-day activities without seeking out or creating these situations. Some women may be so used to higher levels of stress that when life becomes a little more settled without the use of alcohol and drugs, they may experience a sense of boredom, uncomfortable feelings, or a sense of being down or depressed. In recovery, women may place themselves in circumstances that are high risk for relapse by returning to old risk-taking behaviors or by creating stressful situations to offset these feelings.

As a clinician, it is important to anticipate these behaviors and reactions and to begin teaching strategies to manage these experiences. Using anxiety management strategies can be invaluable, but it is important to teach these techniques as early as possible to help build an arsenal of coping skills. Women need to learn about their accustomed risk-taking levels and premorbid levels of stress and the subsequent consequences if they engage in sensation-seeking behaviors. By developing alternative, healthy behaviors, some women will discover they don't need to maintain the same level of stress to function as in the past, while other women will learn they can exchange their destructive desire for excitement with other recovery-oriented activities; e.g., enrolling in an exercise class (with medical clearance) or telling their recovery story at a 12-Step speakers meeting.

defend herself, alter her judgment, and draw her into unsafe environments.

Kilpatrick and colleagues (1997) speak of the "vicious cycle" of substance abuse and violence, in which violence is both a risk factor and a consequence of substance abuse. TIP 25, *Substance Abuse Treatment and Domestic Violence* (CSAT 1997b), defines domestic violence as "the use of intentional emotional, psychological, sexual, or physical force by one family member or intimate partner to control another" and provides an array of means of abuse: "verbal, emotional, and physical intimidation; destruction of the victim's possessions; maiming or killing pets; threats; forced sex; and slapping, punching, kicking, choking, burning, stabbing, shooting, and killing victims" (p. 1).

The actual introduction to substances by a significant other can be a way of increasing control and establishing power over some women. While rates of domestic violence vary across studies, it is evident that there is a significant relationship between violence and substance initiation, abuse, and dependence. In one survey study assessing the prevalence of domestic violence among women in substance abuse treatment, 60 percent of women reported either current or past domestic violence, 47 percent reported current domestic violence at treatment intake, and 39 percent reported either physical or emotional abuse in the past year leading up to treatment (Swan et al. 2000). Moreover, the prevalence of interpersonal violence and substance use extends to pregnant women who are drug dependent. In another study on prevalence of violence and pregnant women, 73 percent reported a lifetime history of physical abuse. Approximately 33 percent of women in substance abuse treatment who were pregnant reported having physical fights with their current partner in the past year (Velez et al. 2006). In the first analysis of evaluating the role of substance use as a means of coping among women who have experienced domestic violence (Kaysen et al. 2007), the results support the self-medication hypothesis in that women use alcohol as a means of managing painful affect.

Co-Occurring Substance Use and Mental Disorders

Women are more likely than men to have co-occurring mental and substance use disorders (see chapter 8 and TIP 42, *Substance Abuse Treatment for Persons With Co-Occurring Disorders* [CSAT 2005e]). According to the National Comorbidity Study of women diagnosed with alcohol abuse, 72.4 percent have lifetime co-occurring mental disorders and 86 percent of women diagnosed with alcohol dependence have co-occurring disorders (Kessler et al. 1997). In comparison to men, women are more likely to have multiple comorbidity (three or more psychiatric diagnoses in addition to substance use disorder; Zilberman et al. 2003). Various literature on co-occurring disorders highlights the role of substance abuse as a means of self-medicating distressing affect. While differences are noted in prevalence rates of co-occurring disorders among women of specific ethnic populations, Corcoran and Corcoran (2001) assert, based on their retrospective study, that gender (specifically female), appears to play a more salient role than ethnicity in endorsing the use of substances to manage negative affect.

For women, anxiety disorders and major depression are positively associated with substance use, abuse, and dependence and are the most common co-occurring diagnoses (Agrawal et al. 2005). Other common mental disorders in women with substance use disorders are eating disorders and PTSD, a common sequel to violence and trauma. In a study screening women veterans for substance abuse and psychiatric disorders, 57 percent of the women who screened positive for depression,

Protective Factor—Coping Skills: Engaging in problemsolving skills, mobilizing support from others, and learning to cope with one's feelings are key protective ingredients (Mrazek and Haggerty 1994).

eating and panic disorders, and PTSD also screened positive for substance abuse (including tobacco use). This sample demonstrated that women with a positive screen for psychiatric conditions were twice as likely to have abused drugs in the last year (Davis et al. 2003). While it is likely that mental disorders can play a primary role in initiating substance use to gain relief, it is as important to acknowledge that psychiatric disorders may occur as a consequence of substance use or develop independently, yet concurrently, of the current pattern of substance use.

Preliminary investigations and discussions suggest that some co-occurring mental disorders may be likely risk factors for the initiation of substance use and the subsequent development of substance use disorders (such as anxiety disorders and major depression), while other co-occurring disorders may be more likely to occur after the development of substance use disorders (Conway and Montoya 2007). For many women, the onset of the mental illness may precede the substance abuse, particularly in cases of PTSD (Brady and Randall 1999). One study reveals that women with PTSD were five times more likely than women without PTSD to have substance use disorders (Brady et al. 2000). A review of several studies reveals that current PTSD rates among women who abuse substances range between 14 and 60 percent (Brady 2001; Najavits et al. 1998; Triffleman 2003), and that women who use substances are still more than twice as likely to have PTSD than men (Najavits et al. 1997). The planned TIP, *Substance Abuse and Trauma* (CSAT in development *h*), provides more information on this topic.

Regarding eating disorders (anorexia nervosa and bulimia nervosa), women who are diagnosed with these disorders are more likely to develop alcohol use disorders later on (Franko et al. 2005). Specifically, the behavioral pattern of purging, but not bingeing, appears to be associated more strongly with substance use. This finding is consistent with a theory that overeating or bingeing competes with substance use for the reward sites in the brain (Kalarchian et al. 2007; Kleiner et al. 2004; Warren et al. 2005), and that obesity may be a protective

factor against developing substance use disorders.

Discrimination

Discriminatory acts range from mundane slights to devastating violent acts. Women may experience varied levels of discrimination—based on gender, race, ethnicity, language, culture, socioeconomic status, sexual orientation, age, and disability—that affect their substance use and may affect their recovery (see chapter 6). For some women, substance abuse may become a way of coping with the additional stresses of discrimination. When women experience more than one type of discrimination, the effect can be compounded (Krieger 1999). Discrimination can result in fewer educational and employment opportunities, lower socioeconomic status, fewer choices in housing, and poorer health outcome (Mays et al. 2007). Less access to health care and difficulty in funding treatment due to a lack of health insurance can result in later referral for substance abuse treatment. These circumstances can lead directly and indirectly to negative health consequences and psychological distress, requiring special considerations during treatment (Krieger 1999).

Acculturation

Studies have found that as immigrants become increasingly acculturated into American society, and even as African Americans move closer to mainstream European/Caucasian lifestyles, alcohol and drug use increases. Acculturation can involve intergenerational conflict and feelings of disconnection, a struggle for cultural identity, and feelings of grief and loss related to the life left behind—all of which can put a woman at risk for substance abuse. For example, foreign-born Mexican Americans and foreign-born non-Hispanic Caucasians are at significantly lower risk for substance use disorders than are their American-born counterparts (Grant et al. 2004). Second- and third-generation Hispanics/Latinas are more likely than their mothers to use alcohol and illicit drugs (Mora 2002). A

When working with individuals with co-occurring disorders, it is often a challenge to understand the history and development of symptoms and the chronological relationship between each disorder. While it would be valuable to understand the temporal relationship between disorders and to determine which set of symptoms and disorder came first, it is generally information that is difficult to obtain. Nonetheless, clinicians can help clients gain awareness of the interrelationship between disorders and symptoms and how one disorder may exacerbate the other or serve as a coping mechanism to manage symptoms. To lay the groundwork to help clients understand this relationship, a simple timeline exercise can be implemented to highlight the prevalence and presenting symptoms across time.

Directions: On a piece of paper, draw a straight line from birth to current age. Mark the line either in 1-year or 5-year increments depending on the age of the client and the duration of the disorders. Start with one disorder and mark the approximate onset of the initial symptoms, then write in the symptoms starting with the initial occurrence (approximate) and add the subsequent symptoms across the timeline. Once you have completed one disorder, go back (use a different color pen or marker) and do the same for the next. Use the timeline as a tool to promote discussion. Don't forget to process feelings that may surface during this exercise. **Note**: As a clinician, it can be enticing to add other variables from the start, but usually it is better to start out simple and then return to the timeline in the next individual or group session to explore other issues, such as rating severity of use on the timeline

A sample timeline is provided below. This timeline was developed for a patient with a history of an eating disorder (anorexia nervosa) and alcohol dependence. Not all symptoms have been noted on this timeline for either disorder.

Clinical Activity: Sample Timeline

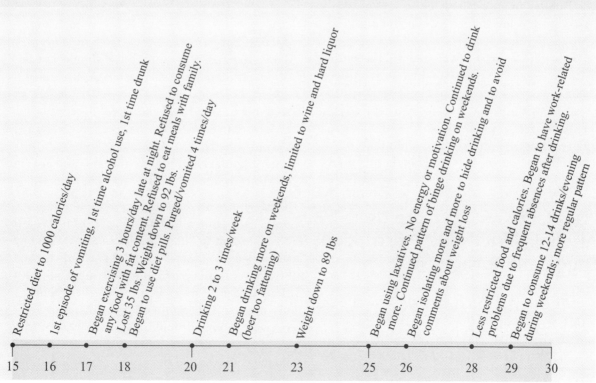

suggested explanation for this increase in use among younger Latinas is conflicting cultural expectations; their mothers and grandmothers are more constrained by traditional cultures.

Socioeconomic Status

Women with substance use disorders are more likely to have lower incomes and less education and are less likely to be employed. Employment status appears to be a factor associated with alcohol and drug abuse and dependence. Drug abuse and dependence are higher among women who are unemployed; in 2003, 12.5 percent of women aged 18 to 49 who were unemployed abused or were dependent on alcohol or an illicit drug compared with 8 percent of women who were employed full time (SAMHSA 2004). The temporal relationship between unemployment and the development of substance use disorders is rather complex and not well understood.

Patterns and Prevalence of Substance Use Among Women

This section covers specific prevalence rates associated with women's initiation of substance use. Similar to males, females initiate use based on, but not limited to, alcohol and drug availability, level of ease in obtaining the substances, price of substances, the ratio between perceived drug benefit versus perceived risk associated with use, and general attitude toward substance use. Yet, women typically display different patterns of use with alcohol, illicit and prescription drugs, and tobacco. The following segment highlights these unique patterns.

Prevalence of Substance Use: Alcohol, Illicit Drugs, Prescription Drugs, and Tobacco

Alcohol and illicit drugs
SAMHSA's National Survey on Drug Use and Health (NSDUH) interviews yearly more than 67,000 persons ages 12 or older to assess their use of alcohol and illicit drugs and their symptoms of substance abuse or dependence during the past year (SAMHSA 2007). Results of NSDUH for 2006 indicate that 45.2 percent of females ages 12 or older used alcohol during 2006, and 6.2 percent reported current illicit drug use. Figure 2-1 (p. 29) provides more specific information about the use of illicit drugs, alcohol, and tobacco by females ages 12 and older.

Prescription drugs
An analysis of data from the National Medical Expenditures Survey shows women not only use significantly more prescription drugs than men, they also use significantly more prescription drugs with addictive properties. Compared with men, women are 48 percent more likely to use a prescription drug that can be abused (Simoni-Wastila 2000). According to the NSDUH 2004 survey, between 2003 and 2004, the number of persons aged 12 or older with lifetime nonmedical use of pain relievers increased from 31.2 million to 31.7 million including the use of Vicodin, Lortab, Lorcet, Percocet, Percodan, Tylox, hydrocodone products, OxyContin, and oxycodone products (SAMHSA 2005). The NSDUH 2003 survey found that 55 percent of new people who used these prescription drugs were female (SAMHSA 2004).

Tobacco
The importance of tobacco use should not be underestimated in a discussion of substance abuse. The negative physical consequences are well documented and can be fatal—increased risk for cardiovascular disease and stroke; chronic obstructive pulmonary disease; and lung, bladder, and other cancers—and specific risks are related to gender (see chapter 3).

Tobacco use among American women has decreased from a high of 34 percent in 1965 to 23.3 percent in 2006 (SAMHSA 2007). Among females ages 12 or older, 22.2 percent smoked cigarettes in the past month during 2006. Less than 1 percent of women reported current use of a smokeless tobacco product, and 2.1 percent reported smoking cigars. Women who use smokeless tobacco (ST) reported using ST to manage weight and in response to mood states.

Six Patterns Associated with Women's Substance Use

1. Narrowing of the Gender Gap: In comparing male and female rates of alcohol use across 10 years (Grant et al. 2006), there is significant evidence of the gender gap narrowing. Overall, younger adult females are more likely to mirror male patterns of alcohol and illicit drug use than older females. This shrinking gender gap for alcohol and drug use has been noted across ethnic groups, especially among younger women.

2. People of Introduction and Relationship Status: Women are more likely to be introduced to and initiate alcohol and drug use through significant relationships including boyfriends, spouses, partners, and relatives. According to the National Center on Addiction and Substance Abuse and Columbia University (CASA) research report, females are often introduced to substances in a more private setting (2003). In addition, marital status plays an important role as a protective factor in the development of substance use disorders.

3. Drug Injection and Relationships: Even though women are less likely to inject drugs than men, research suggests that women accelerate to injecting at a faster rate than men (Bryant and Treloar 2007). When women inject drugs for the first time, they are more likely than men who are first-time injectors to be introduced to this form of administration by a sexual partner (Frajzyngier et al. 2007). Women are more likely to be involved with a sexual partner who also injects. While various personality and interpersonal factors influence needle sharing among women (Brook et al. 2000), women are more likely to inject with and borrow needles and equipment from their partner, spouse, or boyfriend. Among women who use with their sexual partners, Bryant and Treloar (2007) highlight a division of labor where men are responsible for obtaining, purchasing, and injecting the drug for them. Thus, needle sharing and drug using with a sexual partner may engender a sense of emotional intimacy among women or reflect inequity of power in the relationship. Other "people of introduction" besides sexual partners are groups that are predominantly female. While women may initiate drug injection through relational means, it is important to recognize that some women are as likely to initiate drug injection on their own.

4. Earlier Patterns Reflect Later Problems: Drinking low to moderate levels of alcohol in early adulthood is a predictor of later heavy drinking and alcohol-related substance use disorders among women (Andersen et al. 2003; Morgen et al. 2008). In addition to amount of alcohol intake, frequency of use appears positively associated with risk of alcohol dependence, particularly for women (Flensborg-Madsen et al. 2007). Females who begin smoking at a young age are more likely to initiate alcohol and drug use than females who do not smoke.

5. Responsibilities and Pattern of Use: Women are more likely to temporarily alter their pattern of use in response to caregiver responsibilities. As an example, women are likely to curtail or establish abstinence of alcohol and illicit drugs while pregnant (SAMHSA 2004), even though they are as likely to resume use later on. In addition, some women report that they use stimulants to help meet expectations associated with family responsibilities (Joe 1995).

6. Progression and Consequences of Use: Women experience an effect called telescoping (Piazza et al. 1989), whereby they progress faster than men from initial use to alcohol and drug-related consequences even when using a similar or lesser amount of substances. While extensive research is available pertaining to the telescoping effect of alcohol and alcohol-related consequences among women, more recent research (Hernandex-Avila et al. 2004; Ridenour et al. 2005) supports a preliminary finding—a similar pattern of rapid progression for illicit drugs. While women have a greater biological vulnerability to the adverse consequences of substance use, it is important to note that variations in progression and the biopsychosocial consequences of substance use may also be linked to socioeconomic status, racial/ethnic differences, and age (Johnson et al. 2005). As an example, African Americans generally begin regular alcohol use later than most population groups yet demonstrate more rapid transition from initiation of use to abuse.

In addition, women reported that initiation of use was significantly influenced by other females who use (Cohen-Smith and Severson 1999).

Data from the 1997–1998 National Center for Health Statistics' National Health Interview Survey revealed that among racial or ethnic groups, American-Indian and Alaska-Native women have the highest prevalence of tobacco use with 34.5 percent; Asian- or Pacific-American women have the lowest prevalence at 11.2 percent (Office of the Surgeon General 2001*b*). Women with more education tend to smoke less than women with less education. According to the survey, the lowest rates among people who smoke were for women with more than 16 years of education, and the highest rates were for women with 9 to 11 years of education.

There is increasing evidence that children of parents who smoke cigarettes are more likely to smoke than the children of parents who do not smoke. Although some studies show conflicting results, girls seem to be more influenced by their parents' smoking and are particularly more likely to model maternal behavior. This applies not just to smoking but also to cessation. The Office of the Surgeon General (2001*b*) reports one study that found when mothers stopped smoking, it helped delay or deter smoking in adolescent daughters, but not in sons.

Although there is debate about the relevance of the "gateway" concept (in which use of one substance leads to use of other more "dangerous" substances), many studies show that tobacco use precedes alcohol and drug use. Young women in particular who smoke tobacco are more likely than young women who do not smoke to drink alcohol or use drugs, especially when they begin smoking at a young age (Ellickson et al. 1992; Lai et al. 2000; Torabi et al. 1993). Based on these studies, associated behaviors and environmental factors play a probable role in initiating tobacco, alcohol, and drug use.

Prevalence of Substance Use Patterns Among Women Who Are Pregnant

NSDUH includes questions about the use of alcohol, illicit drugs, tobacco, and pregnancy status among women ages 15 to 44; results show past-month rates for substance use are curtailed substantially during pregnancy (see Figure 2-2 on p. 30; SAMHSA 2008). These rates are likely to be conservative because they reflect only past-month use, not use during the entire pregnancy. They also are limited to women who were aware of their pregnancies at the time of the survey. Responses are affected by an unknown degree of stigma associated with using substances during pregnancy.

Among pregnant women ages 15 to 44 years, 5 percent reported using illicit drugs in the past month, based on combined 2006 and 2007 NSDUH data. This rate is significantly lower than the rate among women ages 15 to 44 who were not pregnant (10.0 percent). The rate of past-month cigarette use was also lower among those who were pregnant (16.4 percent) than it was among those who were not pregnant (28.4 percent). Alcohol use followed a similar pattern among pregnant women ages 15 to 44 with an estimated 11.6 percent reporting past-month alcohol use. This rate was significantly lower than the rate for nonpregnant women in the same age group (53.2 percent).

These data are encouraging, indicating that women tend to reduce their substance use during pregnancy. However, women's reduction of substance use during pregnancy appears to be temporary (SAMHSA 2008). NSDUH data suggest that women ages 15 to 44 use alcohol, tobacco, and illicit drugs less during pregnancy but are likely to resume substance use after pregnancy.

Women who continued to use illicit drugs occasionally or regularly after their last menstrual period are more likely to have a

Figure 2-1

Use of Illicit Drugs, Alcohol, and Tobacco by Females Aged 12 or Older, Past Year and Past Month, Numbers in Thousands and Percentages, 2006

	Past Year Number	Past Year Percent	Past Month Number	Past Month Percent
Any Illicit Drug	15,007	11.8	7,816	6.2
Marijuana (includes hashish)	9,785	7.7	5,162	4.1
Any Illicit Drug Other Than Marijuana	9,310	7.4	4,019	3.2
Cocaine	2,116	1.7	797	0.6
Crack	453	0.4	182	0.1
Heroin	184	0.1	77	0.1
Hallucinogens (LSD, PCP, Ecstasy)	1,593	1.3	428	0.3
Inhalants	875	0.7	257	0.2
Nonmedical Use of Any Psychotherapeutics	7,509	5.9	3,141	2.5
Pain Relievers	5,427	4.3	2,206	1.7
Tranquilizers	2,622	2.1	801	0.6
Stimulants/Methamphetamine	1,677	1.3	599	0.5
Sedatives	519	0.4	250	0.2
Any Tobacco	34,751	27.4	29,484	23.3
Alcohol	79,140	62.5	57,283	45.2
Binge Alcohol Use	—	—	19,276	15.2
Heavy Alcohol Use	—	—	4,172	3.3

Source: SAMHSA 2007.

higher number of pregnancies, less prenatal care, greater likelihood of substance use among family and friends, and greater severity of substance use (Derauf et al. 2007; Shieh and Kraavitz 2006). Continued substance abuse during pregnancy is a major risk factor for fetal distress, developmental abnormalities, and negative birth effects. It is also associated with delayed prenatal care, and it is quite likely that this delay is exacerbated as a result of fears pertaining to potential legal consequences (Jessup et al. 2003). Timely prenatal care for pregnant women who continue to use illicit drugs provides a significant buffer against adverse pregnancy outcomes, including premature births, small for gestational age status, and low birth weight (El-Mohandes et al. 2003; Quinlivan and Evans 2002).

Prevalence of Substance Abuse and Dependence Among Women

The Shrinking Gender Gap of Substance Abuse and Dependence

Even though studies have consistently shown a greater prevalence of substance use disorders among men, evidence is also mounting on the narrowing of the gender gap for these disorders (see Figure 2-3 on p. 31). According to the NSDUH 2006 survey, females were as likely as males to abuse or be dependent on substances between 12 and 17 years of age, while older adolescent males and females continue to show a greater gender gap in percentages of substance-related disorders. In comparing epidemiologic surveys from 1992 to 2002, an analysis found a significant increase in risk for alcohol abuse and dependence among women born after 1944, except for African-American women (Grucza et al. 2008).

Across the Life Span

As women become older, the prevalence of substance abuse and dependence becomes lower (Grant et al. 2006). The 2003 NSDUH estimated that 15.7 percent of women ages 18 to 25 abused or were dependent on alcohol or an illicit drug in the past year compared with 1.5 percent of those ages 50 or older (see Figure 2-4 on p. 32). However, it is important to remember that women remain vulnerable to substance use, abuse, and dependence and its consequences across their life spans. As women encounter major life transitions, they are at a heightened risk for substance use and abuse (Poole and Dell 2005).

	Pregnant, Aged 15–44	Not Pregnant, Aged 15–44
Figure 2-2 **Past-Month Substance Use, Based on Combined 2006 and 2007 Data: National Survey on Drug Use and Health (NSDUH), 2007**		
Any alcohol use	11.6 percent	53.2 percent
Binge alcohol use	3.7 percent	24.1 percent
Any illicit drug use	5.2 percent	9.7 percent
Cigarette use	16.4 percent	28.4 percent

Source: SAMHSA 2008.

Characteristics of Treatment Admissions Among Women

Data from treatment admissions provides considerable information on the patterns of substance use among women. Yet caution needs to be taken when generalizing this information across the entire population of women who have substance use disorders, since most women who have substance use disorders never receive treatment. According to TEDS data (SAMHSA 2004), women are less likely to report alcohol as their primary substance of abuse compared with males. Although alcohol is still the primary substance of abuse, women are more likely than men to be in treatment for drug use. For women, 37 percent report that opiates (20 percent) or cocaine (17 percent) are their primary substances of abuse.

While women often receive other healthcare services prior to identification of substance use disorders, referrals from healthcare providers (other than alcohol and drug use treatment providers) are one of the lowest referral routes to treatment for women. Currently, self-referral, social service agencies, and the criminal justice system are the primary sources of referral to treatment for women (Brady and Ashley 2005; SAMHSA 2004). In comparison to men, women are more likely to be identified with a substance use disorder through child protective services (Fiorentine et al. 1997).

Women who enter treatment are more likely to identify stress factors as their primary problem rather than substance use (Green et al. 2002; Thom 1987). They also exhibit more severity and problems related to substance use upon entering substance abuse treatment, including medical and psychological problems (Arfken et al. 2001). This heightened level of severity and symptomotology may, in part, be a result of delayed access to treatment due to various barriers, a reflection of rapid progression from initiation to alcohol and drug use consequences (telescoping), a manifestation of a woman's tendency to consume alcohol and use cocaine more frequently than men (Pettinati et al. 2000), or the lack of appropriate screening or identification of treatment need until severity is paramount.

In Figure 2-5 (p. 33), the percentage of female admissions to substance abuse treatment

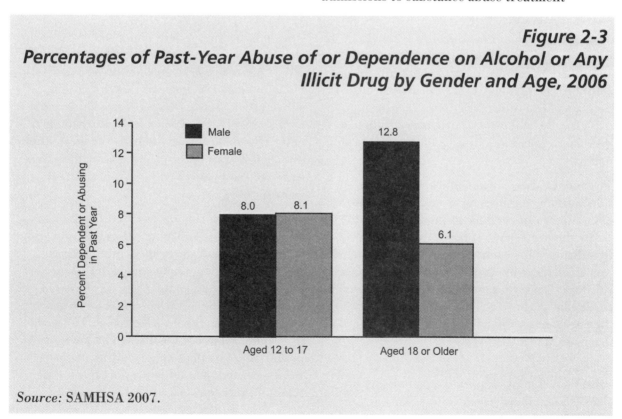

Figure 2-3
Percentages of Past-Year Abuse of or Dependence on Alcohol or Any Illicit Drug by Gender and Age, 2006

Source: SAMHSA 2007.

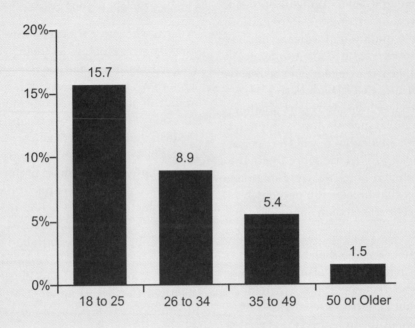

Figure 2-4

Percentages of Past-Year Abuse of or Dependence on Alcohol or Any Illicit Drug Among Women Aged 18 or Older by Age Group: 2003

Source: SAMHSA 2007.

programs by racial/ethnic groups is shown. For more detailed information on ethnicity and substance abuse, refer to chapter 6. In addition, the planned TIP, *Improving Cultural Competence in Substance Abuse Treatment* (CSAT in development *a*) provides additional information on ethnicity and substance abuse patterns.

TEDS data also provide information about substance preferences for women of specific population/ racial/ethnic groups. Figure 2-6 shows the percentage of treatment admissions by substance for each ethnic or racial group of women. Except for the "alcohol plus another substance" category, only the woman's primary substance of abuse is indicated in the table; the prevalence of polydrug abuse cannot be determined (SAMHSA 2004).

As Figure 2-6 (p. 34) indicates, the primary substance of abuse reported on admission of Caucasian and American-Indian/Alaska-Native women is alcohol. Asian- and Pacific-American women reported methamphetamine most often. African-American women were more likely to name crack/cocaine as the primary substance of abuse, whereas some subgroups of Hispanic/Latina women were more likely to enter treatment for heroin use. For most ethnic or racial groups, alcohol and a secondary drug were abused by the next largest percentage of women.

In 2002, women constituted about 30 percent of admissions for substance abuse (Brady and Ashley 2005), but they represented a larger proportion of admissions for prescription and over-the-counter (OTC) drug abuse (46 percent; OAS 2004*b*). Depending on treatment level, admission rates varied from 29 percent in hospital inpatient facilities to 39 percent in outpatient methadone programs. Women were admitted in notable proportions for all types of prescription and OTC drug abuse: 47

percent for prescription narcotics, 44 percent for prescription stimulants, 50 percent for tranquilizers, 51 percent for sedatives, and 42 percent for OTC medications (OTC drugs include aspirin, cough syrup, and any other medication available without prescription). The majority of individuals admitted for prescription and OTC drug treatment were Caucasian (88 percent; OAS 2004b).

According to TEDS data (OAS 2004c), 15,300 (4 percent) of women admitted to substance abuse treatment in 2002 were pregnant at the time of admission. Compared with the women in treatment who were not pregnant at admission, the pregnant women in treatment were more likely to report cocaine/crack (22 versus 17 percent), amphetamine/methamphetamine (21 versus 13 percent), or marijuana (17 versus 13 percent) as their primary substance of abuse. Alcohol was the primary substance of abuse among almost one-third of women aged 15 to 44 (31 percent) who were not pregnant at the time of admission. In contrast, only 18 percent of women who were pregnant at admission reported alcohol as their primary substance of abuse.

Figure 2-5 Percentage of Admissions to Substance Abuse Treatment Programs by Racial/Ethnic Group in 2006	
Group	**Percentage of Total Admissions**
Female Admissions	31.8
Caucasian	20.1
African American	6.4
Hispanic (Mexican Origin)	1.6
Hispanic (Puerto Rican Origin)	0.8
American Indian/Alaska Native	0.9
Asian/Pacific Islander	0.4
Source: HHS, SAMHSA, OAS 2008	

For a woman entering treatment, the tendency to focus on problems or stressors other than her substance abuse is quite normal. Women are socialized to assume more caregiver roles and to focus attention on others. Even if she has not appropriately cared for others (such as her children) during her addiction, it does not mean that she will not see this as an important issue immediately upon entering a detoxification or treatment program. The clinician needs to appreciate this gender difference; instead of assuming that the client's worries and her tendency to be other-focused is a detriment or an issue of resistance for treatment, use the client's concerns as a means of motivation throughout treatment.

Figure 2-6
Primary Substance of Abuse Among Women Admitted for Substance Abuse Treatment by Racial/Ethnic Group by Percentage

Substance of Abuse	Cauca-sian	African American	Hispanic (Mexi-can Origin)	Hispanic (Puerto Rican Origin)	American Indian/ Alaska Native	Asian/ Pacific Island-er	TWO OR MORE RACES
Alcohol	35.5	24.8	22.6	20.4	39.5	26.4	21.7
Cocaine/crack	13.3	35.0	12.0	18.4	8.0	9.2	12.0
Heroin	12.7	16.3	11.8	38.5	9.7	8.2	5.7
Other opioids	7.7	1.3	1.7	1.8	4.7	3.1	4.0
Marijuana/hashish	11.8	17.6	15.6	15.2	10.2	16.3	19.4
Methamphetamines	13.3	1.7	34.0	2.2	25.2	33.1	31.9
Benzodiazepines	1.0	0.2	0.1	0.4	0.4	0.3	0.6
Other amphet-amines	0.6	0.1	0.3	0.1	0.5	0.7	0.8
Other sedatives/ hypnotics	0.4	0.1	0.3	0.1	0.2	0.1	0.2
Hallucinogens	0.1	0.1	0.1	0.1	0.1	0.2	0.1
PCP	0.0*	0.4	0.5	0.3	0.1	0.2	0.2
Inhalants	0.1	0.1	0.2	0.0*	0.2	0.1	0.2
Over-the-counter (OTC) medications	0.1	0.0*	0.1	0.0*	0.1	0.1	0.1

* Less than 0.05 percent

Source: HHS, SAMHSA, OAS 2008.

Advice to Clinicians and Administrators:
Using Patterns of Use as a Clinical Guide

For Clinicians:

- Foremost, it is important to remember that women are as likely as men to become addicted to alcohol and drugs if given an opportunity. By making an assumption that women are less likely to have a substance use disorder, important information may not be obtained in the screening and assessment process, thus leading to misdiagnosis or under diagnosis.

- Depending on the specific drug class, some women may have considerable concerns regarding potential weight gain if they enter treatment and establish abstinence. Among women, weight loss is more likely a major benefit in continuing drug use.

- In assessing risk factors or potential triggers for relapse, don't underestimate that the initial reasons for use may be the same reasons for relapse, even if initial use occurred many years ago. As a clinician, it is important to prepare for a premature termination of treatment and establish an intervention plan tailored to address these initial reasons for use. More times than not, women generally will underestimate the risks associated with these issues. For example, women who initiated use due to a relationship will often deny that relationships are a current risk factor. Nonetheless, the counselor should not immediately follow the client's self-assessment but rather proceed with creating roleplays that simulate possible scenarios to provide practice in how to handle relationship issues before they actually occur in treatment; i.e., roleplay a telephone call from a boyfriend who believes that the client does not have a problem and begs her to come home. More often than not, other women in the treatment group have a better handle on the actual scenarios that are high risk for each other.

- Remember that women are socialized to be other-focused. Just because they may not have attended to some of their responsibilities during active substance use does not mean that they will not be focused on these responsibilities upon entering treatment. Rather than pushing the idea that they need to "get their head into treatment and not be so focused on outside issues," use their ability to be other-focused as a tool in developing motivation for recovery. Assuming that a woman is resistant to treatment because she is other-focused in the program is a form of gender bias. Women are socialized to think about others.

- Because substance abuse tends to run in families, a woman's parents and children as well as her partner need to be considered in planning treatment. As important, a woman needs to be aware of the influence of substance abuse in her family. Using a family geneogram or family tree to mark who has used substances can be a valuable tool in assessing the degree of influence in her family.

- A partner's substance use and attitudes toward substance use can influence a woman's substance use. A woman who uses illicit drugs is more likely to have a partner who also uses illicit drugs. The counselor should work with all individuals who have influence on the client so that each person develops attitudes and behaviors that will be supportive of the client's recovery.

- Remember to assess for personality traits that are more conducive to substance abuse among women, namely sensation-seeking.

Advice to Clinicians and Administrators:
Using Patterns of Use as a Clinical Guide (continued)

- Trauma is both a risk factor for and a consequence of substance abuse. Women with histories of trauma may be using substances to self-medicate symptoms. Subsequently, interventions should be immediately put into place to help build coping strategies to manage strong affect, including relaxation training and other anxiety management skills. Start skills-building immediately rather than waiting for an incident to occur. It is far more difficult to manage symptoms when they are heightened than when they are at lower levels of intensity.
- From the outset, counselors need to be aware of the potential and common occurrence and impact of co-occurring disorders among women with substance use disorders, especially mood, anxiety, and eating disorders.

For Administrators:

- Administrators need to develop and incorporate policies and procedures that support family involvement from the onset. Beginning with the initial contact, staff need to convey the importance of family involvement and the program's expectations regarding the necessity of family participation.
- Administrators need to develop policies and procedures to address co-occurring issues, including screening, assessment, and referral processes. They need to secure funding and endorse programs that are effective with various populations, such as trauma-informed services and culturally responsive programs.

3 Physiological Effects of Alcohol, Drugs, and Tobacco on Women

Overview

Based on human and animal studies, women are more sensitive to the consumption and long-term effects of alcohol and drugs than men. From absorption to metabolic processes, women display more difficulty in physically managing the consequences of use. In general, with higher levels of alcohol and drugs in the system for longer periods of time, women are also more susceptible to alcohol- and drug-related diseases and organ damage.

This chapter provides an overview of the physiological impact of alcohol and drugs on women, with particular emphasis on the significant physiological differences and consequences of substance use in women. It begins with a general exploration of how gender differences affect the way alcohol and drugs are metabolized in the body and then highlights several biopsychosocial and cultural factors that can influence health issues associated with drugs and alcohol. The chapter goes on to explore the physiological effects of alcohol, drugs (both licit and illicit), and tobacco on the female body. A summary of key research on the impact of these substances when taken during pregnancy follows, and the chapter closes with a review of the effect that substance abuse has on women's HIV/AIDS status. Counselors can use the information presented in this chapter to educate their female clients about the negative effects substances can have on their physical health. A sample patient lecture is included that highlights the physiological effects of heavy alcohol use.

Physiological Effects and Consequences of Substance Abuse in Women

Alcohol and drugs can take a heavy toll on the human body. The same general statements can be made for both men and women about their long-term effects—for example, both genders incur liver problems resulting from alcohol abuse, respiratory impairment and lung cancer as a consequence of smoking, HIV/AIDS and hepatitis from injection drug use, and memory difficulties associated with the use of marijuana. Yet women have different physical responses to substances and greater susceptibility to health-related issues. Women differ from men in the severity of the problems that develop from use of alcohol and drugs and in the amount of time between initial use and the development of physiological problems (Greenfield 1996; Mucha et al. 2006). For example, a consequence of excessive alcohol use is liver damage (such as cirrhosis) that often begins earlier in women consuming less alcohol over a shorter period of time. By and large, women who have substance use disorders have poorer quality of life than men on health-related issues.

In addition, women who abuse substances have physiological consequences, health issues, and medical needs related to gynecology (Peters et al. 2003). Specifically, drugs and alcohol affect women's menstrual cycles, causing increased cramping and heavier or lighter periods. Women sometimes use illicit drugs and alcohol as medication for cramping, body aches, and other discomforts associated with menstruation (Stevens and Estrada 1999). On the other hand, women who use heroin and methadone can experience amenorrhea (absence of menstrual periods; Abs et al. 2000), leading them to believe that they are unable to conceive and misreading early signs of pregnancy as withdrawal symptoms. Subsequently, they are unaware that they are pregnant. Women's substance use also poses risks to fetuses and nursing infants.

Limitations of Current Research on Gender Differences in Metabolism

In general, research on the unique physiological effects of alcohol and drugs in women is limited and sometimes inconclusive. Although the differences in the way women and men metabolize alcohol have been studied in some depth, research on differences in metabolism of illicit drugs is limited. For many years, much of the research on metabolism of substances either used male subjects exclusively or did not report on gender differences. Historically, women were omitted due to the potential risk of pregnancy and the possibility that hormonal changes across the menstrual cycle would wreak havoc on the drugs' effects and subsequent results.

Available research is typically based on small sample sizes and has not been replicated. Race and ethnic background can affect metabolism and the psychological effects of alcohol and illicit drugs, as can the psychopharmaceuticals sometimes used in treatment (Rouse et al. 1995), but their effects have not been studied. Similar to men, few women abuse only one substance. Polysubstance use complicates the ability to study and understand the physiological effects of specific drugs on women, while increasing the risk associated with synergistic effects when substances are combined. Significant gaps in knowledge exist regarding physiological effects across the continuum of a woman's life.

Physiological Effects: Factors of Influence

Ethnicity and Culture

The level of acculturation and cultural roles and expectations play a significant role in substance use patterns among women of color (Caetano et al. 2008). The prevalence of substance abuse among ethnic women typically coincides with higher levels of acculturation in the United States, thus leading to greater health issues. Literature suggests that women from ethnically diverse backgrounds who have substance use disorders possess greater risks for developing certain conditions and disorders, such as hypertension, high blood pressure, and HIV/AIDS (Centers for Disease Control [CDC] 2000a, b; Steffens et al. 2006; Vernon 2007). These health disparities arise from many sources, including difficulty in accessing affordable health care, delays in seeking treatment, limited socioeconomic resources, racism, and discrimination (Gee 2002; Mays et al. 2007; Williams 2002). In addition, mistrust of health care providers is a significant barrier to receiving appropriate screening, preventive care, timely interventions, and adequate treatment (Alegria et al. 2002). More recent studies have explored the role of gender in perceived discrimination and health, and some studies have noted differences in the type of stressors, reactions, and health consequences between men and women (Finch et al. 2000; Flores et al. 2008). For example, the Black Women's Health Study found that perceived experiences of racism were associated with an increased incidence of breast cancer (Taylor et al. 2007).

Sexual Orientation

Lesbian/bisexual women exhibit more prevalent use of alcohol, marijuana, prescription drugs, and tobacco than heterosexual women, and they are likely to consume alcohol more frequently and in greater amounts (Case et al. 2004; Cochran et al. 2001, 2004). Based on the Substance Abuse and Mental Health Services Administration's (SAMHSA's) 1996 National Household Survey on Drug Abuse, researchers compared patterns of use between homosexual and heterosexual women and found that lesbians have greater alcohol-related morbidity (Cochran et al. 2001). Likewise, they are less likely to have health insurance and to use preventive screenings, including mammograms and pelvic examinations. With less utilization of routine screenings, lesbians and bisexual women may not be afforded the benefit of early detection across disorders, including substance use disorders, breast cancer, and cardiovascular disease.

Socioeconomic Status and Homelessness

Overall, lower socioeconomic status is associated with higher mortality rates and greater risks for cervical cancer, coronary heart disease, HIV/AIDS, and other health conditions and medical disorders (Adler and Coriell 1997). More than ethnicity, socioeconomic status heavily influences the health risks associated with substance abuse. Research suggests that when the socioeconomic conditions of ethnically diverse populations are similar to those of the White population, consequences of substance use appear comparable (Jones-Webb et al. 1995). Among women, alcohol and drug-related morbidity and mortality are disproportionately higher in individuals of lower socioeconomic status, which is associated with insufficient healthcare services, difficulties in accessing treatment, lack of appropriate nutrition, and inadequate prenatal care. Subsequently, impoverished women who abuse substances often experience greater health consequences and poorer health outcomes.

Similarly, homelessness is associated with higher mortality rates for all life-threatening disorders, including greater risks for infectious diseases. With greater high-risk sexual behaviors and repeated exposure to overcrowded shelters, homeless women who use injection drugs are more likely to be infected with HIV/AIDS and other infectious diseases, including airborne infections such as tuberculosis, thereby leading to greater health consequences (for review, see Galea and Vlahov 2002).

Developmental Issues and Aging

Although little is known regarding the effect of alcohol and drugs on development across the lifespan, there is some evidence in alcohol-related research that there are different vulnerabilities at different ages for women. Even though developmental research on alcohol is not easily transferred to other drugs of abuse, it can give us a glimpse of the potential physiological issues associated with age and aging. For example, adolescent women are more likely than their male counterparts to experience cognitive impairment despite less alcohol consumption. Women of child-bearing age are more likely to experience infertility with heavier drinking (Tolstrup et al. 2003). Postmenopausal women are more likely to exhibit significant hormonal changes with heavy consumption of alcohol, leading to potentially higher risks for breast cancer, osteoporosis, and coronary heart disease (Weiderpass et al. 2001). Older women are more sensitive to alcohol and display a decrease in tolerance and alcohol metabolism (Center for Substance Abuse Treatment [CSAT] 1998d). While research has been more devoted to examining gender differences, limited data are available for other substances and less is known regarding the effect of these substances on development and aging.

Co-Occurring Disorders: A Bidirectional Influence

According to SAMHSA's National Survey on Drug Use and Health (NSDUH) report (Office of Applied Studies [OAS] 2004b), women with co-occurring mental and substance use disorders are likely to experience serious physical health problems. Co-occurring disorders have a bidirectional relationship and often a synergistic effect on one another. As much as substance abuse can increase the risk of, exacerbate, or cause medical conditions, medical disorders can also increase substance abuse as a means of self-medicating symptoms or mental distress associated with the disorder. Similar to men, women who have mental disorders can have more difficulty adhering to health-related treatment recommendations, such as treatment attendance, diet restrictions, or medication compliance.

Physiological Effects of Alcohol

Gender Differences in Metabolism and Effects

Alcohol is a leading cause of mortality and disability worldwide. According to the World Health Organization, alcohol is one of the five most significant risk factors for diseases, with more than 60 percent of alcohol-related diseases being chronic conditions, including cancer, cirrhosis of the liver, diabetes, and cardiovascular disease (Chisholm et al. 2004).

Alcohol's effects on women have been studied more than those of illicit drugs. Compared with men, women become more cognitively impaired by alcohol and are more susceptible to alcohol-related organ damage. Women develop damage at lower levels of consumption over a shorter period of time (for review, see Antai-Otong 2006). When men and women of the same weight consume equal amounts of alcohol, women have higher blood alcohol concentrations. Women have proportionately more body fat and a lower volume of body water compared with men of similar weight (Romach and Sellers 1998). As a result, women have a higher concentration of alcohol because there is less volume of water to dilute it.

In comparison with men, women, at least those younger than 50, have a lower first-pass metabolism of alcohol in the stomach and upper small intestine before it enters the bloodstream and reaches other body organs, including the liver. One researcher concluded that women's lack of a functional gastric protective barrier means that "for an alcoholic woman to drink alcohol is the same as taking the alcohol directly into a vein," contributing to her greater vulnerability to alcohol-related organ damage (Lieber 2000, p. 417).

These factors may be responsible for the increased severity, greater number, and faster rate of development of complications that women experience from alcohol abuse when compared with men, according to reviews of several studies (Blum et al. 1998; Greenfield 1996). Women develop alcohol abuse and dependence in less time than do men, a phenomenon known as telescoping (Piazza et al. 1989). At a rate of consumption of two to three standard drinks per day, women have a higher mortality rate than men who drink the same amount. Men do not experience an increased mortality risk until they consume four drinks daily (Holman et al. 1996).

Women develop other alcohol-related diseases at a lower total lifetime exposure than men, including such disorders as fatty liver, hypertension, obesity, anemia, malnutrition, gastrointestinal hemorrhage, and ulcers that require surgery (Van Thiel et al. 1989). Heavy alcohol use also increases the risk of hemorrhagic stroke, according to one study cited by Nanchahal and colleagues (2000). Older women respond to alcohol somewhat differently than do younger women. They have even less body water, a heightened sensitivity to and decreased tolerance for alcohol, and a decrease in alcohol metabolism in the gastrointestinal tract (CSAT 1998d).

The following sections identify specific physiological effects related to alcohol use by women. These effects are not distinct from one another; rather, they interact in a synergistic way in the body.

Liver and Other Organ Damage

Females are more likely than their male counterparts to experience greater organ damage as a result of consuming similar amounts of alcohol. Compared with men, women develop alcohol-induced liver disease over a shorter period of time and after consuming less alcohol (Gavaler and Arria 1995). Women are more likely than men to develop alcoholic hepatitis and to die from cirrhosis (Hall 1995). One researcher has theorized that women's faster alcohol elimination rate can endanger the liver by subjecting it to high, though transient, levels of acetaldehyde, a toxic byproduct of alcohol metabolism. This exposure may explain the higher liver cirrhosis rates among women (e.g., Thomasson 2000).

Cardiac-Related Conditions

According to current studies, women who drink exhibit a greater propensity to develop alcohol-induced cardiac damage. While light consumption (less than one drink per day) can serve as a protective factor for women who have a risk for coronary artery disease, studies suggest that protection is not evident for younger women, women who drink heavily, and women without risk factors associated with heart disease. Women who are dependent on alcohol or consume heavier amounts are more likely to die prematurely from cardiac-related conditions (Bradley et al. 1998a; Fernandez-Sola and Nicolas-Arfelis 2002; Hanna et al. 1992).

Heavy consumption (more than four drinks per day) is associated with increased blood pressure in both women and men (Bradley et al. 1998a). A major epidemiological study found that women between ages 30 and 64 who consumed 15–21 units of alcohol per week had an increased risk of hypertension compared with those who drank 14 or fewer units; those who drank 1–7 units per week had an overall decrease in 10-year risk of cardiovascular disease compared with those who drank more (Nanchahal et al. 2000). The female heart appears to experience a functional decline at a lower level of lifetime exposure to alcohol than does the male heart (Urbano-Marquez et al. 1995).

What constitutes light, moderate, or heavy drinking?

The U.S. Department of Health and Human Services and U.S. Department of Agriculture's definition of moderate alcohol consumption (2005) varies by gender: In women, moderate drinking is considered to be no more than one drink per day, compared with no more than two drinks per day for men. These differences stem from gender differences in body composition and metabolism.

Reproductive Consequences

Research into the adverse impact of alcohol consumption on fertility is growing. While numerous studies have shown a consistent relationship between heavy drinking and infertility (Eggert et al. 2004; Tolstrup et al. 2003), additional studies examining moderate consumption are more inconsistent. Nevertheless, findings suggest a need to educate and screen women for alcohol use while they are seeking infertility treatment (Chang et al. 2006). In addition, heavy drinking is associated with painful and/or irregular menstruation (Bradley et al. 1998a). The reproductive consequences associated with alcohol use disorders range from increased risk for miscarriage to impaired fetal growth and development (Mello et al. 1993).

There are considerable variations among women in their capacity to consume and metabolize alcohol. Early literature suggests that variations in alcohol metabolism among women may be linked to the different phases of the menstrual cycle, but more recent reviews suggest that there are no consistent effects of the menstrual cycle on the subjective experience of alcohol intake or alcohol metabolism (Terner and de Wit 2006). Studies reviewed by Romach and Sellers (1998) found that significant hormonal changes are reported in postmenopausal women who consume alcohol. Women taking hormone replacement therapy (HRT), now referred to as menopausal hormone therapy, and consuming 14 or more standard drinks weekly had significantly higher estradiol levels. These high levels are associated with a greater risk of breast cancer and coronary heart disease.

Breast and Other Cancers

Numerous studies have documented associations and suggested causal relationships between alcohol consumption and breast cancer risk (Key et al. 2006; Li et al. 2003; Zhang et al. 2007). A review of data from more than 50 epidemiological studies from around the world revealed that for each drink of alcohol consumed daily, women increased their risk of breast cancer by 7 percent (Hamajima et al. 2002). Postmenopausal women have an increased risk of breast cancer as well if they currently drink alcohol (Lenz et al. 2002; Onland-Moret et al. 2005). Women who drink alcohol have elevated estrogen and androgen levels, which are hypothesized to be contributors to the development of breast cancer in this population (Singletary and Gapstur 2001). In addition, postmenopausal women who are moderate alcohol drinkers (one to two drinks a day) and who are using menopausal hormone therapy have an increased risk of breast cancer, with even greater risk at higher rates of alcohol consumption (Dorgan et al. 2001; Onland-Moret

et al. 2005).

While the risk for in situ and invasive cervical cancer and cancer of the vagina may be associated with other environmental factors including high-risk sexual behavior, human papilloma viruses, smoking, hormonal therapy, and dietary deficiency, Weiderpass and colleagues (2001) concluded, based on 30 years of retrospective data, that women who are alcohol dependent are at a higher risk for developing these cancers. Similarly, Bagnardi et al. (2001) conducted a meta-analysis of more than 200 studies whereby they found that alcohol significantly increased the risks for cancers of the oral cavity, pharynx, esophagus, larynx, stomach, colon, rectum, liver, and ovaries. Although further investigation is needed to explore the role of alcohol consumption on gastric cancer, preliminary findings suggest that the type of alcoholic beverage, namely medium-strength beer, creates an increased risk of gastric cancer (Larsson et al. 2007). Based on a multiethnic cohort study, the risk of endometrial cancer increases when postmenopausal women consume an average of two or more drinks per day (Setiawan et al. 2008). Additional risks are associated with tobacco use, particularly for cancers of the upper digestive and respiratory tract.

Osteoporosis

According to Bradley and colleagues (1998a), evidence suggests "decreased bone formation and abnormal vitamin D metabolism may predispose alcohol-dependent premenopausal women to osteoporosis" (p. 631). Heavy alcohol use clearly has been shown to harm bones and to increase the risk of osteoporosis by decreasing bone density. These effects are especially striking in young women, whose bones are developing, but chronic alcohol use in adulthood also harms bones (Sampson 2002). In addition, animal studies suggest that the damaging effects of early chronic alcohol exposure are not overcome even when alcohol use ceases (Sampson 1998). Tobacco use also may increase the risk of osteoporosis and fractures; people who drink are 75 percent more likely to smoke, and people who

Clinical Activity: Sample Client-Educating Lecture Outline for Counselors Physiological Effects of Alcohol

This 60-minute lecture provides a general outline highlighting the physiological effects of moderate-to-heavy alcohol use. Refer to this TIP chapter for additional information to support your lecture. To increase participation, first ask women in the group to identify medical problems they believe to be related to their alcohol use. The format of this lecture can also be used with illicit and prescription drugs. Many conditions do occur in men, but it is important to emphasize the enhanced risk and the earlier appearance of these diseases and conditions among women. The list of physiological consequences identifies the most common disorders; it is not intended as a comprehensive review.

I.   Rationale: Women's positive response to health education

II. Objectives:

   A. To review what constitutes moderate-to-heavy drinking among women

   B. To describe physiological differences in how alcohol is metabolized in a woman's body

   C. To explore the long-term consequences of drinking, with emphasis on specific consequences unique to women

III. Equipment: Using an easel with newspaper print or a board, draw a human body. As you lecture, write in the effects of alcohol on the body to demonstrate how dramatically alcohol affects women. At the end of the lecture, the body should be covered with physiological consequences.

IV. Definition: In women, moderate drinking is considered to be no more than one drink per day (U.S. Department of Health and Human Services and U.S. Department of Agriculture [2005]).

V.   Alcohol Metabolism and Women:

   A. Women have higher blood alcohol concentrations after drinking the same amount of alcohol as men.

   B. Women have more body fat and a lower volume of body water than men of equal weight. Consequently, women are less able to dilute alcohol once it enters the body, and this leads to a higher concentration of alcohol in the bloodstream and organs.

   C. Women have a lower concentration of gastric dehydrogenase, an enzyme responsible for metabolism. Because alcohol takes longer to metabolize in women, it has more deleterious effects on major organs for a longer period of time. Longer metabolism and less dilution is a potent mixture for women! In addition, women have smaller organs than men, causing greater vulnerability to the long-term effects of alcohol.

VI. Long-Term Consequences: Women experience negative physical consequences and complications from alcohol sooner and at lower levels of consumption than men. Evidence suggests that women progress significantly faster in developing dependence, organ damage, and diseases with much lower levels of alcohol consumption. Women are more likely to die many years earlier from alcohol abuse and dependence.

   A. Liver and Other Gastrointestinal Disorders

      1. Fatty Liver

      2. Alcohol Hepatitis

      3. Cirrhosis

      4. Liver Cancer

      5. Ulcers/Gastritis

      6. Pancreatitis

      7. Diabetes

   B. Cardiac-Related Conditions

      1. High Blood Pressure (hypertension)

      2. Cardiomyopathy

      3. Stroke

      4. Arrhythmia

   C. Nutritional Deficiencies

      1. Malnutrition

      2. Vitamin and Mineral Deficiencies

   D. Reproductive Consequences

      1. Fetal Alcohol Spectrum Disorders: Fetal alcohol syndrome, alcohol-related birth defects (ARBD), partial fetal alcohol syndrome (pFAS), and alcohol-related neurodevelopmental disorder (ARND)

      2. Low Birth Weight

      3. Miscarriage

      4. Painful/Irregular Menstruation

      5. Underproduction of Hormones

Clinical Activity: Sample Client-Educating Lecture Outline for Counselors Physiological Effects of Alcohol (continued)

E. Breast and Other Cancers

   1. Breast Cancer

   2. Throat and Mouth Cancer

   3. Stomach and Colon Cancer

   4. Other Cancers

F. Osteoporosis

G. Cognitive and Other Neurological Effects

   1. Brain Shrinkage

   2. Peripheral Neuritis/Neuropathy

   3. Dementia

   4. Korsakoffs/Wernickes

   5. Cerebellar Degeneration

H. Infections: Greater Susceptibility and Progression

   1. HIV/AIDS

   2. Tuberculosis

   3. Pneumonia

I. Other Disorders and Conditions

smoke are 86 percent more likely to drink (Shiffman and Balabanis 1995). Women in menopause who enter treatment need bone density assessment, nutritional guidelines, and medication consultations.

Neurological Effects

Starting with adolescence, women appear to be more susceptible to the toxic effects of alcohol or its metabolites on the nervous system and more vulnerable to alcohol-induced brain damage than men (Bradley et al. 1998a; Hommer et al. 1996; Mann et al. 2005; Mumenthaler et al. 1999). Research supports that adult and adolescent women who are alcohol dependent experience greater declines in cognitive and motor function than men despite less alcohol consumption, shorter history of overall use, and shorter duration of alcohol dependence (Acker 1986; Flannery et al. 2007; Sullivan et al. 2002).

In comparison with men who are alcohol dependent and female controls (women who are not dependent on alcohol), women who are alcohol dependent exhibit deterioration in planning, visuospatial ability, working memory, and psychomotor speed. They also show brain abnormalities and shrinkage after a shorter drinking history and lower peak consumption than do men. Studies demonstrate that in general, women with alcohol dependence disorders have significantly smaller volumes of gray and white matter, less hippocampal volume (memory), and greater peripheral neuropathy than either men who abused alcohol or women who did not abuse alcohol (Ammendola et al. 2000; Hommer et al. 2001; Romach and Sellers 1998; Schweinsburg et al. 2003).

Women appear to be at greater risk than men for Alzheimer's disease, although women's longer life spans may contribute to this higher risk (Sohrabji 2002). Heavy alcohol consumption is known to result in memory deficits and may increase the risk for Alzheimer's disease in both genders, but particularly in women, who appear to be more vulnerable than men to alcohol-induced brain damage (Sohrabji 2002).

Physiological Effects of Licit and Illicit Drugs

Gender Differences in Metabolism and Effects

Research (Hernandez-Avila et al. 2004) supports the concept of an accelerated progression to treatment entry among women dependent on opioids, cannabis, or alcohol, and suggests the existence of a gender-based vulnerability to the adverse consequences of these disorders. No gender difference was noted for age at onset of regular use, but the women had used opioids, cannabis, and alcohol for fewer years before entering treatment. The severity of drug and alcohol dependence did not differ by gender, but women reported more severe psychiatric, medical, and employment complications than did men. In one substance abuse treatment study focused on urban outpatient clinics, women had more symptoms than men across substances (Patkar et al. 1999). They reported more cardiovascular, mood, nose and throat, neurological, skin, and gastrointestinal symptoms than did men. In addition, there is evidence that women who use injection drugs are more susceptible to medical disorders and conditions (Zolopa et al. 1994). Similarly, women who

use cocaine, heroin, or injection drugs have a heightened risk of developing herpes, pulmonary tuberculosis, and/or recurrent pneumonia (Thorpe et al. 2004).

To date, little is known regarding the consequences of specific drug use among women. Complicated by polysubstance use, studies are often unable to obtain adequate sample sizes of women who abuse only one drug. The following section highlights specific physiological effects of licit and illicit drugs that are unique to women. This is not a general primer on drugs, but rather a compendium of known physiological effects that are gender-specific.

Cocaine, Amphetamine, and Methamphetamine

Hormonal changes across the menstrual cycle have the greatest effect on stimulant drugs, particularly cocaine and amphetamine. Literature highlights a consistent and greater mood-altering effect of stimulant use during the follicular phase of the cycle (for review, see Terner and de Wit 2006), and the fluctuations in progesterone levels may account, in part, for this sex difference (Evans 2007; Evans and Foltin 2006). More specifically, Evans and colleagues (2002) investigated whether cocaine effects vary as a function of menstrual cycle phase; they found that heart rate and ratings such as "good drug effect" were increased more during the follicular phase than the luteal phase. Conversely, injection drugs and/or crack cocaine appear to produce changes in the menstrual cycle, including the development of amenorrhea, degree of blood flow, and the intensity of cramps (Stevens and Estrada 1999). Overall, women who use cocaine report more positive subjective drug effects, including greater euphoria and desire to use, while physiological responses to the drug did not change (McCance-Katz et al. 2005).

Methamphetamine use has an array of possible adverse effects (for review, see Winslow et al. 2007), but data regarding specific gender differences are limited. Psychoactive effects of methylenedioxy- methamphetamine (ecstasy) have been found to be more intense in women than in men; women report experiencing a higher degree of perceptual changes, thought disturbances, and fear of the loss of control of their bodies. Acute adverse effects, such as jaw clenching, dry mouth, and lack or loss of appetite, are more common among women (Liechti et al. 2001).

Heroin and Other Opioids

Research is lacking that would allow definitive conclusions about gender similarities or differences in the following effects of heroin use: scarred and collapsed veins, bacterial infections of blood vessels and heart valves, abscesses, cellulitis, and liver or kidney disease (National Institute on Drug Abuse [NIDA] 2000).

Research suggests that there are no menstrual cycle differences in women's subjective experience or physiological reaction to opioids (Gear et al. 1996), but women using heroin or methadone do experience menstrual abnormalities, particularly amenorrhea or an irregular menstrual cycle (Abs et al. 2000; Santen et al. 1975; Smith et al. 1982). It can take up to a year for regular menstrual cycles to resume after drug use is stopped. Deficits in sexual desire and performance are also consequences of heroin use (Smith et al. 1982). These symptoms probably are related to the lower levels of luteinizing hormone, estradiol, and progesterone found in these women (Abs et al. 2000). Amenorrhea and other symptoms often make women believe they are permanently sterile, a fear that can be lessened with education. TIP 43 *Medication-Assisted Treatment for Opioid Addiction in Opioid Treatment Programs* (CSAT 2005b) provides more information.

Marijuana

Studies on marijuana effects have not focused specifically on gender differences; therefore, little is known about how marijuana affects men and women differently. In studies evaluating hormonal changes and the physiological and psychological effects of marijuana use, findings suggest that the effects of marijuana do not vary markedly across the menstrual cycle (Block et al. 1991; Griffin et al. 1986; Lex et al. 1984).

Effects of marijuana on birth outcomes are discussed below.

Prescription and Over-the-Counter Medications

Women are significantly more likely to use and abuse prescription medications, including anxiolytics (antianxiety medications) and narcotic analgesics (pain medications), than are men (Simoni-Wastila 2000). Little research is available, however, on the gender differences and differential physiological effects of abuse of prescription medications. Moreover, research into the influence of hormonal changes across the menstrual cycle on subjective, behavioral, and physiological effects is limited to benzodiazepines, and findings are minimal (Bell et al. 2004; Kamimori et al. 2000).

Over-the-counter (OTC) medications include cold remedies, antihistamines, sleep aids, and other legally obtained nonprescription medications. It is not uncommon for individuals with eating disorders, particularly those diagnosed with bulimia nervosa, to abuse laxatives, diuretics, emetics, and diet pills. Misuse of these medications can result in serious medical complications for those with eating disorders, who primarily are women (U.S. Department of Health and Human Services, Office on Women's Health 2000). Complications can involve the gastrointestinal, neuromuscular, and cardiac systems and can be lethal. Many prescription and OTC medications interact negatively with alcohol and drugs.

Gender Differences and OTC Drugs

Across studies, prevalence rates comparing the use and misuse of OTC medications among men and women vary according to age and race/ethnicity. For individuals 65 years of age and older, women are more likely to use OTC drugs (Halon et al. 2001). NSDUH evaluated the misuse of OTC cough and cold medications among persons aged 12 to 25 (SAMHSA 2007) and found that women aged 12 to 17 were more likely than men to have misused OTC cough and cold medications in the past year, while men between 18 and 25 years of age were more likely to have misused these medications. Whites and Hispanics had higher rates of misuse than African Americans. Similar to men, women who had ever misused OTC cough and cold medications also had lifetime use of marijuana and inhalants. In evaluating prescription and OTC drug treatment admissions, women represented a larger proportion of prescription and OTC medication admissions (46 percent) than treatment admissions for all substances (30 percent; SAMHSA 2004).

> "Every woman is different. No amount of drinking is 100 percent safe, 100 percent of the time, for every individual woman" (National Institute on Alcohol Abuse and Alcoholism [NIAAA] 2003).

Physiological Effects of Tobacco Use

The health risks associated with nicotine use are considerable, particularly among women. In comparison with men, women who smoke show higher disease risk regardless of smoking level or intensity (Mucha et al. 2006). Currently, cancer is the second leading cause of death among women, with mortality rates higher for lung cancer than breast cancer. According to the Office of the Surgeon General (2001b), women who smoke:

- Have an increased risk of peptic ulcers and Crohn's disease.
- Have an increased risk of estrogen deficiency; difficult, irregular or painful menstruation; and amenorrhea.
- Are more likely to be diagnosed with cancer, including cancer of the lung, bladder, cervix, pancreas, kidney, larynx, esophagus, liver, and colon.

- Have a higher risk for delayed conception and infertility.
- Are more likely to deliver premature and low-birth-weight infants.
- Have an increased risk for ischemic stroke, subarachnoid hemorrhage, peripheral vascular atherosclerosis, and an abdominal aortic aneurysm rupture.
- Are more likely to have premature decline in lung function, chronic obstructive pulmonary disease, and coronary heart disease.
- Have an increased risk of developing cataracts and macular degeneration.
- Reach menopause at a younger age.
- Have lower bone densities and an increased risk for hip fracture after menopause.

Effects of Alcohol, Drugs, and Tobacco Use on Pregnancy and Birth Outcomes

The use of alcohol, drugs, and tobacco can affect a pregnant woman in a variety of ways. Substance use can result in obstetric complications, miscarriage, or significant problems for the fetus. It is difficult to tease out individual effects of licit and illicit substances on fetal and infant development because women who abuse these substances typically abuse more than one, and the substance abuse can be accompanied by psychological distress, victimization, and poverty. A detailed discussion of alcohol- and drug-related problems in infants and children is beyond the scope of this TIP except insofar as these problems create additional demands and stressors for women as well as guilt and shame about the use of alcohol, drugs, and/or tobacco during pregnancy. This section highlights specific effects of alcohol and drugs during the course of pregnancy.

Alcohol Use and Birth Outcomes

Above all other drugs, alcohol is the most common teratogen (any agent that interrupts development or causes malformation in an embryo or fetus) in pregnancy (Randall 2001).

In utero, alcohol use is associated with an increased risk of spontaneous abortion and increased rates of prematurity and abruptio placentae (premature separation of the placenta from the uterus). A study found that women who consumed five or more drinks per week were three times as likely to deliver a stillborn baby compared with those who had fewer than one drink per week (Kesmodel et al. 2002).

Maternal alcohol use during pregnancy contributes to a wide range of effects on exposed offspring, known as fetal alcohol spectrum disorders (FASDs), and the most serious consequence is fetal alcohol syndrome (FAS). FAS is characterized by abnormal facial features, growth deficiencies, and central nervous system problems (Jones and Smith 1973). Symptoms can include hyperactivity and attention problems, learning and memory deficits, and problems with social and emotional development. Infants who show only some of these features were previously identified as having fetal alcohol effects (FAE). Since 1996, the term FAE has been replaced by alcohol-related birth defects (ARBD), partial fetal alcohol syndrome (pFAS), and alcohol-related neurodevelopmental disorder (ARND; Stratton et al. 1996). Children with ARBD have problems with major and sensory organs, as well as structural abnormalities; children with ARND have central nervous system abnormalities (Green 2007). Despite alcohol-related birth defects being completely preventable, FASDs are the most common nonhereditary causes of mental retardation (CDC 2002).

Another risk factor associated with alcohol exposure in utero is the potential of substance use disorders. Alati et al (2006) found an association of early-onset of alcohol disorders among children exposed to alcohol prenatally; this association was more pronounced with early pregnancy exposure. While little is known about the prevalence of FASD among individuals with substance use disorders, this co-occurring condition is likely to further challenge recovery effects. For guidelines in identifying and referring persons with FAS, see CDC (2005).

Women who drink during breastfeeding pass alcohol on to the baby. Although numerous studies of laboratory animals have demonstrated a variety of adverse outcomes in breastfed offspring during periods when their mothers are consuming alcohol, human data are limited. A review of empirical literature on women who drink while breastfeeding provides evidence that maternal alcohol consumption does not promote lactation and may affect infant sleep patterns. (for review, see Giglia and Binns 2006)

Cocaine Use and Birth Outcomes

According to reviews of several studies conducted during the late 1980s and early 1990s, there are a variety of adverse effects of cocaine use during pregnancy (Zuckerman et al. 1995; Burkett et al. 1994). Studies reported that cocaine-exposed infants had smaller head circumference; lower birth weight and length; irritability; poor interactive abilities; and an increased incidence of stillbirth, prematurity, and sudden infant death syndrome (SIDS; Bell and Lau 1995). Other studies dispute many previously reported severe effects of prenatal exposure of cocaine on the offspring. Frank and colleagues' review (2001) of the literature found that the most consistent effects were small size and less-than-optimal motor performance. Eyler and colleagues (2001) found no evidence of the previously reported devastating effects of prenatal cocaine exposure. Hurt and colleagues

The SAMHSA FASD's Center for Excellence Web site provides information and resources about FASD and related information on legislation, treatment and training curricula, and community awareness (http://www.fascenter.samhsa.gov/).

(1995) followed a cohort of cocaine-exposed infants from birth to age 6; although they found lower weight and head circumference, they found no difference in developmental scores between cocaine-exposed and non–cocaine-exposed infants. However, other evidence suggests that children exposed to cocaine during the first trimester were smaller on all growth parameters at 7 and 10 years of age compared with children who were not exposed to cocaine (Richardson et al. 2007). This longitudinal analysis indicated that the disparity in growth between both groups did not converge over time.

An extensive review by Frank and colleagues (2001) of all studies published in English from 1984 to 2000 (N = 74) that met rigorous methodological criteria (N = 36) concluded that many apparent adverse outcomes of cocaine use during pregnancy "can be explained … by other factors, including prenatal exposure to tobacco, marijuana, or alcohol and the quality of the child's environment" (p. 1624). Other studies (Hurt et al. 2001; Kaltenbach 2000; Lewis et al. 2004b; Messinger et al. 2004) have supported this conclusion. Singer et al. (2004) reported that the quality of the caregiving environment was the strongest independent predictor of cognitive outcomes among children exposed to cocaine.

Nonetheless, the effects of cocaine on the fetus may be dose and timing dependent, and significant cocaine use during pregnancy, with or without other drug use, is associated with negative consequences for the offspring and the mother (Thaithumyanon et al. 2005). Birth weight, length, and head circumference of infants with high exposure to cocaine differed from those with low or no exposure (Bateman and Chiriboga 2000). Heavily cocaine-exposed infants were found to have more jitteriness and attention problems than infants with light or no exposure to cocaine and lower auditory comprehension than unexposed infants (Singer et al. 2000). Evidence suggests that subtle deficits exist in cognitive and attentional processes in cocaine-exposed preschool and 6-year-old children (Leech et al. 1999; Mayes et al. 1998). In addition, infants exposed to cocaine during pregnancy had more infections, including hepatitis and HIV/AIDS exposure (Bauer et al. 2005). Much is still unknown about the effects of prenatal cocaine exposure. However, cocaine use by a pregnant woman should be viewed as an indication of multiple medical and social risk factors (Eyler and Behnke 1999; Tronick and Beeghly 1999); her ability to access prenatal care, gain supportive and effective case management services, and obtain substance abuse treatment can make all the difference in outcome.

Opioid Use and Birth Outcomes

Opioid use in pregnant women presents a difficult situation because of the many medical complications of opioid use, such as infections passed to the fetus by the use of contaminated needles. Obstetric complications in pregnant

Since timely treatment for HIV/AIDS can virtually eliminate the chance of a pregnant woman passing the infection to her fetus, all women with substance use histories should have an HIV/AIDS evaluation at the first sign of any possible pregnancy.

women who use opioids often are compounded by lack of prenatal care. Complications include spontaneous abortion, premature labor and delivery, premature rupture of membranes, preeclampsia (high blood pressure during pregnancy), abruptio placentae, and intrauterine death. The fetus is at risk for morbidity and mortality because of episodes of maternal withdrawal (Kaltenbach et al. 1998).

Reviews of several studies recommend methadone maintenance treatment (MMT) as the only treatment for the management of opioid dependence during pregnancy because, when methadone is provided within a treatment setting that includes comprehensive care, obstetric and fetal complications, including neonatal morbidity and mortality, can be reduced (Jarvis and Schnoll 1995; Kaltenbach et al. 1998). Effective MMT prevents the onset of withdrawal, reduces or eliminates drug craving, and blocks the euphoric effects of illicit self-administered opioids (Dole et al. 1966*a*, *b*; Kreek 1988). The use of methadone in pregnancy prevents erratic maternal opioid levels and protects the fetus from repeated episodes of withdrawal. Because needle use is eliminated, MMT reduces the risk of infectious diseases. The mandatory link to prenatal care, frequent contact with program staff, and elimination of the stress of obtaining opioids daily to feel "normal" are additional benefits from MMT (Burns et al. 2006).

Reviews of the literature note that studies consistently have found that fetuses exposed to opioids (i.e., heroin and methadone) have lower birth weights than unexposed fetuses and usually undergo neonatal abstinence syndrome (NAS) at birth. NAS is a generalized disorder characterized by signs and symptoms of central nervous system irritability, gastrointestinal dysfunction, respiratory distress, vomiting, and fever, among other symptoms. NAS can be more

severe and prolonged with methadone exposure than heroin exposure, but with appropriate pharmacotherapy, NAS can be treated effectively (Kaltenbach 1994; Kaltenbach et al. 1998).

Although findings among studies are diverse, most suggest that methadone-exposed infants and children through age 2 function well within the normal range of development and that methadone-exposed children between ages 2 and 5 do not differ in cognitive function from a population that was not drug exposed and was of comparable socioeconomic and racial background (Kaltenbach 1996). Data suggest that such psychosocial factors as environment and parenting can have as much of an effect on development as prenatal exposure to opioids (Johnson et al. 1987; Lifschitz et al. 1985).

In more recent years, buprenorphine treatment has been examined as an alternative to maintenance therapy for opioid dependence during pregnancy. Nonetheless, research is limited and only two randomized, double-blind studies have been conducted comparing methadone with buprenorphine (Fischer et al. 2006; Jones et al. 2005; Kayembe-Kay's and Laclyde 2003; Raburn and Bogenschultz 2004). For additional information on maintenance therapies during pregnancy, see TIP 43 *Medication-Assisted Treatment for Opioid Addiction in Opioid Treatment Programs* (CSAT 2005*a*) and TIP 40 *Clinical Guidelines for the Use of Buprenorphine in the Treatment of Opioid Addiction* (CSAT 2004*a*).

Marijuana Use and Birth Outcomes

The limited research on the effects of prenatal exposure to marijuana shows somewhat inconsistent results (Bell and Lau 1995).

Longitudinal studies by Day and colleagues (1992) found marijuana to be associated with reduced length at birth, but it did not affect weight or head circumference. Hurd et al. (2005) found that exposed fetuses had significantly reduced body weight and length, even when the data were adjusted to account for maternal alcohol consumption and smoking. Children prenatally exposed to marijuana functioned above average on the Bayley Scale of Infant Development (BSID) at 9 months, but third-trimester marijuana use was associated with decreased BSID mental scores. Followup assessment of these children at age 10 found that prenatal marijuana exposure was associated with higher levels of behavior problems (Goldschmidt et al. 2000). In a review of existing data, Fried and Smith (2001) reported that although global IQ is unaffected by prenatal marijuana exposure, aspects of executive function appear to be negatively associated with prenatal exposure in children beyond the toddler stage.

Amphetamine and Methamphetamine Use and Birth Outcomes

Exposure to amphetamines in utero has been associated with both short- and long-term effects, including abnormal fetal growth, withdrawal symptoms after birth, and impaired neurological development in infancy and childhood (Wagner et al. 1998). Both animal and human studies have shown that fetal exposure to amphetamines increases the risk of reduced fetal growth, cardiac anomalies, and cleft lip and palate (Winslow et al. 2007). Unfortunately, knowledge of the effects of methamphetamine during pregnancy is limited. While there is evidence of increased rates of premature delivery, placental abruption, reduced fetal growth, and heart abnormalities, studies are confounded by other issues, including polysubstance abuse among participants and methodological issues in the research design. In one study, which took into account several confounding variables, findings suggest that methamphetamine exposure in utero is

associated with decreased growth (including lower birth weight) and smaller gestational age for exposed neonates (Smith et al. 2006).

Tobacco Use and Birth Outcomes

Women who smoke tobacco increase their chances of ectopic pregnancy (development of a fetus outside the uterus), spontaneous abortion, premature rupture of membranes, abruptio placentae, placenta previa, preeclampsia, and preterm delivery. Infants born to women who smoke are more likely to have lower birth weights and have an increased risk of SIDS (Office of the Surgeon General 2001b; Visscher et al. 2003). Children of parents who smoke heavily can be affected adversely in their auditory, language, and cognitive performance; hyperactivity and attention deficit disorders are also common, according to the literature (Bell and Lau 1995). Studies have also drawn an association between maternal smoking during pregnancy and disruptive behavior earlier in development (NIDA 2008; Wakschlag et al. 2006; Wakschlag et al. 2002).

Effects of Alcohol and Illicit Drugs on HIV/AIDS Status

People who inject drugs have a high prevalence of co-infection with tuberculosis, hepatitis, and HIV (Cohn 2002; Martin et al. 2000). Evidence suggests that women who inject drugs often incur added risk by injecting after men, who often procure the drugs and injection equipment (Pugatch et al. 2000). According to CDC (2002), 57 percent of HIV infections among women are attributable to use of injection drugs or intercourse with a person who injects drugs.

Some substances make women more vulnerable to STDs because of physiological changes. For example, women who abuse large amounts of alcohol tend to have drier mucous membranes, which results in abrasions and small tears that allow HIV easier access to the bloodstream during intercourse (Norris and Hughes 1996).

Douching increases vulnerability to HIV by removing protective bacteria (Cottrell 2003; Funkhouser et al. 2002).

Since timely treatment for HIV/AIDS can virtually eliminate the chance of a pregnant woman passing the infection to her fetus, all women with substance use histories should have an HIV/AIDS evaluation at the first sign of any possible pregnancy.

Although highly active antiretroviral therapy (HAART) has extended survival time, evidence suggests that the gains are not equal when comparing gender and status as a person who uses injection drugs. Poundstone and colleagues (2001) concluded that women who inject drugs do not benefit as much as men and women who do not use injectable drugs. CDC (1998) reports that antiretroviral drugs administered to pregnant women and their newborns have been shown to reduce greatly the risk of perinatal mother-to-child HIV/AIDS transmission. Aggressive combinations of drugs currently are recommended, but the specific regimens that can both treat a client's HIV/AIDS infection and reduce perinatal transmission depend on many factors. The ability to provide effective health care to women who are HIV positive can be influenced significantly by their use of substances and adherence to therapy (Lucas et al. 2006). Once women are in treatment, counselors need to ensure that they are provided with or referred for medical and prenatal care as soon as possible to prevent medical complications. For more detailed information regarding HIV/AIDS, refer to TIP 37 *Substance Abuse Treatment for Persons with HIV/AIDS* (CSAT 2000c).

HCV and Women

The hepatitis C virus (HCV) is the primary cause of cirrhosis and liver cancer in United States. An estimated 4.1 million people in the United States are infected with HCV. Of these, 80 to 85 percent will develop chronic hepatitis C, but the rate is lower for women. In 2006, the rate of HCV in women was 0.25 cases per 100,000 (CDC 2008).

HCV can remain silent for many years; most people infected with chronic hepatitis C thus may not be aware that they are infected because they are not chronically ill (Heintges and Wands 1997). For some, the only sign of an infection is found in blood test results. A positive result can occur when the liver enzyme ALT is abnormally high. Women's ALT levels are naturally lower than men's, yet the cutoff number for abnormal liver tests is the same for both sexes. This can result in women being misdiagnosed as having a normal ALT level. If a woman's liver enzymes are on the high side of normal or she has any risk factors for HCV, testing is recommended for HCV (Porter 2008).

Approximately 250,000 women are infected with HCV due to blood they received after a cesarean section prior to 1992 (Porter 2008). Since 1992, screening and regulations on U.S. blood supplies ensure that the recipient is free from risks of contracting any blood-borne illness. Currently, risk factors for contracting HCV are generally the same for men and women, yet women are at higher risk of contracting HCV from sexual contact with an HCV-positive partner, and women are more likely to be initiated into drug use or share equipment for injection drugs with a sexual partner. Below is a list of risk factors for acquiring HCV:

- Injection drug use (56 percent of HCV cases in men and women reported in 2006; CDC 2008).
- Sexual contact with HCV positive partner (0–3 percent for women in monogamous heterosexual relationships; the risk increases with multiple partners, the presence of a sexually transmitted disease, hepatitis B virus [HBV], or open sores, cuts, or wounds [Porter 2008]; 1–12 percent among female prostitutes [The C. Everett Koop Institute 2008]).
- Occupational exposure (1.5 percent of HCV cases reported in 2006; CDC 2008) through the use of razors, needles, nail files, a barber's scissors, tattooing equipment, or body piercing or acupuncture needles if these items are contaminated by blood from an infected person.

- Perinatal or vertical transmission (5 percent in children of mothers with HCV monoinfection; 18.7 percent rate in mothers with HIV/HCV co-infection; Bell et al. 2004). Almost one out of four newly diagnosed cases of HIV in the United States is a woman, and approximately 20 percent of these newly diagnosed women with HIV are co-infected with HCV (Orenstein and Tsogas 2001). Among pregnant and nonpregnant women, HCV and HIV co-infection is significantly associated with injection drug use (Nikolopoulou et al. 2005). The rate of HIV/HCV co-infection may be as high as 50 to 90 percent for those who contracted HIV through injection drug use. HIV co-infection with HCV appears to raise the risk of mother-to-child transmission to 18.7 percent. The risk for transmission from a woman with HCV monoinfection to her infant is 5.4 percent (Bell et al. 2004).

Prevention and intervention

Prevention strategies are gender neutral and include screening blood, plasma, organ, tissue, and sperm donors; effective infection control practices; identification, testing, and counseling of at-risk persons; and medical management of infected persons (Bell 2004).

Although this is by no means an overview of the disease or its treatment process, a review of interventions can prove beneficial when working with clients who are infected with HCV. Gender-specific guidelines for intervention are minimal.

Early medical intervention is helpful even though people infected with HCV infection often experience mild symptoms and subsequently do not seek treatment. Not everyone with hepatitis C needs medical treatment. Treatment is determined by HCV genotype, viral load, liver enzyme levels, and extent of liver damage. There are many elements to consider when undergoing treatment for chronic hepatitis C virus. Women are slightly more likely to respond favorably to HCV treatment; however, there are gender-specific issues that factor into the decision to start treatment.

Issues of treatment specific to women

- Women should not get pregnant during and up to 6 months following HCV treatment; for those who are in treatment after childbirth, breastfeeding should be avoided.
- Autoimmune conditions occur more often in women than men. One of the HCV medications, interferon, can aggravate autoimmune diseases.
- Women have less hemoglobin (a component of red blood cells that carries oxygen to the cells) than men. Menstruating women have even lower hemoglobin levels because of monthly blood loss, which can sometimes cause anemia. HCV-positive women undergoing treatment should talk to their medical advisor about ribavirin (one of the treatment medications for HCV) and its connection to hemolytic anemia—a type of anemia that causes red blood cells to burst before the body has a chance to use them. Women, especially menstruating women, are vulnerable to this kind of anemia and need to be monitored with regular blood tests during treatment.

In general, women are two times more likely than men to have depression. Depression is a common side effect of HCV treatment medications. Some providers recommend starting an antidepressant prior to starting treatment for HCV (Porter 2005).

Women are less likely to need HCV treatment because they tend to have less severe liver damage due to the virus (Highleyman 2005). Approximately 3 to 20 percent of clients with chronic HCV will develop cirrhosis over a 20- to 30-year period (CDC 1998). Alcoholic beverage consumption accelerates HCV-associated fibrosis and cirrhosis. A study by Chen et al. (2007) reveals that heavy alcohol use affects females more strongly than males, resulting in a higher mortality rate. This difference may be due to the more detrimental effect of alcohol on the progression of liver injury among women than among men with a similar level of alcohol use (Becker et al. 1996). Current guidelines strongly recommend that HCV patients be vaccinated for hepatitis A and B if they have not yet been exposed to these viruses, as these would radically worsen their liver disease.

Some ways addiction counselors can contribute to treatment are (for review, see Sylvestre 2007):

- Providing education and lifestyle guidelines.
- Distributing information on HCV in substance abuse treatment programs.
- Providing information on intervention programs such as the Healthy Liver Group. The Healthy Liver Group, launched in 2005, is an hour-long intervention comprising a 30-minute group educational session followed by an individualized meeting with the attending registered nurse to discuss laboratory results (Hagedorn et al. 2007).
- Teaching coping skills for side effects to clients undergoing medical therapy.
- Promoting self-care by urging clients to abstain from alcohol, to get vaccinated for hepatitis A and hepatitis B, and to inform themselves of HCV and its risk factors.

- Providing moral support and hope to clients of obtaining the best possible results by maintaining treatment.

Accessing screening and care on behalf of addicted clients with HCV can take persistence. Although the HCV antibody screening test is relatively inexpensive, the HCV viral test is not, but most county medical clinics and hospitals will provide it (Sylvestre 2007). Substance abuse treatment providers are more apt to spot the signs of depression or mania in those patients on medical therapy for HCV. Early detection and stabilization of any psychiatric side effect should not interrupt the progression of treatment. People with a substance use disorder can participate successfully in HCV therapy. For more information, see the planned TIP *Viral Hepatitis and Substance Use Disorders* (CSAT in development *j*).

4 Screening and Assessment

Overview

Understanding the extent and nature of a woman's substance use disorder and its interaction with other life areas is essential for careful diagnosis, appropriate case management, and successful treatment. This understanding begins during the screening and assessment process, which helps match the client with appropriate treatment services. To ensure that important information is obtained, providers should use standardized screening and assessment instruments and interview protocols, some of which have been studied for their sensitivity, validity, and accuracy in identifying problems with women.

Hundreds of screening instruments and assessment tools exist. Specific instruments are available to help counselors determine whether further assessment is warranted, the nature and extent of a client's substance use disorder, whether a client has a mental disorder, what types of traumatic experiences a client has had and what the consequences are, and treatment-related factors that impact the client's response to interventions. This TIP makes no specific recommendations of screening and assessment tools for women and does not intend to present a comprehensive discussion of this complex topic. Rather, the TIP briefly describes several instruments that providers often use to examine areas of female clients' lives. Attention is given to instruments that have gender-specific normative data or are useful in attending to the biopsychosocial issues unique to women. Several of the screening and assessment instruments discussed in this chapter are provided in Appendix C.

This chapter introduces and provides an overview of current screening and assessment processes that may best serve women across the continuum of care. It covers several areas for which to screen, such as acute safety risk, mental disorders, sexual victimization, trauma, and eating disorders. The chapter also discusses factors that may influence the overall assessment, and reviews screening for substance abuse and dependence in settings other than substance abuse treatment facilities.

It provides information about instruments for use by drug and alcohol counselors, primary healthcare providers, social workers, and others. The assessment section includes general principles for assessing women, the scope and structure of assessment interviews, and selected instruments. Finally, other considerations that apply to screening and assessment are discussed, including women's strengths, coping styles, and spirituality.

The Difference Between Screening and Assessment

The purpose of screening is to determine whether a woman needs assessment. The purpose of assessment is to gather the detailed information needed for a treatment plan that meets the individual needs of the woman. Many standardized instruments and interview protocols are available to help counselors perform appropriate screening and assessment for women.

Screening involves asking questions carefully designed to determine whether a more thorough evaluation for a particular problem or disorder is warranted. Many screening instruments require little or no special training to administer. Screening differs from assessment in the following ways:

- *Screening* is a process for evaluating the possible presence of a particular problem. The outcome is normally a simple yes or no.
- *Assessment* is a process for defining the nature of that problem, determining a diagnosis, and developing specific treatment recommendations for addressing the problem or diagnosis.

Screening and Assessment: Factors of Influence

Ethnicity and Culture

The treatment field depends on tools or questionnaires that, for the most part, have been found valid and reliable with two populations of women—Caucasians and African Americans. Although translations of some instruments for non–English-speaking populations have been made, the validity of the adapted instruments is not always documented.

Women need a thorough explanation of the screening and assessment process. Some women from diverse ethnic groups may find the process threatening, intrusive, and foreign. In some cultures, for example, questions about personal habits can be considered unnecessarily intrusive (Paniagua 1998). Many immigrant women have little experience with American medical care and do not understand the assessment process. Some women may have had negative experiences with human service agencies or other treatment programs and felt they were stereotyped or treated with disrespect.

Screening and assessment must be approached with a perspective that affirms cultural relevance and strengths. An understanding of the cultural basis of a client's health beliefs, illness behaviors, and attitude toward and acceptance of treatment provides a foundation for building a successful treatment program for the client. Whenever possible, instruments that have been normed, adapted, or tested on specific cultural and linguistic groups should be used. Instruments that are not normed for the population being evaluated can contain cultural biases and produce misleading results and perhaps inappropriate treatment plans and misunderstandings with clients.

Counselors and intake personnel may hold preconceived beliefs concerning the prevalence of substance abuse among women from particular ethnic groups. For example, counselors may overlook the need to screen and assess Asian women (Kitano and Louie 2002). All assessment staff members should receive training about the cultural and ethnic groups they serve; the appropriate interpersonal and communication styles for effective interviews; and cultural beliefs and practices about substance use and abuse, mental health, physical health, violence, and trauma. Through training, counselors can learn what cultural factors need to be considered to test accurately.

Acculturation and Language Issues

Acculturation level may affect screening and assessment results. The counselor may need to replace standard screening and assessment approaches with an in-depth discussion with the client and perhaps family members to understand substance use from the client's personal and cultural points of view. The migration experience needs to be assessed; some immigrants may have experienced trauma in their countries of origin and will need a sensitive trauma assessment.

Specifically, the counselor may begin by asking the client about her country of birth and, if she was not born in the United States, the length of time she has lived in this country. Several screening tools are available to determine general acculturation level. The Short Acculturation Scale for Latinos (Marin et al. 1987) is a

12-item acculturation scale available in English and Spanish. Acculturation, as measured by this scale, correlates highly with respondents' generation, length of residence, age at arrival, and ethnic self-identification. The scale can be adapted easily for other groups. Two other useful scales are the Acculturation Rating Scale for Mexican Americans II (ARSMA; Cuéllar et al. 1980) and the Oetting and Beauvais Questionnaire, available at www.casaa.unm.edu, which assesses cultural identification for Caucasian Americans, Hispanics, American Indians, and African Americans. Scales also have been developed for Asian-American groups (Chung et al. 2004).

Counselors should be aware that although a client speaks English relatively well, she still may have trouble understanding assessment tools in English. It is not adequate to simply translate items from English into another language. Some words, idioms, and examples do not translate directly into other languages but need to be adapted. Ideally, interviews should be conducted in a woman's preferred language by trained staff who speak the language or by professional translators from the woman's culture. Differences in literacy level may require that some clients be screened and assessed by interview or that self-administered questions be adapted to appropriate reading levels. For women with low literacy levels, language comprehension problems, or visual impairments, screening personnel can read the questions to them; however, results may not be as accurate. Self-administered questionnaires should be available in a woman's preferred language if possible.

Socioeconomic Status

Counselors may have conscious or subconscious expectations based on socioeconomic status. Such perceptions have led to failures to diagnose drug or alcohol abuse in pregnant middle- and upper-class women, with tragic consequences for their infants. For example, primary care providers are much less apt to ask private middle-income patients about their use of drugs. Some healthcare providers may fear offending their patients by asking them about their substance use. Weir and colleagues (1998) found that clients with more than a high school education are less apt to disclose the use of drugs or alcohol during pregnancy.

Specific Populations: Other Noteworthy Considerations

Cognitive and learning disabilities

Prior to screening and assessment, the counselor should inquire about current or past difficulties in learning, past participation in special education, a diagnosis of a learning disability, prior involvement in testing for cognitive functioning or learning disability, and problems related to self-care and basic life management skills.

Depending on the type and severity of the disability or impairment, these women will likely need more assistance throughout the screening

and assessment process. Moreover, women with developmental disabilities or cognitive impairments are more likely to respond to items they do not understand by stating "yes" or by responding in a manner they think the assessment counselor will approve of instead of asking for clarification.

Sexual orientation

The Institute of Medicine's (IOM) report on lesbian health identifies substance abuse as one of the primary heath concerns among lesbians (Solarz 1999). While research has concluded that the CAGE instrument has similar reliability and concurrent validity among lesbian and heterosexual women, very few studies have addressed the issue of validity and reliability in screening and assessment tools for lesbians (Johnson and Hughes 2005). Consequently, counselors need to cautiously interpret screening and assessment results.

Screening

Screening often is the initial contact between a woman and the treatment system, and the client forms her first impression of treatment during screening and intake. For women, the most frequent points of entry from other systems of care are obstetric and primary care; hospital emergency rooms; social service agencies in connection with housing, child care, disabilities, and domestic violence; community mental health services; and correctional facilities. How screening is conducted can be as important as the actual information gathered, as it sets the tone of treatment and begins the relationship with the client.

Screening processes always should define a protocol or procedure for determining which clients need further assessment (i.e., screen positive) for a condition being screened and for ensuring that those clients receive a thorough assessment. That is, a professionally designed screening process establishes precisely how to score responses to the screening tools or questions and what constitutes a positive score for a particular possible problem (often called a "cutoff" score). The screening protocol details the actions taken after a client scores in the positive range and provides the standard forms for documenting the results of the screening, the actions taken, the assessments performed, and that each staff member has carried out his or her responsibilities in the process. Although a screening can reveal an outline of a client's involvement with alcohol, drugs, or both, it does not result in a diagnosis or provide details of how substances have affected the client's life. The most important domains to screen for when working with women include:

- Substance abuse
- Pregnancy considerations
- Immediate risks related to serious intoxication or withdrawal
- Immediate risks for self-harm, suicide, and violence
- Past and present mental disorders, including posttraumatic stress disorder (PTSD) and other anxiety disorders, mood disorders, and eating disorders
- Past and present history of violence and trauma, including sexual victimization and interpersonal violence
- Health screenings, including HIV/AIDS, hepatitis, tuberculosis, and STDs

Substance Abuse Screening

The goal of substance abuse screening is to identify women who have or are developing alcohol- or drug-related problems. Routinely, women are less likely than men to be identified as having substance abuse problems (Buchsbaum et al. 1993); yet, they are more likely to exhibit significant health problems after consuming fewer substances in a shorter period of time.

Screening for substance use disorders is conducted by an interview or by giving a short written questionnaire. While selection of the instrument may be based on various factors, including cost and administration time (Thornberry et al. 2002), the decision to use an interview versus a self-administered screening tool should also be based upon the comfort level of the counselor or healthcare professional (Arborelius and Thakker 1995; Duszynski et al.

> Substance abuse screening and assessment tools, in general, are not as sensitive in identifying women as having substance abuse problems.

Advice to Clinicians:
Substance Abuse Screening and Assessment Among Women

- How screenings and assessments are conducted is as important as the information gathered. Screening and assessment are often the initial contact between a woman and the treatment system. They can either help build a trusting relationship or create a deterrent to engaging in further services.
- Self-administered tools may be more likely to elicit honest answers; this is especially true regarding questions related to drug and alcohol use.
- Face-to-face screening interviews have not always been successful in detecting alcohol and drug use in women, especially if the counselor is uncomfortable with the questions.
- Substance abuse screening and assessment tools, in general, are not as sensitive in identifying women as having substance abuse problems.
- Selection of screening and assessment instruments should be examined to determine if they were developed using female populations. If not, counselors need to explore whether or not there are other instruments that may be more suitable to address specific evaluation needs.

1995; Gale et al. 1998; Thornberry et al. 2002). If the healthcare staff communicates discomfort, women may become wary of disclosing their full use of substances (Aquilino 1994; see also Center for Substance Abuse Prevention [CSAP] 1993).

Many instruments have been developed to screen for alcohol consumption, and several measures have been adapted to screen for specific drugs. While numerous screening tools are available, information about the reliability and validity of these instruments with women is limited. The following listing, while not exhaustive, individually reviews tools with available gender-specific information.

General Alcohol and Drug Screening

AUDIT
The Alcohol Use Disorder Identification Test (AUDIT; Babor and Grant 1989) is a widely used screening tool that is reproduced with guidelines and scoring instructions in TIP 26 *Substance Abuse Among Older Adults* (CSAT 1998*d*). The AUDIT is effective in identifying heavy drinking among nonpregnant women (Bradley et al. 1998*c*). It consists of 10 questions that were highly correlated with hazardous or harmful alcohol consumption. This instrument can be given as a self-administered test, or the questions can be read aloud. The AUDIT takes about 2 minutes to administer. **Note:** Question 3, concerning binge drinking, should be revised for women to refer to having 4 (not 6) or more drinks on one occasion.

TCUDS II
The Texas Christian University Drug Screen II (TCUDS II) is a 15-item, self-administered substance abuse screening tool that requires 5–10 minutes to complete. It is based in part on Diagnostic Interview Schedule and refers to *Diagnostic and Statistical Manual of Mental Disorders, 4th Edition, Text Revision* (DSM-IV-TR; American Psychiatric Association [APA] 2000*a*) criteria for substance abuse and dependence. TCUDS II is used widely in criminal justice settings. It has good reliability among female populations (Knight 2002; Knight et al. 2002). This screen, along with related instruments, is available at www.ibr.tcu.edu.

CAGE
CAGE (Ewing 1984) asks about lifetime alcohol or drug consumption (see Figure 4-1). Each "yes" response receives 1 point, and the cutoff point (the score that makes the test results positive) is either 1 or 2. Two "yes" answers results in a very small false-positive rate and the clinician will be less likely to identify clients as potentially having a substance use disorder when they do not. However, the higher cutoff of 2 points decreases the sensitivity of CAGE for women—that is, increases the likelihood that some women who are at risk for a substance problem will receive a negative screening score (i.e., it increases the false-negative rate). **Note:** It is recommended that a cutoff score of 1 be employed in screening for women. This measure has also been translated and tested for Hispanic/Latina populations.

Figure 4-1
The CAGE Questionnaire

- Have you ever felt you ought to Cut down on your drinking [or drug use]?
- Have people Annoyed you by criticizing your drinking [or drug use]?
- Have you ever felt bad or Guilty about your drinking [or drug use]?
- Have you ever had a drink [or used drugs] first thing in the morning (Eye opener) to steady your nerves or get rid of a hangover [or get the day started]?

Source: Mayfield et al. 1974.

A common criticism of the CAGE is that it is not gender-sensitive—that is, women who have problems associated with alcohol use are less likely than male counterparts to screen positive when this instrument is used. One study of more than 1,000 women found that asking simple questions about frequency and quantity of drinking, coupled with a question about binge drinking, was better than the CAGE in detecting alcohol problems among women (Waterson and Murray-Lyon 1988).

The CAGE is "relatively insensitive" with Caucasian females, yet Bradley and colleagues report that it "has performed adequately in predominantly black populations of women" (1998c, p. 170). Johnson and Hughes (2005) conclude that CAGE has similar reliability and concurrent validity among women of different sexual orientations. The CAGE-AID (CAGE Adapted to Include Drugs) modifies the CAGE questions for use in screening for drugs other than alcohol. This version of the CAGE shows promise in identifying pregnant, low-income women at risk for heavier drug use (Midanik et al. 1998).

Screening for Tobacco Use

Similar to other substances, women pay an exceptional price for using tobacco. The second leading cause of death in women is cancer (CDC 2004), with tobacco accounting for 90 percent of all lung cancers, according to the Surgeon General's Report on Women and Smoking (2001). Yet, women are less likely to be referred to smoking cessation programs or provided smoking cessation products (Steinberg et al. 2006). Therefore, screening for tobacco use and referral for nicotine cessation should be standard practice in substance abuse treatment. Counselors can simply screen for tobacco use beginning with current and past patterns of use, including type of tobacco, number of cigarettes smoked per day, frequency of use, circumstances surrounding use, and specific times and locations. For individuals who currently smoke, a more comprehensive assessment needs to be completed with recommendations incorporated into the woman's treatment plan.

Screening Instruments for Pregnant Women

Considering the devastating impact of substances on the developing fetus, routine screening for drug, alcohol, and tobacco use among pregnant women is imperative. Face-to-face screening interviews are not always successful in detecting alcohol and drug use, especially in pregnant women. However, self-administered screening tools have been found to be more likely to elicit honest answers (Lessler and O'Reilly 1997; Russell et al. 1996; Tourangeau and Smith 1996). Three screening instruments for use with pregnant women are TWEAK, T-ACE, and 5Ps Plus (CSAP 1993; Morse et al. 1997).

> Women who smoked in the month before pregnancy are nine times more likely to be currently using either drugs or alcohol or both while pregnant (Chasnoff et al. 2001).

TWEAK

TWEAK (Russell et al. 1991) identifies pregnant women who are at risk for alcohol use (Figure 4-2). It consists of five items and uses a 7-point scoring system. Two points are given for positive responses to either of the first two questions (tolerance and worry), and positive responses to the other three questions score 1 point. A cutoff score of 2 indicates the likelihood of risk drinking. In a study of more than 3,000 women at a prenatal clinic, the TWEAK was found to be more sensitive than the CAGE and Michigan Alcohol Screening Test (MAST), and more specific than the T-ACE (Russell et al. 1996). The tolerance question scores 2 points for an answer of three or more drinks. However, if the criterion for the tolerance question is reduced to two drinks for women, the sensitivity of TWEAK increases, and the specificity and predictive ability decrease somewhat (Chang et al. 1999). In comparison with T-ACE, TWEAK had higher sensitivity and slightly lower specificity (Russell

How many drinks does it take for you to feel high? [Tolerance] (2 or more drinks = 2 points)

Does your partner (or do your parents) ever **W**orry or complain about your drinking? (yes = 2 points)

Have you ever had a drink first thing in the morning to steady your nerves or get rid of a hangover? (**E**ye opener) (yes = 1 point)

Have you ever **A**wakened the morning after some drinking the night before and found that you could not remember part of the evening? (yes = 1 point)

Have you ever felt that you ought to **K**/cut down on your drinking? (yes = 1 point)

Source: Morse et al. 1997.

et al. 1994, 1996). It can also be used to screen for harmful drinking in the general population (Chan et al. 1993).

T-ACE

The T-ACE is a 4-item instrument appropriate for detecting heavy alcohol use in pregnant women (Sokol et al. 1989). T-ACE uses the A, C, and E questions from CAGE and adds one on tolerance for alcohol (see Figure 4-3). The first question assesses tolerance by asking if it takes more than it used to to get high. A response of two or more drinks is scored as 2 points, and the remaining questions are assigned 1 point for a "yes" response. Scores range from 0 to

5 points. A total of 2 or more points indicates risk drinking (Chang et al. 1999). T-ACE has sensitivity equal to the longer MAST and greater than CAGE (Bradley et al. 1998*c*). It has been validated only for screening pregnant women with risky drinking (Russell et al. 1994).

In a study with a culturally diverse population of pregnant women, Chang and colleagues (1998) compared T-ACE with the MAST (short version) and the AUDIT. The study found T-ACE to be the most sensitive of the three tools in identifying current alcohol consumption, risky drinking, or lifetime alcohol diagnoses (Chang et al. 1998). Although T-ACE had the lowest specificity of the three tests, it is argued

How many drinks does it take you to feel high? [Tolerance] (2 or more drinks = 2 points)

Have people **A**nnoyed you by criticizing your drinking? (yes = 1 point)

Have you ever felt you ought to **C**ut down on you drinking? (yes = 1 point)

Have you had an **E**ye opener (a drink first thing in the morning) to steady your nerves? (yes = 1 point)

Source: Sokol et al. 1989

that false positives are of less concern than false negatives among pregnant women (Chang et al. 1998).

Prenatal substance abuse screen (5Ps)

This screening approach has been used to identify women who are at risk for substance abuse in prenatal health settings. A "yes" response to any item indicates that the woman should be referred for assessment (Morse et al. 1997). Originally, four questions regarding present and past use, partner with problem, and parent history of alcohol or drug problems were used (Ewing 1990). However, several adaptations have been made, and recently a question about tobacco use in the month before the client knew she was pregnant was added (Chasnoff 2001). Chasnoff and colleagues (2001) reported that women who smoked in the month before pregnancy were 11 times more likely to be currently using drugs and 9 times more likely to be currently using either drugs or alcohol or both while pregnant. This version, the 5Ps, is shown in Figure 4-4.

In a study evaluating prevalence of substance use among pregnant women utilizing this screening tool, the authors suggest that it not only identified pregnant women with high levels of alcohol and drug use but also a larger group of women whose pregnancies were at risk from smaller amounts of substance use (Chasnoff et al. 2005). For a review on how to improve screening for pregnant women and motivate healthcare professions to screen for risk, refer to the Alcohol Use During Pregnancy Project (Kennedy et al. 2004).

Acute Safety Risk Related to Serious Intoxication or Withdrawal

Screening for safety related to intoxication and withdrawal at intake involves questioning the woman and her family or friends (with client's permission) about current substance use or recent discontinuation of use, along with past and present experiences of withdrawal. If a woman is obviously severely intoxicated, she needs to be treated with empathy and firmness, and provision needs to be made for her physical safety. If a client has symptoms of withdrawal, formal withdrawal scales can be used by trained personnel to gather information to determine whether medical intervention is required. Such tools include the Clinical Institute Withdrawal Assessment for Alcohol Withdrawal (Sullivan et al. 1989; See Appendix C for specific

---

Figure 4-4
5Ps Screening

Peers: Do any of your friends have a problem with drug or alcohol use?

Partner: Does your partner have a problem with alcohol or drugs?

Parents: Did either of your parents ever have a problem with alcohol or drugs?

Past Use: Before you knew you were pregnant, how often did you drink beer, wine, wine coolers, or liquor? *Not at all, rarely, sometimes, or frequently?*

Present Use: In the past month, how often did you drink beer, wine, wine coolers, or liquor? *Not at all, rarely, sometimes, or frequently?*

Smoke: How many cigarettes did you smoke in the month prior to pregnancy?

Source: Morse et al. 1997; Chasnoff et al. 2001

information) and the Clinical Institute Narcotic Assessment for Opioid Withdrawal (Zilm and Sellers 1978). While specific normative data are unavailable, it is important to screen for withdrawal to assess risk and to implement appropriate medical and clinical interventions.

Not all drugs produce physiological withdrawal; counselors should not assume that withdrawal from any drug of abuse requires medical intervention. Only in the case of opioids, sedative-hypnotics, or benzodiazepines (and in some cases of alcohol), is medical intervention likely to be required. Nonetheless, specific populations may warrant further assessment and assistance in detoxification, including pregnant women, women of color, women with disabilities or co-occurring disorders, and older women. (Review TIP 45 *Detoxification and Substance Abuse Treatment*, [CSAT 2006a], pp. 105–113.) Specific to women who are pregnant and dependent on opioids, withdrawal during pregnancy poses specific medical risks including premature labor and mortality to the fetus. **Note:** Women who are dependent on opioids may misinterpret early signs of pregnancy as opioid withdrawal symptoms (review TIP 43 *Medication-Assisted Treatment for Opioid Addiction in Opioid Treatment Programs* [CSAT 2005a], pp. 211–224).

Mental Illness Symptoms and Mental Disorders

Considering that women are twice as likely as men to experience mood disorders, excluding bipolar and anxiety disorders (Burt and Stein 2002), all women entering substance abuse treatment should be screened for co-occurring mental disorders. If the screening indicates the possible presence of a disorder, a woman should be referred for a comprehensive mental health assessment and receive treatment for the co-occurring disorder, as warranted. Depression, anxiety, eating disorders, and PTSD are common among women who abuse substances (McCrady and Raytek 1993).

Because certain drugs as well as withdrawal symptoms can mimic symptoms of mental disorders, the continual reassessment of mental illness symptoms is essential to ensure accurate diagnosis and treatment planning. TIP 42 *Substance Abuse Treatment for Persons With Co-Occurring Disorders* (CSAT 2005e) contains information on screening and treatment of persons with co-occurring substance use and mental disorders.

General mental disorder screening instruments

Symptom screening involves questions about past or present mental disorder symptoms that may indicate the need for a full mental health assessment. Circumstances surrounding the resolution of symptoms should be explored. For example, if the client is taking psychotropic medication and is no longer symptomatic, this may be an indication that the medication is effective and should be continued. Often, symptom checklists are used when the counselor needs information about how the client is feeling. They are not used to screen for specific disorders, and responses are expected to change from one administration to the next. Symptom screening should be performed routinely and facilitated by the use of formal screening tools.

Basic mental health screening tools are available to assist the substance abuse treatment team. The 18 questions in the Mental Health Screening Form-III (MHSF-III) screen for present or past symptoms of most mental disorders (Carroll and McGinley 2001). It is available at no charge from the Project Return Foundation, Inc., and is reproduced in TIP 42 *Substance Abuse Treatment for Persons With Co-Occurring Disorders* (CSAT 2005e), along with instructions and contact information (a Spanish-language form and instructions can be downloaded from www.asapnys.org/resources.html). MHSF-III was developed in a substance abuse treatment setting and is referred to as a *"rough screening device"* (Carroll and McGinley 2001, p. 35).

The Mini-International Neuropsychiatric Interview (M.I.N.I.) is a brief, structured interview for more than 20 major psychiatric and substance use disorders (Sheehan et al. 2002). Administration time is 15–30 minutes. Scoring is simple and immediate. M.I.N.I. can be administered by clinicians after brief training and by lay personnel with more extensive training. M.I.N.I. can be downloaded from www.medical-outcomes.com and used for no cost in nonprofit or publicly owned settings.

The Brief Symptom Inventory is a research tool that can be adapted for use as a screening checklist. This tool's 53 items measure 9 primary symptom dimensions as well as 3 global indices of distress. Respondents rate the severity of symptoms on a 5-point scale ranging from "Not at all" (0 points) to "Extremely" (4 points) (Derogatis and Melisaratos 1983).

Depression and anxiety disorders

Many formal tools screen for depression, including the Beck Depression Inventory-II (Beck et al. 1996a, b; Smith and Erford 2001; Steer et al. 1989), the Center for Epidemiologic Study Depression Scale (Radloff 1977), and the General Health Questionnaire—a self-administered screening test to identify short-term changes in mental health (depression, anxiety, social dysfunction, and somatic symptoms)—are available.

Programs that screen for depression should ensure that "yes" answers to these questions are followed by a comprehensive assessment, accurate diagnosis, effective treatment, and careful followup. Asking these two questions may be as effective as using longer instruments (U.S. Preventive Services Task Force 2002). Little evidence exists to recommend one screening method over another, so clinicians can choose the method that best fits their preference, the specific population of women, and the setting. Refer to TIP 48 *Managing Depressive Symptoms in Substance Abuse Clients During Early Recovery* (CSAT 2008) for more guidance in working with clients who have depressive symptoms. **Note:** Women who are depressed are more likely to report bodily symptoms, including fatigue, appetite and sleep disturbance, and anxiety (Barsky et al. 2001; Kornstein et al. 2000; Silverstein 2002).

The U.S. Preventive Services Task Force (2002) recommends two simple questions that are effective in screening adults for depression:

1. Over the past 2 weeks have you felt down, depressed, or hopeless?

2. Over the past 2 weeks have you felt little interest or pleasure in doing things?

An example of an instrument that can detect symptoms of anxiety is the 21-item Beck Anxiety Inventory (BAI; Beck 1993; Hewitt and Norton 1993). Among a group of psychiatric patients with a variety of diagnoses, women's BAI scores indicated higher levels of anxiety than men's BAI scores. However, the nature of the anxiety reported appears similar for women and men (Hewitt and Norton 1993).

Assessing Risk of Harm to Self or Others

Suicidal attempts and parasuicidal behavior (nonfatal self-injurious behavior with clear intent to cause bodily harm or death; Welch 2001) are more prevalent among women. The greatest predictor of eventual suicide is prior suicidal attempts and deliberate self-harm inflicted with no intent to die (Joe et al. 2006). While substance dependence and PTSD are associated with self-harm and suicidal behavior (Harned et al. 2006), the most frequent diagnoses associated with suicide are mood disorders, specifically depressive episodes (Kessler et al. 1999). Considering the prevalence of suicidal attempts, self-injurious behavior, and depression among women, employing safety screenings should be a standard practice. From the outset, clinicians should specifically ask the client and anyone else who is providing information whether she is in immediate danger and whether she has any immediate intention to engage in violent or self-injurious behavior. If the answer is "yes," the clinician should obtain more information about the nature and severity of the thoughts, plan, and intent, and then arrange for an in-depth risk assessment by a trained mental health clinician. The client should not be left alone.

No tool is definitive for safety screening. Clinicians should use safety screening tools only as an initial guide and proceed to detailed questions to obtain relevant information. In addition, care is needed to avoid underestimating risk because a woman is using substances or has frequently engaged in self-injurious behavior. For example, a woman who is intoxicated might seem to be making empty threats of self-harm, but all statements about harming herself or others must be taken seriously. Overall, individuals who have suicidal or aggressive impulses when intoxicated are more likely to act on those impulses; therefore, determination of the seriousness of threats requires a skilled mental health assessment, plus information from others who know the client very well. Screening tools and procedures in evaluating risk are discussed in depth in TIP 50 *Addressing Suicidal Thoughts and Behaviors in Substance Abuse Treatment* (CSAT 2009a).

Substance abuse treatment programs need clear mental health referral and follow-up procedures so that clients receive appropriate psychiatric evaluations and mental health care. The American Association of Community Psychiatrists (AACP) developed the Level of Care Utilization System for Psychiatric and Addiction Services (LOCUS) that evaluates clients along six dimensions and defines six levels of resource intensity. It includes an excellent tool for helping the counselor determine the risk of harm (AACP 2000; See Appendix C for specific information on the LOCUS). The potential risk of harm most frequently takes the form of suicidal intentions, and less often the form of homicidal intentions. The scale has five categories, from minimal risk of harm to extreme risk of harm. It is available at www.comm.psych.pitt.edu/finds/LOCUS2000.pdf and can be easily adapted for use in treatment facilities.

Trauma and Posttraumatic Stress Disorder

PTSD can follow a traumatic episode that involves witnessing, being threatened, or experiencing an actual event involving death or serious physical harm, such as auto accidents, natural disasters, sexual or physical assault, war, and childhood sexual and physical abuse (APA 2000a). During the trauma, the individual experiences intense fear, helplessness, or horror. PTSD has symptoms that last longer than 1 month and result in a decline in functioning in several life areas, such as work and relationships. A diagnosis of PTSD cannot be made without a clear history of a traumatic event (Figure 4-5 presents sample screening questions for identifying a woman's history of trauma). General symptoms of PTSD include persistently re-experiencing the traumatic event, numbness or avoidance of cues associated with the trauma, and a pattern of increased arousal (APA 2000a).

Historically, women have not been routinely screened for a history of trauma or assessed to determine a diagnosis of PTSD across treatment settings (Najavits 2004). Among women in substance abuse treatment, it has been estimated that 55–99 percent have experienced trauma—commonly childhood physical or sexual abuse, domestic violence, or rape (Najavits et al. 1997; Triffleman 2003). Studies have reported that current PTSD rates among women who abuse substances range between 14 to 60 percent (Brady 2001; Najavits et al. 1998; Triffleman 2003). In comparison to men, women who use substances are still more than twice as likely to have PTSD (Najavits et al. 1997). Brief screening is paramount in not only establishing past or present traumatic events but in identifying PTSD symptoms. Upon identification of traumatic stress symptoms, counselors need to refer the women for a mental health evaluation in order to further assess the presenting symptoms, to determine the appropriateness of a PTSD diagnosis, and to assist in establishing an appropriate treatment plan and approach. Brief screenings are used to identify clients who are more likely to have

Figure 4-5
Questions to Screen for Trauma History

Responses include yes, no, or maybe. Maybe is used if the client is unsure (e.g., she was too young to remember but suspects it happened). If answering these questions is upsetting, the counselor may need to stop the interview or redirect the questions, provide support and reassurance to the client, and seek consultation from a clinical supervisor.

In your lifetime, have you suffered any of the following experiences or seen them happen to someone else? (Answers are yes, no, or maybe.)

- Child physical abuse (e.g., hitting that caused bruises or injury)
- Child sexual abuse (e.g., being molested, touched, or forced into any sexual activity)
- Child neglect (e.g., not enough to eat, inadequate shelter)
- Domestic violence (e.g., a partner who hurt you physically)
- Crime victimization (e.g., rape, holdup)
- Serious accident (e.g., car crash, chemical spill, or fire)
- Life-threatening illness (e.g., cancer)
- Natural disaster (e.g., hurricane, earthquake)
- War
- Captivity or kidnapping
- The *threat* of any of the events listed above, even if it wasn't completed (e.g., threat of being raped or murdered)
- Violence by you (e.g., you physically hurt someone, such as abusing a child, murdering someone, or attacking someone with a weapon)
- Other upsetting events (make a list)

Source: Najavits 2002a.

PTSD. A positive response to any PTSD screen does not necessarily indicate that a patient has PTSD, but it does warrant further investigation.

Numerous screening and assessment tools are available to assess lifetime traumatic events, traumatic stress symptoms, and diagnostic criteria for PTSD. Screening and assessment for trauma-related symptoms and disorders are discussed in depth in the planned TIP *Substance Abuse and Trauma* (CSAT in development *h*). One specific screening tool that coincides with the symptoms and criteria listed in the DSM-IV-TR is the PTSD Checklist – Civilian Version (PCL-C) and the PCL-Military Version (Weathers et al. 1993). The PTSD Checklist is a 17-item, self-report rating scale. It was initially developed and validated for male Vietnam veterans; further empirical data support the reliability, validity, and diagnostic utility among women and among mixed-gender civilian groups (Andrykowski et al. 1998; Blanchard et al. 1996; Dobie et al. 2004). This instrument requires no formal training to administer and can be downloaded from the National Center for PTSD (http://www.ptsd.va.gov).

Sexual Victimization, Childhood Abuse, and Interpersonal Violence

Sexual victimization and childhood abuse

Women entering treatment for substance use disorders have consistently reported high rates of sexual abuse. Approximately two-thirds of all women entering treatment have specifically reported a history of sexual violence (Gil-Rivas et al. 1996; Lincoln et al. 2006). In 1998, Bassuk reported higher rates of lifetime occurrence of physical and sexual violence among women who are poor and homeless (82 percent and 92 percent, respectively; Bassuk 1998). More recent research focuses on sociocultural factors supporting the belief that socioeconomic status contributes more to women's vulnerability to abuse and stress symptoms than does ethnicity (Vogel and Marshall 2001).

During the intake process, many women are reluctant to reveal their sexual abuse before trust is established with the counselor. Some women may not realize that their experiences

Note to Clinicians

So often, clients who have PTSD have a difficult time in distinguishing between the past feelings of danger associated with the trauma(s) and their current surroundings when discussing trauma-related material during interviews and counseling. Therefore, it is important for counselors to remember that discussing the occurrence or consequences of traumatic events and subsequent PTSD symptoms can feel as unsafe, dangerous, and helpless to the client as if the event were occurring now. While the counselor does not want to encourage avoidance or reinforce the belief that discussing trauma-related material is dangerous, it is important to be sensitive when gathering information about a woman's history of trauma in the initial screening.

Initial questions about trauma should be general and gradual. While ideally you want the client to control the level of disclosure, it is important as a counselor to mediate the level of disclosure. At times, clients with PTSD just want to gain relief; they disclose too much, too soon without having established trust, an adequate support system, or effective coping strategies. Preparing a woman to respond to trauma-related questions is important. By taking the time with the client to prepare and explain how the screening is done and the potential need to pace the material, the woman has more control over the situation. Overall, she should understand the screening process, why the specific questions are important, and that she can choose not to answer or to delay her response. From the outset, counselors need to provide initial trauma-informed education and guidance with the client.

were not normal and were abusive. Some women do not remember the abuse. Therefore, a negative finding on abuse at an intake screening should not be taken as a final answer. The Substance Abuse and Mental Health Services Administration (SAMHSA)-funded Women, Co-Occurring Disorders and Violence Study includes questions about sexual abuse in its baseline interview protocol, presented in Figure 4-6. In addition, SAMHSA's CSAT has developed a brochure for women that defines childhood abuse and informs the reader of how to begin to address childhood abuse issues while in treatment (CSAT 2003*a*). TIP 36 *Substance Abuse Treatment for Persons With Child Abuse and Neglect Issues* (CSAT 2000*b*) includes detailed information on this topic.

Interpersonal violence

Studies estimate that between 50 to 99 percent of women with substance use disorders have a history of interpersonal violence (Miller et al. 1993; Rice et al. 2001). In one study focused on sensitivity and specificity of screening questions for intimate partner violence, Paranjape and Liebschutz (2003) concluded that when three simple screening questions were used together, identification of lifetime interpersonal violence was effectively identified for women. This screening tool, referred as the STaT, is presented in Figure 4-7 (p. 72). Along with a sample personalized safety plan, additional screening tools, including the Abuse Assessment Screen (English and Spanish version), Danger Assessment, The Psychological Maltreatment of Women Inventory, and The Revised Conflict Tactics Scale (CTS2), are available in TIP 25 *Substance Abuse Treatment and Domestic Violence* (CSAT 1997*b*). **Note:** It is important to assess for interpersonal violence in heterosexual

---

Figure 4-6
Questions Regarding Sexual Abuse

Have you ever been bothered or harassed by sexual remarks, jokes, inappropriate touching, or demands for sexual favors by someone at work or school?
- How often has this happened?
- How old were you when this first happened?
- Has this happened in the past 6 months?

Were you ever touched or have you ever touched someone else in a sexual way because you felt forced or coerced or threatened by harm to yourself or someone else?
- How old were you when this first happened?
- How often did this happen before age 18?
- How often has this happened since you turned 18?
- Has this happened in the past 6 months?

Did you ever have sex because you felt forced or threatened by harm to yourself or someone else?
- How old were you when this first happened?
- How often did this happen before age 18?
- How often has this happened since you turned 18?
- Has this happened in the past 6 months?

Have you ever had sex when you did not want to in exchange for money, drugs, or other material goods such as shelter or clothing?
- How often has this happened?
- How old were you when this first happened?
- Has this happened in the past 6 months?

Source: SAMHSA n.d.

and homosexual relationships.

Interpersonal violence and disabilities

Women with disabilities are at a significantly greater risk for severe interpersonal violence and neglect (Brownridge 2006). As a counselor, additional screening questions tailored to address unique vulnerabilities associated with the specific physical disability may be warranted. For example,

- Has anyone ever withheld food or medication from you that you asked for or needed?
- Has anyone ever refused to let you use your wheelchair or other assistive devices at home or in the community?
- Has anyone ever refused to assist you with self-care that you needed, such as getting out of bed, using the toilet, or other personal care tasks?
- Has anyone used restraints on you to keep you from getting out of bed or out of your wheelchair?

Initial questions about trauma should be general and gradual. While ideally you want the client to control the level of disclosure, it is important as a counselor to mediate the level of disclosure. At times, clients with PTSD just want to gain relief; they disclose too much, too soon without having established trust, an adequate support system, or effective coping strategies.

Preparing a woman to respond to trauma-related questions is important. By taking the time with the client to prepare and explain how the screening is done and the potential need to pace the material, the woman has more control over the situation. Overall, she should understand the screening process, why the specific questions are important, and that she can choose not to answer or to delay her response. From the outset, counselors need to provide initial trauma-informed education and guidance with the client.

Eating Disorders

Eating disorders have one of the highest mortality rates of all psychological disorders (Neumarker 1997; Steinhausen 2002). Approximately 15 percent of women in substance abuse treatment have had an eating disorder diagnosis in their lifetimes (Hudson 1992). Three eating disorders are currently included in the DSM-IV-TR: anorexia nervosa, bulimia nervosa, and eating disorder not otherwise specified (APA 2000a). Compulsive eating, referred to as binge-eating disorder, is not included as a diagnosis in the DSM. Currently, it is theorized that substance use disorders and compulsive overeating are competing disorders, in that compulsive overeating (binge-eating) is not as likely to appear at the same time as substance use disorders. Consequently, disordered eating in

> Be aware that weight gain during recovery can be a major concern and a relapse risk factor for women.

the form of compulsive overeating is more likely to appear after a period of abstinence, thus enhancing the risk of relapse to drugs and alcohol to manage weight gain.

Bulimia nervosa, characterized by recurrent episodes of binge and purge eating behaviors, has the highest incidence rates in the general population for eating disorders (Hoek and van Hoeken 2003), and it is the most common eating disorder among women in substance abuse treatment (Corcos et al. 2001; Specker et al. 2000; APA 2000*a*). For specific information regarding the co-occurring disorders of eating and substance use disorders, counselors should refer to TIP 42 *Substance Abuse Treatment for Persons With Co-Occurring Disorders* (CSAT 2005*e*).

Screening for eating disorders in substance abuse treatment is based on the assumption that identification of an eating disorder can lead to earlier intervention and treatment, thereby reducing serious physical and psychological complications and decreasing the potential risk for relapse to manage weight. Eating disorder screenings are not designed to establish an eating disorder diagnosis but instead to identify the need for additional psychological and medical assessments by a trained mental health

clinician and medical personnel. The EAT-26 (Garner et al. 1982), or Eating Attitudes Test, is a widely used screening tool that can help identify behaviors and symptoms associated with eating disorder risk (Garner et al. 1998). It is recommended that a two-stage process be employed using the EAT-26: screening followed by a clinical interview. Specifically, if the woman scores at or above a cutoff score of 20 on the EAT-26, she should be referred for a diagnostic interview. For a copy of the screening tool and scoring instructions, refer to Appendix C.

Figure 4-8 lists questions that probe for an eating disorder. A woman with an eating disorder often feels shame about her behavior, so the general questions help ease into the topic as the counselor explores the client's attitude toward her shape, weight, and dieting.

Screening by Healthcare Providers in Other Settings

Healthcare providers such as nurse practitioners, physicians, physicians' assistants, and social service professionals have opportunities to screen women to determine whether they use or abuse alcohol, drugs, or tobacco. The most frequent points of entry

---

Figure 4-8
General and Specific Screening Questions for Persons With Possible Eating Disorders

General Screening Questions

- How satisfied are you with your weight and shape?
- How often do you try to lose or gain weight?
- How often have you dieted?
- What other methods have you used to lose weight?

Specific Screening Questions

- Have you ever lost weight and weighed less than others thought you should weigh?
- Have you had eating binges in which you eat a large amount of food in a short period of time?
- Do you ever feel out of control when eating?
- Have you ever vomited to lose weight or to get rid of food that you have eaten?
- What other sorts of methods have you used to lose weight or to get rid of food?

Source: CSAT 2005*e*.

> Our own preconceived images of women who are addicted, coupled with a myth that women are less likely to become addicted, can undermine clinical judgment to conduct routine screenings for substance use.

from other systems of care are obstetric and primary care; hospital emergency rooms; probation officer visits; and social service agencies in connection with housing, child care, and domestic violence.

Between 5 and 40 percent of people seeing physicians and/or reporting to hospital emergency rooms for care have an alcohol use disorder (Chang 1997), but physicians often do not identify, refer, or intervene with these patients (Kuehn 2008). Even clinicians who often use the CAGE or other screening tools for certain patients are less likely to ask women these questions because women—particularly older women, women of Asian descent, and those from middle and upper socioeconomic levels—are not expected to abuse substances (Chang 1997). Volk and colleagues (1996) found that, among primary care patients who were identified as "at risk" for alcohol abuse or dependence by a screening questionnaire, men were 1.5 times as likely as women to be warned about alcohol use and three times as likely to be advised to stop or modify their consumption. Women may be less likely to have problems with alcohol or drugs than men (Kessler et al. 1994, 1995); however, when women have substance use disorders, they experience greater health and social consequences.

Screening must lead to appropriate referrals for further evaluation and treatment in order to be worthwhile. Missed opportunities can be especially unfortunate during prenatal care. In one study of ethnically diverse women reporting to a university-based obstetrics clinic, 38 percent screened positive for psychiatric disorders and/or substance abuse. However, only 43 percent of those who screened positive had symptoms recorded in their chart, and only 23 percent of those screening positive were given treatment. This low rate of treatment is of great concern, given the untoward consequences of substance use for maternal and infant health (Kelly et al. 2001).

To address the disconnection that often happens (beginning with the lack of identification of substance-related problems of the patient and extending to the failure of appropriate referrals and brief interventions), SAMHSA has invested in the Screening, Brief Intervention, and Referral to Treatment Initiative (SBIRT)—research, resources development, training, and program implementation across healthcare settings. Although studies have not focused on gender comparisons, SBIRT programs have yielded short-term improvements in individual health (for review, see Babor et al. 2007). Specifically, some SBIRT programs on the State level have tailored SBIRT to provide assistance to pregnant women (Louisiana Department of Health and Hospitals 2007).

Assessment

The assessment examines a client's life in far more detail so that accurate diagnosis, appropriate treatment placement, problem lists, and treatment goals can be made. Usually, a clinical assessment delves into a client's current experiences and her physical, psychological, and sociocultural history to determine specific treatment needs. Using qualified and trained clinicians, a comprehensive assessment enables the treatment provider to determine with the client the most appropriate treatment placement and treatment plan (CSAT 2000c). Notably, assessments need to use multiple avenues to obtain the necessary clinical information, including self-assessment instruments, clinical records, structured clinical interviews, assessment measures, and collateral information. Rather than using one method for evaluation, assessments should include multiple sources of information to obtain a broad perspective of the client's history, level of functioning and impairment, and degree of distress.

Assessment should be a fluid process throughout treatment. It is not a once-and-done event. Considering the complexity of withdrawal and the potential influence of alcohol and drugs on physical and psychological functioning, it is very important to reevaluate as the client engages into recovery. Periodic reassessment is critical to determine the client's progress and her changing treatment needs. In addition, reassessment is an opportunity to solicit input from the client on what is and is not working for her in treatment and to alter treatment accordingly.

The following section reviews core assessment processes tailored for women, including gender-specific content for biopsychosocial histories and assessment tools that are either appropriate or possess normative data for women in evaluating substance use disorders and consequences. It is beyond the scope of this chapter to provide

specific assessment guidelines or tools for other disorders outside of substance-related disorders.

The Assessment Interview

To provide an accurate picture of the client's needs, a clinical assessment interview requires sensitivity on the part of the counselor and considerable time to complete thoroughly. While treatment program staff may have limited time or feel pressure to conduct initial psychosocial histories quickly, it is important to portray to clients that you have sufficient time to devote to the process. The assessment interview is the beginning of the therapeutic relationship and helps set the tone for treatment.

Initially, the interviewer should explain the reason for and role of a psychosocial history. It is equally important that the counselor or intake worker incorporate screening results into the interview, and make the appropriate referrals within and/or outside the agency to comprehensively address presenting issues. The notion that the women's substance use is not an isolated behavior but occurs in response to,

Advice to Administrators:
General Guidelines for Selecting and Using Screening and Assessment Tools

- What are the goals of the screening and assessment?
- Is the screening and assessment process appropriate for the particular setting with women?
- What costs are associated with the screening process; e.g., training, buying the screening/assessment instruments or equipment (computer), wages associated with giving and scoring the instrument, and time spent providing feedback to the client and establishing appropriate referrals?
- What other staff resources are needed to administer and score the instrument, interpret the results, review the findings with the client, arrange referrals, or establish appropriate services to address concerns highlighted in the screening and assessment process?
- While screening measures can be completed in just a few minutes, positive screenings involve more work. Does staff see a need for and value of the additional work? Did you prepare and train staff? What strategies did you employ to obtain staff or administrative buy-in? What other obstacles have you identified if the screening is implemented? Have you developed strategies to target their specific obstacles?
- Do you have a system in place to manage the results of the screening and assessment process?

Note: While formal assessment tools are consistently used in research associated with substance use disorders, treatment providers and counselors are less likely to use formalized tools and more likely to only use clinical interviews (Allen 1991). The standardization of formal assessment measures offers consistency and uniformity in administration and scoring. If the implementation of these tools is not cost prohibitive and staff maintain adherence to administration guidelines, formal assessment tools can be easily adopted regardless of diverse experience, training, and treatment philosophy among clinicians. Using psychometrically sound instruments can offset clinical bias and provide more credibility with clients.

and affects, other behaviors and areas of her life is an important concept to introduce during the intake phase. This information can easily disarm a client's defensiveness regarding use and consequences of use.

The focus of the assessment may vary depending on the program and the specific issues of an individual client. A structured biopsychosocial history interview can be obtained by using The Psychosocial History (PSH) assessment tool (Comfort et al. 1996), a comprehensive multidisciplinary interview incorporating modifications of the Addiction Severity Index

(ASI) designed to assess the history and needs of women in substance abuse treatment. Investigators have sought to retain the fundamental structure of ASI while expanding it to include family history and relationships, relationships with partners, responsibilities for children, pregnancy history, history of violence and victimization, legal issues, and housing arrangements (Comfort and Kaltenbach 1996). PSH has been found to have satisfactory test-retest reliability (i.e., the extent to which the scores are the same on two administrations of the instrument with the same people) and concurrent validity with the ASI (Comfort et al. 1999).

Psychosocial and Cultural History

Treatment programs have their own prescribed format for obtaining a psychosocial history that coincides with State regulations as well as other standards set by Joint Commission on Accreditation of Healthcare Organizations (JCAHO) and Commission on Accreditation of Rehabilitation Facilities (CARF). While many States require screening and assessment for women, specific guidelines and specificity in incorporating women-specific areas vary in degree (CSAT 2007). **Note:** When using information across State standards, the following psychosocial and cultural subheadings should be included in the initial assessment for women, and these areas need to be addressed in more depth as treatment continues. **Keep in mind that the content within each subheading does not represent an entire psychosocial and cultural history. Only biopsychosocial and cultural issues that are pertinent to women were included in the list below.**

Medical History and Physical Health: Review HIV/AIDS status, history of hepatitis or other infectious diseases, and HIV/AIDS risk behavior; explore history of gynecological problems, use of birth control and hormone replacement therapy, and the relationship between gynecological problems and substance abuse; obtain history of pregnancies, miscarriages, abortions, and history of substance abuse during pregnancy; assess need for prenatal care.

Substance Abuse History: Identify people who initially introduced alcohol and drugs; explore reasons for initiation of use and continued use; discuss family of origin history of substance abuse, history of use in previous and present significant relationships, and history of use with family members or significant others.

Mental Health and Treatment History: Explore prior treatment history and relationships with prior treatment providers and consequences, if any, for engaging in prior treatment; review history of prior traumatic events, mood or anxiety disorders (including PTSD), as well as eating disorders; evaluate safety issues including parasuicidal behaviors, previous or current threats, history of interpersonal violence or sexual abuse, and overall feeling of safety; review family history of mental illness; and discuss evidence and history of personal strengths and coping strategies and styles.

Interpersonal and Family History: Obtain history of substance abuse in current relationship, explore acceptance of client's substance abuse problem among family and significant relationships, discuss concerns regarding child care needs, and discuss the types of support that she has received from her family and/or significant other for entering treatment and abstaining from substances.

Family, Parenting, and Caregiver History: Discuss the various caregiver roles she may play, review parenting history and current living circumstances.

Children's Developmental and Educational History (applicable to women and children programs): Assess child safety issues; explore developmental, emotional, and medical needs of children.

Sociocultural History: Evaluate client's social support system, including the level of acceptance of her recovery; discuss level of social isolation prior to treatment; discuss the role of her cultural beliefs pertaining to her substance use and recovery process; explore the specific cultural attitudes toward women and substance abuse; review current spiritual practices (if any); discuss current acculturation conflicts and stressors; and explore need or preference for bilingual or monolingual non-English services.

Vocational, Educational, and Military History: If employed, discuss the level of support that the client is receiving from her employer; review military history, then expand questions to include history of traumatic events and violence during employment and history of substance abuse in the military; assess financial self-reliance.

Legal History: Discuss history of custody and current involvement with child protective services, if any; obtain a history of restraining orders, arrests, or periods of incarceration, if any; determine history of child placement with women who acknowledge past or current incarceration.

Barriers to Treatment and Related Services: Explore financial, housing, health insurance, child care, case management, and transportation needs; discuss other potential obstacles the client foresees.

Strengths and Coping Strategies: Discuss the challenges that the client has faced throughout her life and how she has managed them, review prior attempts to quit substance use and identify strategies that did work at the time, identify other successes in making changes in other areas of her life.

Assessment Tools for Substance Use Disorders

Addiction Severity Index (ASI): The ASI (McLellan et al. 1980) is the most widely used substance abuse assessment instrument in both research and clinical settings. It is administered as a semi-structured interview and gathers information in seven domains (i.e., drug use, alcohol use, family/social, employment/finances, medical, psychiatric, and legal). The ASI has demonstrated high levels of reliability and validity across genders, races/ethnicities, types of substance addiction, and treatment settings (McCusker et al. 1994; McLellan et al. 1985; Zanis et al. 1994; See Appendix C for specific information on the ASI).

ASI-F (CSAT 1997c): The ASI-F is an expanded version of ASI; several items were added relevant to the family, social relationships, and psychiatric sections. Additional items refer to homelessness; sexual harassment; emotional, physical, and sexual abuse; and eating disorders. The supplemental questions are asked after the administration of ASI. Psychometric data for ASI-F are limited.

Texas Christian University Brief Intake, the Comprehensive Intake, and Intake for Women and Children: These instruments are available electronically and are administered by a counselor. The seven problem areas in the Brief Intake Interview were derived from

> Since women are more likely to experience greater consequences earlier than men, using an instrument that highlights specific consequences of use is crucial.

the ASI: drug, alcohol, medical, psychological, employment, legal, and family/social. Scoring is immediate, and the program generates a one-page summary of the client's functioning in 14 domains (Joe et al. 2000). The Comprehensive Intake has an online version for women (Simpson and Knight 1997.

Drinker Inventory of Consequences (DrinC): This measurement is a self-administered 50-item, true-false questionnaire that elicits information about negative consequences of drinking in five domains: physical, interpersonal, intrapersonal, impulse control, and social responsibility (Miller et al. 1995). This instrument has normative data for women, men, inpatient and outpatient, and has good psychometric properties. Since women are more likely to experience greater consequences earlier than men, using an instrument that highlights specific consequences of use is crucial. A version that assesses drug use consequences is also available (Tonigan and Miller 2002). For a copy of the assessment tool, scoring, and gender profile in interpreting severity of lifetime consequences, see Appendix C.

Available screening and assessment tools: Language availability

Figure 4-9 (p. 80) provides available information on screening and assessment versions in languages other than English. This is not an exhaustive list, and counselors and administrators should not assume language availability is a sign that the instrument is appropriate for a particular culture, ethnic, or racial group.

Other Considerations in Assessment: Strengths, Coping Styles, and Spirituality

Looking at women's strengths

Focusing on a woman's strengths instead of her deficits improves self-esteem and self-efficacy. Familiarity with a woman's strengths enables the counselor to know what assets the woman can use to help her during recovery. In the *Woman's Addiction Workbook* (Najavits 2002*a*), the author provides a self-assessment worksheet that focuses on individual strengths. In addition to assessing strengths, coping styles and strategies should be evaluated (see Rotgers 2002).

Measurements of spirituality and religiousness

Spirituality and religion play an important role in culture, identity, and health practices (Musgrave et al. 2002). In addition, women are more likely to embrace different coping strategies (including emotional outlets and religion) to assist in managing life stressors (Dennerstein 2001). Practices such as consulting religious leaders or spiritual healers (*curanderas*, medicine men) and attending to spiritual activities (including sweats and prayer ceremonies, praying to specific saints or ancestors) are common. The consensus panel believes it is important that programs assess the spiritual and religious beliefs and practices of women and incorporate this component into their treatment with sensitivity and respect.

A challenge in determining the effect of spirituality on treatment outcomes is how to assess the extent and nature of a person's spirituality or religiousness. Several assessment tools are available; however, they are more often used for research. They include, but are not limited to, the Religious Practice and Beliefs measurement (CASAA 2004), a 19-item self-assessment tool that reviews specific activities associated with religious practices; the Multidimensional Measure of Religiousness/ Spirituality, an assessment device that examines domains of religious or spiritual activity such as

Figure 4-9
Available Screening and Assessment Tools in Multiple Languages

Instrument	Language
Addiction Severity Index	Spanish
Alcohol Use Disorders Identification Test (AUDIT)	Numerous language versions including Spanish, French, German, Russian, Chinese, etc.
Beck Depression Inventory (BDI)	Numerous language versions including Spanish, French, German, Swedish, Chinese, Korean, etc.
Brief Symptom Inventory (BSI)	Spanish and French
CAGE	Numerous language versions including Spanish, Flemish, French, Hebrew, Japanese, etc.
Eating Attitudes Test (EAT-26)	Numerous language versions including Spanish and Japanese
General Health Questionnaire (GHQ)	Numerous language versions including Spanish, Japanese, Chinese, Farsi, etc.
Mini International Neuropsychiatric Interview (MINI)	Available in 43 languages including Spanish
Spiritual Well-Being Scale	Spanish
Texas Christian University Drug Screen II (TCUII)	Spanish
TWEAK	Spanish

daily spiritual experiences, values and beliefs, and religious and spiritual means of coping (Fetzer Institute 1999); and the Spiritual Well-Being Scale, a 20-item scale that examines the benefits of spirituality for African-American women in recovery from substance abuse (Brome et al. 2000; See Appendix C for specific information on the Spiritual Well-Being Scale).

Health Assessment and Medical Examination

Because women develop serious medical problems earlier in the course of alcohol use disorders than men, they should be encouraged to seek medical treatment early to enhance their chances of recovery and to prevent serious medical complications. Health screenings and medical examinations are essential in women's treatment. In particular, women entering substance abuse treatment programs should be referred for mental health, medical, and dental examinations. In many cases, they may not have had adequate health care because of lack of insurance coverage or transportation, absence of child care, lack of time for self-care, chaotic lifestyle related to a substance abuse, or fear of legal repercussions or losing custody of children. The acute and chronic effects of alcohol and drug abuse, the potential for violence, and other physical hardships (e.g., homelessness) greatly increase the risk for illness and injury.

Women may practice behaviors that put them at high risk for contracting sexually transmitted diseases (STDs) and other infectious diseases

Advice to Clinicians:
General Guidelines of Assessment for Women

- Similar to the screening process, women should know the purpose of the assessment.
- To conduct a good quality assessment, counselors need to value and invest in the therapeutic alliance with the client. Challenging, disagreeing, being overly invested in the outcome, or vocalizing and assuming a specific diagnosis without an appropriate evaluation can quickly erode any potential for a good working relationship with the client.
- The assessment process should include various methods of gathering information: clinical interview; assessment tools including rating scales; behavioral samples through examples of previous behavior or direct observation; collateral information from previous treatment providers, family members, or other agencies (with client permission); and retrospective data including previous evaluations, discharge summaries, etc.
- Assessment is only as good as the ability to follow through with the recommendations.
- Assessments need to incorporate sociocultural factors that may influence behavior in the assessment process, interpretation of the results, and compliance with recommendations.
- The assessment process should extend beyond the initial assessment. As the woman becomes more comfortable, additional information can be gathered and incorporated into the revised assessment. Subsequently, this new information will guide the reevaluation of presenting problems, treatment priorities, and treatment planning with input and guidance from the client.
- Reassessments help monitor progress across the continuum of care and can be used as a barometer of effective treatment. Moreover, the presenting problems and symptoms may change as recovery proceeds.

(Greenfield 1996). Testing for HIV/AIDS, hepatitis, and tuberculosis is important; however, it is as essential to have adequate support services to help women process test results in early recovery. Anticipation of the test results is stressful and may place the client at risk for relapse. Residential centers may offer medical exams onsite, but outpatient service providers may need to refer patients to their primary care provider or other affordable health care to ensure that each client has a thorough medical exam. Healthcare professionals may benefit in using the Women-Specific Health Assessment (Stevens and Murphy 1998), which assesses health and wellness and addresses gynecological exams, HIV/AIDS, drug use, STDs, pregnancy/child delivery history, family planning, mammography, menstruation, disease prevention, and protection behaviors.

5 Treatment Engagement, Placement, and Planning

Overview

Women often encounter numerous obstacles and barriers prior to and during the treatment process. While these hurdles may not be entirely unique to women, they are often more common for women due to the myriad pressures associated with assuming various caregiver roles, intrinsic socioeconomic and health conditions (particularly for women with substance use disorders), and societal bias and stigma associated with substance abuse. These challenges often interfere with treatment initiation and engagement.

This chapter is devoted to the exploration of treatment barriers as well as to the engagement strategies conducive to supporting treatment initiation for women. Considerations in treatment placement and the importance of client involvement are reviewed. The chapter ends with an overview of American Society of Addiction Medicine (ASAM) placement criteria for each treatment level with emphasis on issues specific to women, pregnant women, and women and children.

Barriers to Treatment Engagement

Making a decision to change is an essential step toward fulfilling any goal, but is only one ingredient of a successful outcome. Many times, the idea of making a change is shortsighted: How often has a decision been made without looking beyond the initial necessity or enthusiasm for the change? To support change across time, obstacles need to be anticipated and strategies need to be developed either to decrease the occurrence of the barriers or to find alternative routes around the potential obstacles.

Barriers to treatment are not exclusive to women (for review, see Appel et al. 2004), yet identifying potential challenges and obstacles can help enable successful treatment engagement and outcome. Historically, women have identified multiple factors as barriers to entering treatment, to engaging and continuing the utilization of treatment services across the continuum of care, and in maintaining connections with community services and self-help groups that support long-term recovery (see Figure 5-1 for an overview of barriers identified in the Substance Abuse and Mental Health Services Administration's (SAMHSA's) National Survey on Drug Use and Health [NSDUH]).

While the identification of barriers is essential to effective case management and treatment planning, it is equally important to develop specific strategies to address each barrier as early as possible. As highlighted in the Center for Substance Abuse Treatment's (CSAT's) *Comprehensive Substance Abuse Treatment Model for Women and Their Children* (for review, see Appendix B; HHS 2004), strategies to overcome these barriers need to focus on three core areas: clinical treatment services, clinical support services, and community support systems. Without a proactive plan to address barriers, women will not be as able to engage in or benefit from substance abuse treatment.

At the outset, barriers may exist on several levels:

- *Intrapersonal*: Individual factors including health problems, psychological issues, cognitive functioning, motivational status, treatment readiness, etc.
- *Interpersonal*: Relational issues including significant relationships, family dynamics, support systems, etc.
- *Sociocultural*: Social factors including cultural differences; the role of stigma, bias, and racism; societal attitudes; disparity in health services; attitudes of healthcare providers toward women; and others.
- *Structural*: Program characteristics including treatment policies and procedures, program design, and treatment restrictions.

- *Systemic:* Larger systems including Federal, State, and local agencies that generate public policies and laws; businesses including health insurance companies; and environmental factors such as the economy, drug trafficking patterns, etc.

Intrapersonal Obstacles

Various individual factors impede interest in and commitment to entering treatment. The anticipation of not being able to use substances to cope with stress, to manage weight, or to deal with symptoms associated with other mental disorders creates considerable apprehension in making a commitment to treatment. While the level of motivation and the degree of treatment readiness may also obstruct a woman's commitment to treatment (Miller and Rollnick 2002), there are other individual characteristics that may serve as a barrier to treatment, including feelings related to previous treatment failures, feelings of guilt and shame regarding use and behavior associated with use, fear of losing custody of children if the drug or alcohol problem is admitted and treatment is sought, feelings of helplessness, and a belief that change is not possible (Allen 1995; Greenfield 1996).

Moreover, health issues can serve as a powerful roadblock for women. Depending on the medical diagnosis and severity of the disorder, women may encounter difficulties in accessing treatment, securing appropriate services, and coordinating medical and substance abuse treatment needs. Many women neglect their health while they are actively using substances, hence treatment entry may be delayed or difficult to coordinate due to the additional burden imposed by health issues (including HIV/AIDS, viral hepatitis and other infectious diseases, mental disorders, and gynecological and obstetric needs). Thus, poor physical health may hinder entry into treatment (Jessup et al. 2003).

Interpersonal Obstacles

Because women are usually the primary caregivers of children as well as of other family members, they are often unable or not

Figure 5-1

Percentages of Reasons for Not Receiving Substance Use Treatment in the Past Year Among Women Aged 18 to 49 Who Needed Treatment and Who Perceived a Need for It: 2004–2006

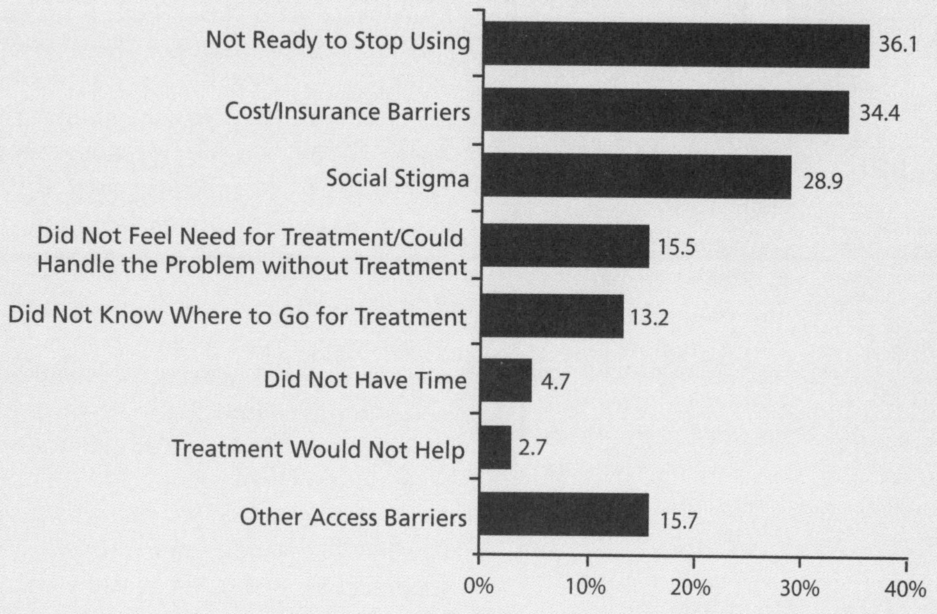

Reason	Percentage
Not Ready to Stop Using	36.1
Cost/Insurance Barriers	34.4
Social Stigma	28.9
Did Not Feel Need for Treatment/Could Handle the Problem without Treatment	15.5
Did Not Know Where to Go for Treatment	13.2
Did Not Have Time	4.7
Treatment Would Not Help	2.7
Other Access Barriers	15.7

Sources: SAMHSA 2004, 2005, 2006.

encouraged to enter and remain in treatment. Also, sometimes their families and friends are involved with substance use and abuse. Further, women may share a social network in which drug or alcohol use is a central activity. This group of family and friends may see no benefit in and offer no encouragement for becoming alcohol and drug free (Amaro and Hardy-Fanta 1995; Finkelstein 1993; Salmon et al. 2000). While women report fear of losing their partner during treatment, they are particularly vulnerable to losing their partner upon entering treatment (Lex 1991). In addition, women generally fear family or partner reactions or resistance to asking for help outside the family.

Sociocultural Obstacles

Women are more stigmatized by alcohol and illicit drug use than men, being characterized sometimes as morally lax, sexually promiscuous, and neglectful as mothers. In addition, women who have children often fear that admitting a substance use problem will cause them to lose custody of their children. They worry that they will be perceived as irresponsible or neglectful—as "bad mothers" if they admit to substance abuse or dependence. These fears and stereotypes compound a woman's shame and guilt about substance use (Finkelstein 1994) and subsequently interfere with help-seeking behavior.

To compound the issue, women in some cultural groups experience more negative attitudes toward their substance use in general and may express more difficulty in engaging in help-seeking behavior and treatment services based on gender roles and expectations. For example, Asian women, in conjunction with cultural practices and level of acculturation, may have considerable difficulty in engaging in mix-gender groups due to the value placed upon male offspring, gender role expectations, and patriarchal family hierarchy (Chang 2000). African-American and Native-American women

> The barriers
> that exist before
> treatment are often
> the same obstacles
> that interfere
> with successfully
> completing treatment
> or maintaining
> abstinence.

are likely to mistrust treatment services. Specifically, Jumper Thurman and Plested (1998) reported that Native-American women list mistrust as one of the primary barriers to engaging in treatment services. A more recent study evaluating barriers among African-American women identified staff attitudes as a significant obstacle in maintaining treatment engagement and retention (Roberts and Nishimoto 2006).

Similar to men, women may face language and cultural barriers that impede involvement or retention in substance abuse treatment. Women whose first language is not English may have language difficulties (Mora 2002). Women with specific needs or from specific groups can face social indifference, lack of culturally appropriate programming, and limited cultural competence among staff. For example, lesbians who are seeking treatment may not trust the service provider or treatment staff to appropriately handle their personal information in a group setting—fearing their sexual orientation will be prematurely disclosed.

Structural Obstacles

According to SAMHSA's 2005 National Survey of Substance Abuse Treatment Services, 87 percent of these programs accepted women as clients, but only 41 percent provided special programs or groups for women. Overall, only 17 percent of treatment facilities offered groups or programs for pregnant or postpartum women (SAMHSA 2006). Being responsible for the care of dependent children is one of the biggest barriers to women entering treatment (Wilsnack 1991). Women who do not have access to a treatment program that provides child care or who cannot arrange alternative child care may

have to choose between caring for their children or entering treatment.

Unfortunately, few residential programs have provisions that allow mothers to have their children with them, and outpatient programs often do not provide services for children or child care (Drabble 1996; Finkelstein 1994; Finkelstein et al. 1997). Only 8 percent of substance abuse treatment facilities provided child care in 2003, and only 4 percent provided residential beds for clients' children (SAMHSA 2004). Even when children are accepted into residential treatment, programs often impose age restrictions and limit the number of children a mother is permitted to bring to treatment.

Treatment resources for pregnant women who abuse substances are also scarce. Few programs can simultaneously combine the necessary prenatal care with substance abuse treatment and services for older children (Amaro and Hardy-Fanta 1995; Finkelstein 1993). Finkelstein (1993) stresses that the major barriers to providing resources for pregnant women are based on administrative concerns about medical issues for mothers, infants, and children; fear of program liability; inability to care for infants and lack of services for other children while mothers are in treatment; lack of financial resources; and limited staff training and knowledge about pregnancy and substance use.

Substance abuse treatment providers may not fully understand the needs and the types of interventions most conducive to assisting women in recovery. Vannicelli (1984) found that treatment staff attitudes and unsubstantiated myths about women actually may act as barriers to successful treatment completion among women. In addition, programs may lack cultural competence in addressing treatment issues for women from different cultural or language backgrounds; thus ethnic women may be reluctant to seek treatment if treatment staff or the programs feel foreign, judgmental, hostile, or indifferent.

Even women who are highly motivated for treatment face additional program barriers that may produce significant challenges. These barriers include waiting lists, delayed admission, limited service availability, and preadmission requirements (e.g., paperwork requirements, detoxification). Other barriers are related to program structure, policies, and procedures and include program location, lack of case management services, limited funding sources, and lack of transportation (Wechsberg et al. 2007). Because women are more likely to be poor, their ability to obtain transportation may make it difficult to receive treatment (Lewis et al. 1996). Also, women may have to travel with their children and use public transportation to reach treatment agencies; this can be a hindrance for women in rural areas and for those who have limited income.

Treatment services continue to struggle to effectively broaden the scope of clinical services, secure adequate resources, and adopt gender-responsive policies to address co-occurring disorders. While more programs have endorsed trauma-informed services in conjunction with programming for women, the coordination and integration of these specific services remains limited. In addition to the barriers mentioned above, others may exist regarding compliance with the Americans with Disabilities Act, such as no translators for women who are deaf, lack of materials for individuals who are visually impaired, and lack of treatment program policies and procedures and acceptance of women who are using methadone maintenance.

Systems Obstacles

Many women in need of treatment are involved in multiple social service systems that have different expectations and purpose. According to Young and Gardner (1997), the co-occurrence of a substance use disorder and involvement in the child welfare system ranges from 50 to 80 percent. Moreover, collaboration among substance abuse treatment, child welfare, and welfare reform systems is challenging and often not integrated because of differences in timetables, definition of clients, complexity of client needs, staff education and training, and funding streams (Goldberg 2000; Young et al. 1998).

Services may be fragmented, requiring a woman to negotiate a maze of service agencies to obtain assistance for housing, transportation, child care, substance abuse treatment, vocational training, education, and medical care. In addition, many agencies have requirements that conflict with each other or endorse repetitive intake processes, including different forms that gather the same information. Overall, these simultaneous demands can discourage a woman, particularly when seeking treatment or during early recovery.

Women who have substance use disorders often fear legal consequences. In entering treatment, they sometimes risk losing custody of their children as well as public assistance support (Blume 1997). Likewise, women who have substance use disorders often fear prosecution and incarceration if they seek treatment during pregnancy. The public debate over privacy and the fetus's right to be born free from harm fuels a legal focus on pregnant women who smoke, drink alcohol, or use illicit drugs. "These conflicts have impeded the diagnosis of women with substance abuse problems, the availability of services, and access to appropriate care" (Chavkin and Breitbart 1997, p. 1201).

Treatment Engagement Strategies

Treatment engagement approaches are important regardless of gender, yet women are likely to benefit from services that support the initiation of treatment and address the diverse challenges that often hamper treatment involvement. Engagement services include an array of strategies that begin in the initial intake and can extend across the continuum of care. Ultimately, they are designed to promote appropriate access to treatment, to increase treatment utilization, to promote treatment retention, and to enhance treatment outcome. Promising engagement practices have evolved by integrating and centralizing services to meet the wide range of treatment needs and social services for women and children (Niccols and Sword 2005). Today, some programs and

Challenges in Maintaining a Therapeutic Alliance: Child Welfare and Issues of Confidentiality

State law can require substance abuse treatment providers to report individuals for child abuse and neglect and to supersede Federal confidentiality laws that cover substance abuse treatment. It is critical, therefore, that admissions staff, program materials, and counselors clearly present and discuss the limits of confidentiality as regulations require. Without this explicit discussion, women in treatment may have questions and feel uneasy with regard to mandated reporting. For instance, when counselors intervene to protect a client's children, this may seem contradictory to the client and raise questions about confidentiality.

A great barrier to treatment for women is fear of losing their children, a fear that engenders intense mistrust on the part of clients who are mothers. Therapeutic alliance and trust are vital to the treatment process, yet treatment providers must protect children. To resolve this, women must understand that although providers will report their concerns for the safety of children, providers are advocates for the women and their families (CSAT 1996; Lopez 1994; U.S. Department of Health and Human Services, Office for Civil Rights 2002).

communities provide very formal strategies such as comprehensive case management and incentive programs to promote engagement (Jones et al. 2001). Other engagement strategies include more specific services such as transportation and escorts to appointments, phone calls to initiate services and to remind clients of appointments, and child care during scheduled appointments or sessions (for review, see Comfort et al. 2000).

Women who are offered services during the intake period are more likely to engage in similar services throughout the treatment process than women from a comparison group (Comfort et al. 2000). Three core engagement strategies that are particularly beneficial for women are outreach services, pre-treatment intervention groups, and comprehensive case management.

Outreach Services

Women are more likely to gain awareness of substance abuse treatment if outreach services are implemented. Outreach and engagement services can be clinically effective in increasing the likelihood of entering substance abuse treatment, particularly for those individuals who are less likely to access treatment services (Gottheil et al. 1997). Effective outreach programs, such as the one described in Figure

5-2 (p. 91), are designed to connect women to substance abuse treatment regardless of point of service entry. For example, programs that address domestic violence, HIV/AIDS, or crisis intervention can be a vital conduit for helping women take the first step in connecting to substance abuse services.

Gross and Brown (1993) outlined three major components of outreach: (1) identifying a woman's most urgent concerns and addressing those first, until she is ready to take on other issues; (2) empathizing with the woman's fears and resistances, while assisting her in following through on commitments; and (3) assisting the woman in negotiating the human service system, particularly when the decision to seek drug or alcohol treatment is stymied by the lack of adequate, appropriate, or accessible programs or when relapse alienates the woman from institutional connections. Although outreach appears to benefit women—in that they are more likely to initiate contact with treatment providers—women's response to outreach services appears related to level of readiness, history of trauma, and degree of support. For instance, Melchior et al. (1999) reported that women who have a history of trauma are more reluctant to follow through with referrals than men.

Strategy: Success Stories

To counter stigma, counselors might provide clients with stories or information about women who have achieved and maintained recovery, such as Marty Mann (www.ncadd.org) or Betty Ford. These stories can be used to stimulate group discussions or could be a part of regular client readings.

Strategy: Barriers to Treatment Assessment Tool

Counselors can gain significant information pertaining to current, potential, or perceived barriers through evaluation. Beyond a comprehensive psychosocial history, counselors and administrators can gain insight into the current obstacles to treatment (for review, see *Allen's Barriers to Treatment*, Appendix D).

Strategy: Decisional Balancing Exercise

The decisional balancing exercise was designed to identify cognitive appraisals associated with benefits and costs of substance use (Cunningham et al. 1997). Both cognitive–behavioral therapy and motivational interviewing endorse this strategy. By easily adapting this activity to analyze pros and cons associated with entering treatment or not entering treatment, counselors are more likely to discover barriers that were not identified in the initial assessment. Counselors may want to demonstrate the activity by using examples, such as the pros and cons of going on a diet or not smoking. This exercise is not a simple pros-and-cons list for one side of the argument, but rather it involves looking at the benefits and costs for both sides of the argument; e.g., pros and cons for going on a diet as well as pros and cons for not going on a diet. This is an important aspect of this exercise. While many issues can be identified with one side of the argument, there are often other subtle issues that are acknowledged by discussing both sides of the argument. Following is the format for the decisional balancing exercise involving the pros and cons of entering or not entering substance abuse treatment.

	Pros (Benefits)	Cons (Costs)
Entering Treatment	Better role model for my children Knowing that I can quit Maybe I can do some things that I haven't been able to do while I have been using, e.g., working toward a GED	Boyfriend may leave Don't like other people watching my children
Not Entering Treatment	Don't have to think about my use Don't have to worry about leaving my family Can continue to use	May end up having more legal problems May lose my children Not HIV positive now, but it may happen if I continue to use

Strategy: Finishing the Story Exercise

Counselors can "reframe" a woman's misgivings about treatment so she may see that the feared outcome of seeking or staying in treatment is, in reality, the likely outcome of ending or not starting treatment. For example, a woman who fears she will lose her children if she enters or stays in treatment should be asked to look into the future. This exercise might clarify for her that continued addiction virtually guarantees that she will lose her children in the long run, whereas treatment and recovery will most likely ensure a long-term and stable relationship with her children. By asking the woman to imagine how her story will end if she continues to use substances, she is less likely to glorify her current use and more likely to withstand the common hassles associated with initiating and engaging in treatment.

Strategy: Caregiver Portrait

Women typically assume caregiver roles that may prevent, complicate, or interfere with treatment. They may feel they should not leave their spouse or significant other and fear the consequences of doing so. In entering treatment, they may express worry because they carry the burden of primary caretaker for their parents, children, or other relatives. They may feel that they are being disloyal to friends and family members for leaving them—believing the message that their substance abuse problem is "not that bad." Women may also maintain primary financial responsibilities for housing and food for others and fear they will not be able to provide support during treatment. In addition, they may worry about child care during treatment regardless of treatment level. Hence, beyond identifying these concerns and potential barriers, it is important to provide a way to discuss these as well as to determine their level of importance based on their perception.

In a group setting, first introduce the idea that everyone has specific and perceived obstacles that can interfere with treatment and it is important to give a voice to these challenges. Next, state that at least one or two people will have an opportunity to create a visual picture of these obstacles—similar to taking a family picture. Next, ask a woman to identify each current or potential obstacle to treatment and assign each obstacle to a particular group member. Emphasize to group members that if they are selected to participate, they don't need to say anything in this assigned role. This decreases anxiety and hesitancy in participating.

After the obstacles are assigned, ask the client to arrange the obstacles (group members) as if she were a photographer setting up a family portrait. Remind her to arrange (only verbally directing other group members) the portrait in one area of the room according to how important she perceives the obstacles, e.g., placing the most challenging or fearful barriers in front of others. Next, have the client discuss each obstacle and the rationale for her placement. As the exercise unfolds, obstacles may end up being rearranged in the picture. In addition, counselors may want to help the client identify feelings related to specific obstacles in the picture by walking around the portrait. Other strategies may be used in conjunction with this activity including problemsolving, cognitive restructuring, or motivational interviewing strategies. However, it is often best to keep it simple and to encourage other group members to do the same exercise. You can involve the entire group through discussion or by using a paper-pencil drawing that demonstrates their barriers. While this exercise is ideal for group, you can modify it by using a paper-pencil drawing for individual sessions.

Note: To reinforce appropriate boundaries, remind participants not to touch others during the exercise.

Pretreatment Intervention Groups

Early identification and intervention may prevent more significant alcohol- and drug-related consequences. Pretreatment intervention groups are typically designed to initially provide personalized or structured feedback to clients about their alcohol and drug use, to provide information regarding available treatment services and treatment processes, and to utilize strategies to enhance motivation and to decrease alcohol and drug use. Specific to women, pretreatment groups are designed to address certain psychosocial barriers, including the stigma that is associated with women's substance use. Similar to frequent misconceptions held by clients that detoxification is treatment, pretreatment can be perceived as treatment rather than an initial step. This is particularly the case with women who are either reluctant or suspicious to use treatment services or who are unable to use treatment services at the time (Wechsberg et al. 2007). While research reports that brief interventions are not consistently helpful for women (Chang 2002), more specific research is needed to examine differences in factors that influence early intervention outcomes, including client-matching studies targeting gender.

Case Management

Comprehensive case management helps bridge the gap between services and agencies. It is based on the premise that services need to match the client's needs rather than force the client to fit into the specific services offered by the agency. With the wide range of services often warranted for most women (especially for women who are pregnant or who have children), comprehensive case management that involves medical and social case management is an essential ingredient (Sorensen et al. 2005). According to Brindis and Theidon (1997), case management serves several functions and provides numerous services for the client,

---

Figure 5-2
PROTOTYPES

The PROTOTYPES Outreach Program in Culver City, California, is a pretreatment program that helps women form therapeutic alliances by providing outreach services that help women enter treatment.

PROTOTYPES began in 1987 in Los Angeles County with outreach to women who used substances and were at risk for HIV/AIDS. The pretreatment program staff grew to include more than two dozen outreach workers. PROTOTYPES staff see outreach as a strategy of sustained contact and support that helps women move from contemplation to action.

Outreach workers learned that even though PROTOTYPES provided a healing and nurturing environment, a large treatment program of this type could be frightening to women contemplating treatment, especially women coming from the streets or other difficult environments. To allay their fears, women were brought in for visits before they entered or committed to enter the residential treatment program. In these visits, the women had an opportunity to talk to counselors and other clients, return home, and revisit at will. Every effort was made to make them feel comfortable. The workers learned that it was best that women enter treatment on their own schedules and terms.

Once in treatment, a woman maintained a relationship with her outreach worker, who usually conducted group sessions in the residential setting. The client decided when to move her primary therapeutic relationship from the outreach worker to the in-house counselor, and the outreach worker could withdraw gradually. If a woman did not wish to return to her home community following residential treatment, the outreach worker helped her settle into a new community (Melchior et al. 1999).

including outreach, needs assessment, planning and resource identification, service linkages, monitoring and ongoing reassessment, and client advocacy. In recent years, communities and agencies have shown considerable progress in developing formal linkages, protocols, and integrated care systems. To date, case management services are key to overseeing the appropriate referral and utilization of services. According to OAS (SAMHSA 2004), approximately 55 percent of facilities provide assistance with obtaining social services, 43 percent provide assistance in locating housing, and 69 percent provide case management services. For an in-depth review, see TIP 27 *Comprehensive Case Management for Substance Abuse Treatment* (CSAT 1998a).

Research sheds light on the potential value of case management, in that it may be particularly useful for individuals with complex problems (Havens et al. 2007; Morgenstern et al. 2003). Morgenstern and colleagues (2006) completed a study on intensive case management with women receiving Temporary Assistance for Needy Families (TANF). The results show that women assigned to intensive case management had significantly higher levels of substance abuse treatment initiation, engagement, and retention in comparison to women who received only screening and referral. In addition, alcohol and drug abstinence rates were higher and length of abstinence was longer among women involved in case management. An earlier study showed similar results, emphasizing that women assigned to intensive case management accessed a greater variety of services (Jansson et al. 2005). Improvement in abstinence rates and family and social functioning are also noted when case management services are employed (McLellan et al. 2003).

Considerations in Treatment Placement and Planning

Based on the assessment process, appropriate treatment placement for a client depends on many factors, including the nature and severity of a woman's substance use disorder, the presence of co-occurring mental or physical illnesses or disabilities, and the identification of other needs related to her current situation. Placement decisions are also affected by other psychosocial factors. Once the comprehensive assessment is completed, the placement can be determined.

Women need to be able, whenever possible, to contribute to the planning and placement discussion for their treatment. For example, when residential care is recommended, barriers such as being unable to bring her children may cause a woman to reject the placement option. In this situation, it is critical to work with the woman to make appropriate arrangements to help her enter treatment. Treatment planning must also include assistance in helping her to express needs, make decisions and choices, and recognize that she is the expert on her life. Overall, active client involvement in all aspects of treatment planning significantly contributes to recovery, validates and builds on a woman's strengths, and models collaborative and mutual relationships, including, most importantly, the client–counselor relationship.

To date, limited literature has examined placement criteria specific to women. However, some States have developed criteria for placing women in appropriate treatment options (CSAT 2007). The available State substance abuse treatment standards listed in Figure 5-3, Services Needed in Women's Substance Abuse Treatment, should be considered in placing female clients in specific services.

Levels of Care

The need for appropriate level of care and treatment is not gender specific; both men and women require a range of treatment services at various levels of care. In 1991, ASAM developed patient placement criteria based on matching severity of symptoms and treatment needs with five levels of care. ASAM's Patient Placement Criteria (ASAM's PPC; ASAM 2001) identifies six clinical dimensions: alcohol intoxication and/

Figure 5-3
Services Needed in Women's Substance Abuse Treatment

The following services are recommended by the consensus panel and reinforced by some State standards (CSAT 2007), and these services may be warranted across the continuum of care beginning with early intervention and extending to continuing care services. More than ever, services need to be tailored to women's needs and to address the specific hardships they often encounter in engaging treatment services. Promising practices designed to treat women with substance use disorders include comprehensive and integrated clinical and community services that are ideally delivered at a one-stop location. Note: This list does not incorporate the customary services that are provided in standard substance abuse treatment, but rather services that are more reflective of women's needs.

Medical Services
- Gynecological care
- Family planning
- Prenatal care
- Pediatric care
- HIV/AIDS services
- Treatment for infectious diseases, including viral hepatitis
- Nicotine cessation treatment services

Health Promotion
- Nutritional counseling
- Educational services about reproductive health
- Wellness programs
- Education on sleep and dental hygiene
- Education about STDs and other infectious diseases; e.g., viral hepatitis and HIV/AIDS
- Preventive healthcare education

Psychoeducation
- Sexuality education
- Assertiveness skills training
- Education on the effects of alcohol and other drugs on prenatal and child development
- Prenatal education

Gender-Specific Needs
- Women-only programming; e.g., is the client likely to benefit more from a same-sex versus mix-gender program due to trauma history, pattern of withdrawal among men, and other issues?
- Lesbian services

Cultural and Language Needs
- Culturally appropriate programming
- Availability of interpreter services or treatment services in native language

Life Skills
- Money management and budgeting
- Stress reduction and coping skills training

Family and Child-Related Services

Childcare services, including homework assistance in conjunction with outpatient services

Children's programming, including nurseries and preschool programs

Family treatment services including psychoeducation surrounding addiction and its impact on family functioning

Couples counseling and relationship enrichment recovery groups

Parent/child services, including developmentally age-appropriate programs for children and education for mothers about child safety; parenting education; nutrition; children's substance abuse prevention curriculum; and children's mental health needs, including recreational activities, school, and other related activities

Comprehensive Case Management

Linkages to welfare system, employment opportunities, and housing

Integration of stipulations from child welfare, TANF, probation and parole, and other systems

Intensive case management, including case management for children

Transportation services

Domestic violence services, including referral to safe houses

Legal services

Assistance in establishing financial arrangements or accessing funding for treatment services

Assistance in obtaining a GED or further education, career counseling, and vocational training, including job readiness training to prepare women to leave the program and support themselves and their families

Assistance in locating appropriate housing in preparation for discharge, including referral to transitional living or supervised housing

Mental Health Services

Trauma-informed and trauma-specific services

Eating disorder and nutrition services

Services for other co-occurring disorders, including access to psychological and pharmacological treatments for mood and anxiety disorders

Children's mental health services

Disability Services

Resources for learning disability assessments

Accommodations for specific disabilities

Services to accommodate illiteracy

Services to accommodate women receiving methadone treatment

Figure 5-3
Services Needed in Women's Substance Abuse Treatment (continued)

Staff and Program Development

Strong female role models in terms of both leadership and personal recovery

Peer support

Adequate staffing to meet added program demands

Staff training and gender-competence in working with women

Staff training and program development centered upon incorporating cultural and ethnic influences on parenting styles, attitudes toward discipline, children's diet, level of parenting supervision, and adherence to medical treatment

Flexible scheduling and staff coordination (Brown 2000)

Adequate time for parent–child bonding and interactions

Administrative commitment to addressing the unique needs of women in treatment

Staff training and administrative policies to support the integration of treatment services with clients on methadone maintenance

Culturally appropriate programming that matches specific socialization and cultural practices for women

Source: Consensus Panel.

or withdrawal potential; biomedical conditions and complications; emotional, behavioral, or cognitive conditions and complications; readiness to change; relapse, continued use or continued problem potential; and recovery environment. The levels of care are determined by the presence and severity of issues within each dimension. The current version (PPC-2R) lists five broad levels of care:

- Level 0.5: Early intervention
- Level I: Outpatient treatment/partial hospitalization
- Level II: Intensive outpatient treatment
- Level III: Residential/inpatient treatment
- Level IV: Medically managed intensive inpatient treatment (ASAM 2001)

ASAM's PPC-2R (2001) is used widely and standardizes treatment placement. It is focused on identifying individual treatment needs, but does not focus specifically on the placement of women or treatment needs that extend to children or family. Counselors needing detailed criteria for each level of care should consult ASAM's PPC-2R Manual. The following review

of ASAM's levels of care contains information that is unique and important to women; it is not meant to be a comprehensive overview of ASAM's placement criteria. When there are relevant issues, the specific needs of pregnant women and children are discussed at the end of each level of care.

Early Intervention (ASAM Level 0.5)

Early intervention, or ASAM Level 0.5, can be considered a pretreatment service that provides an opportunity for treatment providers to intervene across a wide variety of settings. It is designed for individuals with risk factors or problems associated with substance abuse but with whom an immediate substance-related disorder cannot be confirmed. Services that represent this level of care include assessment, psychoeducational services, and counseling. In essence, the goals for this level of care are prevention and intervention. For example, educational experiences allow clients to gain further awareness of their current substance use and the expected consequences of this use, along with the future consequences of use if they continue on their present course. This level of care also provides a forum to assist individuals in developing skills associated with behavioral change, in creating strategies to avoid future problems related to substance use, and in establishing a supportive pretreatment environment and therapeutic alliance.

Early intervention approaches can be provided through many channels—a drop-in model, in-home or mobile treatment services, or a pretreatment group in a treatment setting. It can also be provided through involuntary venues such as drug courts, or voluntary settings such as outpatient or primary medical care clinics. Faith-based initiatives can also provide opportunities for early interventions.

> Healthcare providers have a window of opportunity in working with women who abuse substances. Brief interventions can provide an opening to engage women in a process that may lead toward treatment and wellness.

For women, early intervention services appear quite valuable in enhancing motivation, decreasing anxiety and reluctance in initiating current and future treatment services, gaining support, and establishing strategies to address obstacles associated with treatment access and engagement (Wechsberg et al. 2007). Programs that provide flexibility in attendance, easy access to care, and at-home or mobile services are particularly conducive for women, especially those who have the primary role of parenting. TIP 34 *Brief Interventions and Brief Therapies for Substance Abuse* (CSAT 1999a), discusses how to implement brief interventions in substance abuse treatment and other settings.

Early intervention during pregnancy

Pregnancy creates an increased sense of urgency for both clients and counselors because of the temporary upswing in motivation to change and the need for problem resolution. For some women who abuse substances, pregnancy creates a window of opportunity to enter treatment, become abstinent, quit smoking, eliminate risk-taking behaviors, and lead generally healthier lives (Hankin et al. 2000; Nardi 1998). Brief interventions are sometimes effective in helping pregnant women stop using substances (Hankin et al. 2000). Abstinence for pregnant women should be construed to include alcohol, tobacco, caffeine, and many over-the-counter medications, in addition to illicit substances.

Some studies have found that brief interventions using motivational interviewing (MI) in prenatal care can reduce problem drinking by pregnant women (Handmaker and Wilbourne 2001; Miller 2000). Therapists using MI employ a gentle, empathic style to avoid client defensiveness and constructively and compassionately explore ambivalence about change and motivation for recovery (refer to TIP 35 *Enhancing Motivation for Change in Substance Abuse Treatment* [CSAT 1999b]). MI may be more effective for those women who are primarily dependent on alcohol; studies targeting pregnant women identified as primarily abusing drugs have shown no differences between MI and other standard practices in reducing substance use (Winhusen et al. 2007).

Detoxification (ASAM Levels I–IV)

Detoxification is a set of procedures employed to manage acute intoxication and withdrawal symptoms from drug and alcohol dependence. During this process, the body's physiology adjusts to the absence of alcohol or drugs. Detoxification alone is not substance abuse treatment; it is only the beginning of the treatment process. Issues such as retaining clients in detoxification, stabilization, and fostering treatment entry are discussed in TIP 45 *Detoxification and Substance Abuse Treatment* (CSAT 2006a).

Not all communities have detoxification services. Furthermore, women's programs do not often have adequate medical supervision to perform detoxification, hence women must be detoxified at another facility. Typically detoxification from alcohol or addictive drugs has been a 3- to 5-day inpatient procedure, but as more and more health insurers have declined to reimburse inpatient detoxification, it increasingly is done on an outpatient basis. Yet, if severe withdrawal is expected (as from severe alcohol or sedative-hypnotic dependence), detoxification should be done in a medical facility. Withdrawal from severe alcohol use, sedatives, and benzodiazepines can have severe medical complications.

Some women who are dependent on sedative-hypnotics (tranquilizers) may need a 30-day withdrawal regimen with pharmacological medical intervention to prevent seizures. Concerning alcohol, more recent studies have begun to focus on the effects of sex-specific hormones in response to alcohol dependence and withdrawal. Although research on sex-specific hormonal differences in alcohol withdrawal is in its infancy, currently there appears to be a robust sex difference in seizure susceptibility, in that women appear to have less risk for alcohol withdrawal-induced seizures (Devaud et al. 2006). Women also tend to display fewer and less severe alcohol withdrawal symptoms than men. However, even though research reflects less risk associated with withdrawal from alcohol among women, clinicians and health professionals need to maintain vigilance in evaluating withdrawal symptoms and other health concerns. Detoxification can be a vulnerable period for women who have a history of trauma and violence. They may have significant distress associated with not feeling physically or psychologically safe, and anxiety associated with the anticipation of trying to manage their emotions and trauma-related symptoms without being able to self-medicate. From the outset of treatment, women need interventions and education surrounding traumatic stress reactions. Along with supportive and frequent contact with staff, trauma-informed services can help create or increase a sense of safety and a feeling of control.

For all intents and purposes, if a woman's contact with a substance abuse treatment agency stops at detoxification, the treatment system has failed. Women without treatment subsequent to detoxification are likely to relapse and be lost to followup. Thus, detoxification programs should have adequate funding to include case management, brief interventions, and discharge planning. Immediately after detoxification, a woman may be more likely to be ready for treatment, and this opportunity for engaging the woman in treatment should be maximized. Aggressive case management, referral networks, and treatment linkages are needed to prevent women from disengaging from treatment. From initial contact with the client, the ability to follow up, to coordinate care, and to provide comprehensive services (such as transportation and child care), is essential to effective treatment.

Considerations for women who are parents with dependent children

The safety of children often is a chief concern and one of the principal barriers to treatment engagement and retention for parents—especially women—entering detoxification programs. Even if women do not have custody of their children, they often are the ones who continue to care for them. Thus, ensuring that children have a safe place to stay while their mothers are in detoxification is of vital importance. Working with parents to identify supportive family or friends may help identify available temporary child care resources. A consult or referral to the treatment facility's social services while the patient is being detoxified is indicated when the care of children is uncertain (CSAT 2006).

Detoxification and methadone treatment during pregnancy

Some detoxification programs will not treat a pregnant woman because they lack the necessary obstetrical support and are concerned about liability. Detoxification presents critical risks to a fetus, and withdrawal of a pregnant woman from addictive drugs or alcohol should always be accompanied by close medical supervision and monitoring. Risks of detoxification depend on the drug being abused, but the primary drugs of concern are typically opioids and, potentially, sedative-hypnotics. Sudden withdrawal of these drugs results in withdrawal by a fetus and sometimes leads to fetal distress or death. Withdrawal should be done under supervised conditions and with proper substitutes, such as methadone for opioids. TIP 45 *Detoxification and Substance Abuse Treatment* (CSAT 2006a), TIP 43 *Medication-Assisted Treatment for Opioid Addiction in Opioid Treatment Programs* (CSAT 2005b), and TIP 40 *Clinical Guidelines for the Use of Buprenorphine in the Treatment of Opioid Addiction* (CSAT 2004a), have more comprehensive information on this subject.

In general, it is neither recommended nor necessary for pregnant women to cease methadone treatment. In situations where withdrawal is being contemplated, a thorough assessment should be conducted to determine whether the woman is an appropriate candidate for medical withdrawal. It is important to note that relapse rates among women who use heroin are high, thus placing their fetuses at risk for adverse consequences (Jones et al. 2001). Situations in which medically supervised methadone withdrawal during pregnancy may be considered include the following:

- The client moves to an area where methadone maintenance is not available.
- The client has been stable during treatment and requests withdrawal before delivery.
- The client refuses to be maintained on methadone.
- The client plans to detoxify through a structured treatment program (Archie 1998; Kaltenbach et al. 1998).

If withdrawal is elected, it should be conducted under the supervision of physicians experienced in perinatal addiction and under the guidance of a protocol using fetal monitoring. Medical withdrawal usually is conducted in the second trimester because of the danger of miscarriage in the first trimester and because withdrawal-induced stress may cause premature delivery or fetal death in the third trimester (Donaldson

2000; Kaltenbach et al. 1998). While pharmaceutical agents other than methadone have been introduced to treat symptoms of opioid withdrawal, the research is still preliminary (Anderson et al. 1997; Dashe et al. 1998; Jones and Johnson 2001; McElhatton 2001).

Outpatient Treatment (ASAM Level I)

Outpatient, or ASAM Level I, treatment usually consists of one or two weekly sessions of group or individual therapy. Outpatient treatment settings are the most common, are widely available, and are the setting in which most women receive treatment. In general, outpatient treatment is most appropriate for women with less severe substance use problems and with greater social support and resources. While outpatient services are used for less severe symptoms of substance use disorders, this level of treatment can be employed at various points across the continuum of care. Specifically, continuing care services use outpatient treatment to provide support for ongoing recovery and treatment in a less restrictive environment as recovery evolves. (Refer to chapter 8 for review of continuing care services.)

Women who benefit most from outpatient therapy frequently have some stability in their lives, such as housing and employment. Effective outpatient treatment programs for women should be more comprehensive than traditional programs and should provide a constellation of services (refer to Figure 5-3). For example, outpatient services should evaluate the need for and provide child care and children's treatment services.

Although few women-only outpatient programs exist, mix-gender programs can be made more responsive to women's needs by providing comprehensive case management, services, and programs that support more client-provider contact, more opportunities for individual therapy, and referral to other community services. The development of interagency relationships is essential, yet referral alone will not guarantee utilization of these services. Beyond staff support, it is often necessary to initiate the first contact with the agency referral, to assist the client in developing or making the necessary arrangements to access the community service or referral, and to provide followup to obtain the outcome of the referral. Throughout the last two decades, substance abuse programs have acknowledged the necessity of establishing formalized relationships among community agencies to streamline services and to effectively address and manage the diverse needs of women seeking treatment for substance use disorders. TIP 46 *Substance Abuse: Administrative Issues in Outpatient Treatment* (CSAT 2006b), provides more information on this level of care.

Intensive Outpatient Treatment (ASAM Level II)

Intensive outpatient treatment (IOP), or ASAM Level II, provides a higher treatment level than traditional outpatient programs but does not require structured residential living. Generally, IOP provides many of the same services as residential treatment; however, the intensity of treatment, the time of engaging services, and level of counselor involvement are less. IOP appears to have higher completion rates than traditional outpatient services among postpartum women (Strantz and Welch 1995). The flexibility of IOP may help women overcome barriers to treatment, provided the program attends to the unique needs identified during intake (refer to Figure 5-3). Although IOP historically provides more accommodating schedules and offers treatment during the evening, weekends, and other times of the day, it will not be as useful for some women unless child care and transportation are available. TIP 47 *Substance Abuse: Clinical Issues in Intensive Outpatient Treatment* (CSAT 2006c), provides more information on this level of care.

Residential and Inpatient Treatment (ASAM Level III)

Residential treatment, or ASAM Level III, is for women who have multiple and complex needs and require a safe environment for stabilization, intensive treatment, and an intensive recovery

support structure. Professional staff are available 24 hours a day, and the facility is clinically managed. The type of residential or inpatient placement depends in part on the severity and complexity of the woman's conditions, including but not limited to co-occurring medical and psychiatric disorders, history of trauma (including sexual and domestic violence), and pregnancy. Clinical experience has shown that women in residential care frequently require some or all of the services listed in Figure 5-3 in addition to specific substance abuse treatment services.

Residential treatment can take place in various settings, including halfway houses and other extended care facilities, primary residential or inpatient programs, and recovery homes. As an example, SHIELDS for Families (a Los Angeles agency) uses a combination of day treatment and housing to provide comprehensive residential treatment for families. Overall, the effectiveness of residential treatment appears to rely on at least one key element—length of treatment. Greenfield and colleagues (2004) reviewed data about the effectiveness of residential substance abuse treatment for women from CSAT's Residential Women and Children/Pregnant and Postpartum Women (RWC/PPW) Cross-Site Study and two other national studies. Despite differences in treatment programs, client profiles, followup intervals, data collection methods, and other factors, all three studies found high treatment success rates—ranging from 68 to 71 percent abstinence—among women who spent 6 months or more in treatment. Success rates were lower for clients with shorter stays in treatment.

While length of stay seems paramount, residential treatment has several other components that must be in place to meet the various roles, needs, and other presenting issues of women with substance use disorders. Whether short or long term, residential treatment must maintain a healing, nurturing, and safe environment. This may require special accommodations for women, particularly in mix-gender treatment centers. These accommodations include adequate facilities for visits with children, safety precautions, and treatment programming and policies that decrease the likelihood of potential assaults and sexual involvement in mix-gender residential settings and women-only space. Women who are trauma survivors benefit from secure sleeping accommodations where they can maintain their sense of security and control over bedroom access (except staff rounds; Harris 1994).

Children in residential treatment programs

For many women, having their children with them in treatment is essential to their recovery and removes a barrier to treatment entry. Research suggests that allowing children to accompany their mothers to a residential program has a positive effect on engagement, retention, and recovery (Lungren et al. 2003; Szuster et al. 1996). For example, studies have found that length of stay in residential treatment is associated with women being able to bring their children with them (Hughes et al. 1995; Wobie et al. 1997). One study suggested that the earlier a mother's infant resides with her in the treatment setting, the longer the mother's stay in treatment will be (Wobie et al. 1997). Overall, women in residential treatment accompanied by their children showed better outcomes (abstinence, employment, child custody, and involvement with continuing care or support groups) than women not accompanied by their children at 6 months after discharge (Stevens and Patton 1998). Review Appendix B to obtain an overview of CSAT's *Comprehensive Substance Abuse Treatment Model for Women and Their Children*.

Since 2004, CSAT has funded over 50 grants to treatment facilities under its Residential Women and Children/ Pregnant and Postpartum Women (RWC/PPW) programs. This cross-site evaluation found that the 6- to 12-month treatment programs had several positive outcomes. First, alcohol and drug use was much lower 6 months after discharge compared with pretreatment. The percentage of women reporting alcohol use decreased from 65 percent at pretreatment to 27 percent 6 months after discharge, and the percentage of women reporting crack/cocaine use decreased from 51 to 20 percent. Second, 60 percent of the women reported being completely abstinent throughout the 6 months following discharge. Third, criminal involvement dropped markedly, and economic well-being improved. Next, pregnancy outcomes improved (fewer premature deliveries, fewer low-birth-weight babies, and lower infant mortality) compared with expected rates for this population. In addition, 75 percent of the women had custody of one or more children 6 months after discharge, up from 54 percent before initiating treatment, and fewer clients had children in foster care (CSAT 2001a).

Women who completed treatment that allowed children in residence had less psychological distress and improved skills for independent living, parenting, employment, and relationships (Saunders 1993). In fact, one study found that outcomes from a treatment environment that welcomed children were more positive for women both with and without children. Researchers suggest that "living with and helping with other women's children may provide a sense of shared responsibility and community" in a therapeutic community (Wexler et al. 1998, p. 232). Chapter 7 addresses parenting and the need for children services; it also emphasizes the importance of providing assessment and treatment for both mothers and their children.

The amount of responsibility the mother has for her children during her stay needs to be determined on an individual basis; some mothers can keep their children with them almost continually, whereas others may need to attend treatment apart from their children. Specifically, some women may not want the responsibility of parenting at such a stressful time in their lives but may feel social pressure to keep their children with them during treatment. These mothers should be supported in their decision to place their children in the care of others (such as reliable family members) during their treatment. The following questions can be used by agencies to determine some key decisions regarding children:

- How will child care be handled if the mother is hospitalized?

- Are there limits on the severity of illness of mothers or children beyond which they will not be accepted by the program?
- What rule infractions will result in expulsion from the program?
- How will suspected child abuse or neglect be identified and reported?
- Does the program allow overnight home visits? What guidelines and rules need to be in place to permit mothers and their children to leave residential treatment overnight (Metsch et al. 1995)?
- How will children be disciplined?
- How will visitation by the mother's partner be handled when court-ordered visitation privileges have been issued but the partner continues to abuse alcohol and/or drugs?

Maintenance of relationships with noncustodial children is important. Reunification with children in the care of child protective service agencies is a sensitive issue. Staff of residential programs should be knowledgeable about child welfare issues and develop collaborations with child protective services to facilitate an effective and supportive reunification process for mothers and children.

Residential services for pregnant women

Acknowledging the urgency of treating women who are pregnant, Federal law requires that pregnant women receive priority admission into substance abuse treatment programs, allowing them to bypass waiting lists and gain immediate admission when a bed in a residential program is available (42 U.S.C. § 300x-27[a]). The primary treatment provider must secure prenatal care if a pregnant woman is not already receiving such care.

Notably, collaboration among providers of substance abuse treatment, obstetric care, and pediatric care is a necessity. A comprehensive care program for pregnant women that includes prenatal care and substance abuse treatment has been shown to improve birth outcomes and increase the chances of being drug free at delivery for women who used cocaine (Burkett et al. 1998). Corse and colleagues (1995) looked

at innovative possibilities such as bringing primary obstetric care providers (usually a nurse practitioner or certified nurse midwife) onsite. They found that educating nurse midwives about substance use disorders and pregnancy enhanced their effectiveness and level of comfort in working with this population. Foremost, residential staff should learn the danger signs of pregnancy complications and when to triage a woman to an emergency department or to the doctor of the woman's choice. An internal or external medical or nursing resource is helpful to evaluate need for emergency care.

Upon delivery, some infants have withdrawal symptoms that require supportive care. In individual cases, depending on symptom severity, babies may need to be managed pharmacologically, and most experts agree that newborns should remain hospitalized while on medication related to drug withdrawal. In a residential center, public health nursing visits are critical to the evaluation of infant and maternal status. If a program does not have a nursing staff, public health nurses can provide some service.

The consensus panel recommends that residential programs provide a number of specialized services for pregnant women, including:

- Nutrition services
- Prenatal care
- Transportation to obstetric appointments
- Childbirth education and preparation and a coach, if possible

> *Telling Their Stories: Reflections of the 11 Original Grantees That Piloted Residential Treatment for Women and Children for CSAT (CSAT 2001c), provides profiles of residential programs for women and children, along with issues that arose in treatment and management, evaluation information, and lessons learned.*

- Mental health evaluation at least twice during the pregnancy and postpartum periods, and treatment as needed to rule out (or treat) postpartum depression or other disorders
- Education about alcohol and drug use specifically related to pregnancy, including education about neonatal abstinence syndrome and, if possible, a tour of the delivery site's nursery for the woman in anticipation of the need for infant monitoring in the hospital
- Education about HIV/AIDS risk and management during pregnancy, especially because HIV/AIDS transmission to the fetus and infants can be prevented
- Education about breastfeeding and strong support for mothers who nurse their babies unless they are HIV positive

Comprehensive programs for women who are parents or pregnant typically include outreach, family support services, medical care, case management, and continuing care for women and their children (Finkelstein 1993, 1994). Some researchers recommend individual and group counseling services, independent living skills training, and parenting classes (Haskett et al. 1992). Childbirth education and family planning also are recommended for women in treatment at childbirth and postpartum, along with activities that address bonding and attachment. Home visits help in assessing a woman's needs and in identifying family members who can support her in recovery (Grella 1996). Children who accompany their mothers to treatment can benefit from separate, developmental- and age-appropriate programming, health care, and education programs including substance abuse prevention. For an overview of CSAT's *Comprehensive Substance Abuse Treatment Model for Women and Their Children*, refer to Appendix B.

Medically Managed Intensive Inpatient Treatment (ASAM Level IV)

Treatment in a medically managed intensive inpatient setting, or ASAM Level IV, commonly is used for a person who is medically compromised and meets ASAM Level IV criteria. This patient is at high risk for complications associated with withdrawal and requires the full resources provided by a hospital. Typically, this type of acute inpatient treatment lasts between 3 and 5 days; stays of 10 to 14 days are more likely in an acute care psychiatric unit. It most often includes medical detoxification, client education, group therapy, individual therapy, family therapy, and medical treatment.

As discussed in the detoxification section, appropriate referral from inpatient care to subsequent long-term treatment is needed. Repeat assessments are performed to indicate when a client is ready for a less intrusive or less intense setting for treatment. This referral should include case management and linkage to other treatment services, community services, and support groups.

Advice to Clinicians and Medical Staff: The Impact of Trauma and Prenatal Care

Women who have been sexually traumatized may experience considerable emotional discomfort with prenatal care, labor, and delivery in part because of the necessity of frequent vaginal exams and the physical contact necessary to support women during labor and delivery. The optimal situation for many pregnant women with a history of sexual trauma is to have a female prenatal care provider or a female obstetrician. These clients should have a labor coach or a support person to accompany them on all medical visits and during the labor process and delivery.

6 Substance Abuse Among Specific Population Groups and Settings

Overview

Gender-appropriate and culturally responsive health care improves both short- and long-term outcomes, not just for women with substance use disorders but also for clients with almost any type of healthcare problem. The likelihood of good health or the prevalence of certain disorders is, in part, a product of gender. Certain health issues are unique to women; others affect women disproportionately compared to men; and still others have a different effect on women than on men. To add to these gender differences, the National Institutes of Health (NIH) has identified critical racial and ethnic disparities in health that result in different outcomes or consequences in some groups. Other factors such as sexual orientation also have been shown to affect health status (Dean et al. 2000).

The risks of substance abuse, its consequences, and the processes for treatment and recovery also differ by gender, race, ethnicity, sexual orientation, age, and other factors. Women's risks for substance use disorders are best understood in the context in which the influences of gender, race and ethnicity, culture, education, economic status, age, geographic location, sexual orientation, and other factors converge. Understanding group differences across segments of the women's population is critical to designing and implementing effective substance abuse treatment programs for women.

This chapter provides an overview of available substance-related research for women in specific racial and ethnic groups, settings, and special populations in the United States across four domains: demographics, substance abuse patterns, clinical treatment issues, and resiliency factors. It highlights the need for cultural competence in the delivery of substance abuse treatment and suggests specific and culturally congruent clinical, programmatic, and administrative strategies. For more detailed information on substance related disorders and substance abuse treatment across racially and ethnically diverse populations; the influence of culture on substance abuse patterns, help-seeking behavior, and health beliefs; and guidelines for culturally congruent and competent treatment services, see the planned TIP *Improving Cultural Competence in Substance Abuse Treatment* (Center for Substance Abuse Treatment [CSAT] in development *a*).

Main sections of this chapter address clinical issues related to treating women of different racial and ethnic groups, women of different sexual orientations, older women, and women living in rural areas. Although certain elements of their substance use disorders are common to all these groups (such as trauma and/or socioeconomic stresses), each group also has unique features that will further influence their engagement and successful completion of treatment (including cultural values, beliefs about health care, and help-seeking behavior). Each group of women also brings a unique capacity for resiliency and recovery, and these factors are explored as well. The chapter concludes with a brief review of special populations and settings—women with disabilities, women in the criminal justice system, and women who are homeless.

Racially and Ethnically Diverse Women

Hispanic/Latina Women

Demographics
Of the approximately 40 million Hispanic/ Latino people living in the United States and its Territories, Mexican Americans are the largest group (64 percent), followed by Puerto Ricans (10 percent), Central and South Americans (13 percent), Cubans (4 percent), and other Hispanics or Latinos (9 percent) (U.S. Census Bureau 2007). Half the U.S. Hispanic/Latino population is concentrated in California and Texas. An additional 23 percent reside in Florida, Illinois, New Jersey, Arizona, and New York (U.S. Census Bureau 2007). Women of Hispanic origin in the United States numbered 17 million or slightly less than half the total U.S. Hispanic population (U.S. Census Bureau 2001*d*).

The Hispanic/Latino population is a young, rapidly growing ethnic and cultural group in the United States. At 14 percent of the population, Hispanics/Latinos currently are the largest ethnic subpopulation (U.S. Census Bureau 2007). The recent population growth of Hispanics/Latinos is mainly due to the relative youth and high birth rates of this population (Bachu and O'Connell 2001) and, in part, to immigration. Yet, most Hispanics/Latinos are born in the U.S. and are not immigrants (U.S. Census Bureau 2007). By 2050, Hispanics/ Latinos are expected to nearly triple in number (U.S. Census Bureau 2000*b*).

The socioeconomic status of the U.S. Hispanic/ Latino population may reflect the circumstances of immigration; that is, those who immigrated for economic reasons (the vast majority) tend to be poorer, less well educated, and younger than the overall population. More than a quarter of all Hispanics/Latinos lack health insurance coverage for more than 1 year (Cohen et al. 2004). Approximately 40 percent of Hispanic/ Latino families headed by women live in poverty (U.S. Census Bureau 2007), and many of these women are likely to face the combined stresses of poverty, lack of health insurance, and lack of health care (U.S. Census Bureau 2002).

Substance use among Hispanics/ Latinas

Alcohol
Most research on substance abuse among Hispanics/Latinas has focused on alcohol (e.g., Ames and Mora 1988; Canino 1994; Gilbert 1991) and has confirmed the widely held belief that, regardless of national origin, Hispanics/ Latinas generally have higher rates of abstinence from alcohol and drink alcohol less frequently than Hispanic/Latino men. In a survey of 764 Hispanic/Latino men and 817 Hispanic/ Latina women of all ages, 33 percent of the

men reported frequent and/or heavy drinking, compared with 12 percent of the women. Conversely, 57 percent of the women versus 35 percent of the men reported that they abstained from alcohol use. Thirty-one percent of the women reported infrequent drinking (Aguirre-Molina et al. 2001). This phenomenon has been attributed to strict cultural sanctions against drinking by women that are typical throughout Latin America (Mora 1998) and are maintained by many Hispanics/Latinas in the United States.

Research indicates that some Hispanics/Latinas generally maintain the cultural norms of their countries of origin and resist social pressures to engage in substance use (Mora 2002). However, other research (e.g., Caetano 1988, 1989; Caetano et al. 2007) comparing substance abuse both by gender and within and across Hispanic/Latino subgroups suggests a far more complex relationship between Hispanics/Latinas and substance abuse (Mora 2002). For instance, Mexican-American women show higher rates of abstinence than Cuban and Puerto Rican women. However, they also exhibit the highest rates of frequent heavy drinking of all Hispanic/Latina subgroups (Caetano 1989; Mora 1998). Thus, Mexican-American women who consume any alcohol at all tend to drink frequently and heavily. Mora (1998) explains that this paradox originates from differences between immigrant Mexican women and their American-born counterparts. More established generations of U.S. Hispanics/Latinas—in particular young Mexican-American and Puerto Rican women—drink more alcohol than immigrant women of their subgroups. These differences in alcohol use among Hispanics/Latinas appear to depend primarily on age, generational status, level of acculturation, and country of origin (Collins and McNair 2002; Randolph et al. 1998).

Illicit drug use

The pattern of illicit drug use among Hispanics/Latinas is influenced by level of acculturation and country of origin. In one study based on the Hispanic Health and Nutrition Examination Survey (HHANES) data, illicit drug use among Hispanics/Latinas generally increased with acculturation (Amaro et al. 1990). The

2006 Treatment Episode Data Set (TEDS), a Substance Abuse and Mental Health Services Administration (SAMHSA) data set that provides information on treatment completion, length of treatment stay, and discharge demographics, indicated that Hispanic/Latina women admitted to substance abuse treatment were more likely to report opiates (19 percent) as their primary substance of abuse followed by cocaine/crack (18 percent), marijuana (14 percent), and methamphetamine. In addition, the primary substance of abuse varied according to Hispanic origin: Puerto Rican and Cuban-American women reported more opiate use, whereas Mexican-American women reported more methamphetamine use (SAMHSA 2008).

Sociodemographic factors associated with substance use and substance use disorders

Socioeconomic status, age, and length of time in the United States are associated with substance use and substance use disorders among Hispanic/Latina women. Among this population, those with the most notable risks for substance use disorders are women who immigrated to the U.S. at an earlier age (before 7 years of age) or who were born in the U.S. (Canino et al. 2008; Vega et al. 2003). Of particular concern, the 2007 Youth Risk Behavior Survey found a growing prevalence of alcohol and other drug use among adolescent Hispanic/Latina females (Eaton et al. 2008). Studies have also isolated employment, marital status, and educational level as predictors of alcohol consumption and substance use disorders among Hispanics/Latinas. In a study evaluating racial/ethnic differences among women with co-occurring mental and substance use disorders, Hispanic/Latina women possessed significant social vulnerability characterized by lower socioeconomic and educational status, exposure to violent crimes, and higher rates of criminal justice involvement (Amaro et al. 2005).

Gender socialization

In the Hispanic/Latina culture, women often are afforded special status and respect as matriarchs of extended family networks (Mora

2002). Some Hispanics/Latinas, especially those who are more acculturated, may deemphasize or reject these cultural expectations, but early childhood messages (e.g., the "proper role of a señorita") may remain embedded in the cultural and personal identities of many in this group (Mora 1998). The stresses of negotiating and integrating traditional cultural expectations with new cultural values may result in or exacerbate the prevalence of mental and substance use disorders for many Hispanics/Latinas; more research is needed on this subject (Gloria and Peregoy 1996; Mora 1998).

Acculturation

It has been suggested that acculturation, the process of adapting and adjusting to new surroundings while maintaining a cultural identity, more than any other factor, affects Hispanics/Latinas' substance abuse (Caetano 1989, 1994; Gilbert 1991; Keefe and Padilla 1987; Markides et al. 1988). The onset of alcohol and drug abuse among some Hispanics/Latinas may be explained by acculturative and environmental stresses (e.g., new roles, expectations, opportunities) that result in greater exposure to these substances (Gilbert 1991; Mora 1998). HHANES data study revealed that, for women of all ages in three major subgroups (Mexican American, Puerto Rican, and Cuban American), level of acculturation was correlated consistently with both increased frequency of consumption and increased probability of being a drinker at all (Black and Markides 1993).

Studies consistently have shown that acculturation is positively correlated with consumption of greater quantities of alcohol, greater frequency of alcohol use, and higher rates of drug abuse among Hispanics/Latinas (Amaro et al. 1990; Mora 1998). These findings have significant implications in providing substance abuse treatment, in that the role of acculturation and gender socialization should be a central theme in treatment planning. Specifically, Mora (1998) suggests that clinicians explore with Hispanic/Latina clients several key questions: How have their traditional roles changed since immigration or in comparison to their own mothers? How have these changes in roles influenced their substance use behavior? In what ways have educational and employment opportunities influenced or altered their substance use?

Clinical treatment issues

At first glance, the heterogeneity of Hispanics/Latinas in terms of language, values, and backgrounds may seem to challenge the creation of effective, culturally responsive treatment programs for Hispanic/Latina women. Programs committed to serving Hispanics/Latinas, however, can develop effective services by endorsing culturally competent practices, such as culturally specific assessment tools, counseling that endorses the clients' worldviews, staff training to increase cultural awareness and knowledge, and programs that reflect and respect cultural values. For example, substance abuse treatment programs can create a treatment environment that honors cultural heritage and incorporates values such as *familismo* (reliance on and regard for family and family cohesiveness), when appropriate.

Some treatment issues reflect beliefs or traditions more specific to Hispanics/Latinas. A strong cultural prohibition exists against discussing family matters such as substance use or abuse during childhood, thus the use of psychoeducational groups to provide information on these topics may be more effective initially than therapy groups, where experiences are discussed openly. However, substance abuse counseling based on a family model often is well suited and is more culturally congruent for many Hispanics/Latinas. When engaging in family therapy, therapists need to enter the family relationship as a "learner," since Hispanic/Latino families are so diverse. Counselors need to take the time to understand each client's family history within a cultural context (Rotter and Casado 1998), including the initial identification of the country of origin and family members' acculturation history and levels. Counselors also need to embrace a more expansive definition of family that may include extended family members and others. Early on in treatment, counselors need to assess how the current substance-related problems affect the family's culture and how the culture affects the current presenting issues. Because the exalted role of motherhood in Hispanic/Latino culture often makes loss of child custody especially stigmatizing, treatment programs need to provide support for appropriate family reunification. On a more fundamental level, Hispanics/Latinas may benefit from assistance in gaining English language skills, in job training that leads to employment, in finding stable housing, and in negotiating the requirements for treatment entry (Amaro et al. 1999; Kail and Elberth 2002).

Another treatment concern expressed among some Hispanics/Latinas in treatment—particularly those who are highly acculturated or isolated from a larger Hispanic/Latino community—is alienation from their cultural heritage. It may be difficult to address cultural alienation in treatment because a client may be far removed from her cultural background. A therapeutic decision must be made whether a cultural framework for recovery and empowerment should be utilized for all clients or only for those who request or show interest in this approach. Cultural knowledge can be empowering for many women of color, but not for all; care should be taken to adopt this approach only for those who are comfortable with it.

Hispanics/Latinas represent 14 percent of all new HIV/AIDS cases among women (CDC 2007). Among Hispanic women, 65 percent acquired HIV/AIDS through high-risk heterosexual transmission and 33 percent were infected through injection drug use. Since Hispanic women represent the second largest ethnically diverse group of women living with HIV/AIDS at the end of 2005, education and other prevention services should be essential components of substance abuse treatment.

Similar to other population groups of women, Hispanics/Latinas with substance use disorders experience a high rate of co-occurring mental disorders (Amaro et al. 2005). These disorders also need to be identified and treated if substance abuse treatment is to lead to recovery. A study of 66 Hispanics/Latinas enrolled in a residential substance abuse treatment program found that most (80 percent) reported a childhood history of abuse, as well as mental health problems (76 percent) and physical health problems (68 percent) (Amaro et al.

1999). Compared with women who had not experienced childhood abuse, those with such a history experienced more severe health problems and were more likely both to lose custody of their children and to drop out of treatment. To treat these problems adequately, the relationship between a woman's abuse history and substance use or co-occurring mental disorders must be determined. See TIP 36 *Substance Abuse Treatment for Persons With Child Abuse and Neglect Issues* (CSAT 2000b) for more information.

Resiliency factors

The counselor should evaluate and adopt treatment approaches that are strength-based and that build on the resources and strengths of the client's culture, individual traits and experiences, spirituality, and family. Among Hispanic/Latina clients, families are typically an important part of the support network and can function as a resource in recovery. Similarly, the centrality of family ties may provide motivation for treatment and a sense of responsibility to family. In a study that evaluated the role of family in reducing or delaying alcohol use among young Hispanic/Latina females, services that help improve parental connections can have long-term positive effects (Sale et al. 2005).

In addition, culturally defined gender roles can also serve as a strength-based metaphor for the challenges that clients face as they begin their journeys in recovery. These gender roles, if properly acknowledged during treatment, can emphasize the most positive aspects of *marianismo* and *hembrismo* (the counterparts to *machismo*), such as "strength, perseverance, flexibility, and an ability to survive . . . [that can] . . . promote non-use while respecting

Based on the knowledge and experience gained from the Demonstration Grant Program for Residential Women and their Children (RWC) and the Services Grant Program for Residential Treatment for Pregnant and Postpartum Women (PPW), the publication *Lessons Learned: Residential Substance Abuse Treatment for Women and Their Children* (CSAT 2003b) was developed. Along with other important aspects of residential treatment for women and children, this report provides insight into how to integrate culturally congruent services among Hispanic/Latina women in residential substance abuse treatment.

"La Casita" (which means "the little house" in Spanish) is a residential chemical dependency treatment program designed to meet the needs of low-income Hispanic/Latina mothers. The treatment program places emphasis on the importance of family and its critical role in promoting therapeutic change. La Casita integrates culturally relevant strategies and Hispanic/Latina cultural values with other effective treatment approaches, such as, "simpatia" (the promotion of pleasant social relationships), "lineality" (importance of authority figures in the solution of problems), and "reciprocity" (giving back, in some way, what was given). By adapting these cultural values in treatment, women have an opportunity to use their ethnic heritage as a catalyst for recovery (CSAT 2003*b*).

and maintaining the role of the woman within the family" (Gloria and Peregoy 1996; p. 122). Similarly, religion and spiritual practices are very important for many traditional Hispanics/Latinas in the United States and may serve as a source of sustenance in recovery. Religious beliefs may involve a combination of traditional practices and rituals, world religions, and religious practices in and outside the structure of church (Altarriba and Bauer 1998).

African-American Women

Demographics
There are major differences in cultural identification, income, education, marital status, occupation, and lifestyle between African-American women born in the United States and foreign-born women of African descent (Gray and Littlefield 2002; NIH, ORWH 1999). While this section focuses primarily on African-American women born in the United States, further research is needed to identify intragroup variations in substance abuse etiology and effective treatments.

More than 32 million African Americans live in the United States, including sizable numbers of both African and African-Caribbean immigrants. It is a relatively young population: 32 percent of all African Americans are under age 18. More than half live in a central city within a metropolitan area. African Americans represent 12.3 percent of the U.S. population (U.S. Census Bureau 2001*f*). Nineteen million, or more than half, of all African Americans are females (U.S. Census Bureau 2001*d*). Among African-American women, poverty is more prevalent than in the general population (Gray

and Littlefield 2002). Among African-American single mothers, approximately 35 percent live in poverty compared to 19 percent of non-Hispanic single white mothers.

Although genetics account for differential rates of some diseases among African Americans (e.g., sickle cell anemia), biology alone explains very little about the disparities in health status between African Americans and Caucasians. Overall, African Americans have disproportionately higher rates of disease and illness, a wider variety of undetected diseases, more chronic health conditions, and shorter life expectancies than Caucasians. African-American women experience higher morbidity and mortality rates than do Caucasian women for many health conditions (Minino et al. 2002).

Substance use among African Americans
Even though the total substance abuse admissions among African Americans has been steadily declining since the 1990s, TEDS reports that 21 percent of admissions to substance abuse treatment facilities were African American in 2006 in comparison to 12 percent of non-Hispanic population (HHS 2008*a*). The primary source of referral to treatment among African-American women was through self-referral or by family and friends (SAMHSA 2004).

Alcohol
According to TEDS (HHS 2008*a*), alcohol accounted for 25 percent of substance abuse treatment admissions among African-American women. While most research highlights differences in alcohol use patterns between African-American women and men, and between

African-American women and other diverse groups of women, little attention is given in reporting on the diversity of use among African-American women within their cohort group and throughout their lifespan. In one study comparing differences in alcohol prevalence across age groups, ethnicity, and gender, prevalence rates among African-American females from 19 to 29 years of age rose from 2 percent to 4 percent between 1992 and 2002 (Grant et al. 2006). In a study evaluating the correlates of alcohol consumption of African-American women, women age 40 to 49 have shown the highest prevalence of alcohol consumption (Rosenberg et al. 2002).

Illicit drug use

Among African-American women, most admissions to treatment facilities were for cocaine/crack abuse (35 percent; HHS 2008a). From the same data set, opioids, primarily heroin, accounted for 18 percent of substance-related admissions. In a study that focused on severity of alcohol use and crack/cocaine, evidence suggests that as the level of alcohol consumption increases among African-American women, the severity of symptoms associated with comorbid mental disorders, sexual risk behaviors, and consumption of crack/cocaine increases significantly (Zule et al. 2002). Among African Americans identified as individuals who use crack-cocaine, more than 70 percent reported concerns regarding food, clothing, and transportation, and approximately 50 percent reported problems associated with shelter, medical issues, and employment (Zule et al. 2003). With less adequate housing, financial resources, medical care, and higher cumulative stress, African-American women face an increased susceptibility to substance use disorders and other health conditions.

Clinical treatment issues

Beginning in the 1990s, research on African-American women with substance use disorders focused on low-income, urban women who were dependent on cocaine (Roberts et al. 2000). Now, literature on substance abuse and treatment among African-American women has expanded and environmental stressors have been examined, including psychosocial, sociodemographic, and economic disparities. While research remains limited in the area of treatment approaches and strategies, literature is beginning to reflect promising practices for African-American women.

From the outset, it is vital that African-American women have access to services that provide social support during their pursuit of recovery. Research suggests that African-American women are at risk for substance abuse due to the level of exposure to biopsychosocial and economic stressors and the subsequent difficulty in coping with these life circumstances (Gray and Littlefield 2002). They often experience greater emotional distress and more relationship problems (Liepman et al. 1993; Henderson 1994). Similar to all groups of women, African Americans have very high rates of trauma and abuse, so treatment needs to utilize trauma-informed services.

Coupled with direct and indirect effects of historical trauma (including a history of slavery, lynchings, and racism) (Barnes-Josiah 2004), African-American women disproportionately experience negative health and social consequences of alcohol and drug use (Boyd et al. 2006). For example, African-American women are more likely to have their children legally removed from their custody, in part, as a result of societal bias and discrimination (Wallace 1990). Additionally African-American women are 10 times more likely than Caucasian women to have positive drug screens. Yet, this difference may be directly related to a disproportionate percentage of testing among African-American women (Neuspiel 1996). Subsequently, this threat of loss of child custody or legal sanctions for drug use during pregnancy may prevent African-American women from obtaining prenatal care or seeking substance abuse treatment. Nonetheless, once treatment is initiated, issues surrounding pregnancy, child care, parenting, and custody need be addressed in a nonthreatening but constructive manner—showing support and guidance in promoting and nourishing a healthy parent–child relationship.

Other health consequences include a higher risk for developing alcohol-related disorders, including liver cirrhosis, and a greater propensity to experience toxic effects of cocaine that may lead to earlier onset or greater risk for health problems, particularly cardiovascular disease (D'Avanzo et al. 2001). According to the HIV/AIDS Surveillance Report (CDC 2007), African-American women are 23 times as likely to be diagnosed with HIV/AIDS in comparison to white women, and 4 times more likely than Hispanic women. Among African-American women with HIV/AIDS, 74 percent acquired HIV/AIDS through high-risk heterosexual transmission and 24 percent were infected with HIV through injection drug use. To effectively address pertinent health and clinical issues, treatment programs also need to incorporate HIV/AIDS prevention, intervention, and treatment services.

Coupled with these risk factors, there is a common myth that African-American women "can withstand any amount of pain and keep on working" (McGee et al. 1985; p. 7). This myth may have significant consequences for African-American women who have substance use disorders—delaying treatment, sacrificing self to care for others, and negating the need for preventive health care and substance abuse treatment. (For further review of roles and expectations of African-American women, see Reid 2000.)

Once in treatment, African-American women need a gender-responsive, strengths-based model to develop or enhance a sense of empowerment by recognizing their assets and history of fortitude (Roberts et al. 2000; p. 905). This model provides a framework whereby treatment shifts the focus away from individual internal deficits. For African-American women with substance use disorders, treatment approaches need to extend beyond the general parameters of gender-responsive treatment to include interventions that focus on social contexts across multisystems including social networks or groups, family involvement and therapy, and community involvement and interventions (Boyd-Franklin 1989; Bell 2002). Likewise, spiritual components and Afrocentric perspectives need to be incorporated into treatment to ensure a holistic approach and to assist African-American women in recovery (Brome et al. 2000; Rhodes and Johnson 1997; Roberts et al. 2000).

Role of spirituality and faith-based recovery

Although there is no "one size fits all" definition of spirituality, spiritual activities nevertheless offer women in recovery an outlet to express problems, seek guidance from others or from a higher power, and move from disharmony to harmony with self and others without fear of repercussion, shame, or punitive actions (Brome et al. 2000). America has an extensive history of religious movements and spiritually led programs that address substance abuse (White and Whiters 2005). Today, there is more focus on the importance of integrating these faith-based approaches into addiction treatment, and more recognition that African-American churches can be a vital recovery tool.

Spirituality has been an important source of support for many African-American women (Lewis 2004). Historically, spirituality and religion have provided a central organizing framework for self-definition, problemsolving, and connection to self and others, especially among African-American women. Black churches have led the promotion of health care, disease prevention, and psychological well-being (Leong 2006). Overall, women in recovery from substance use disorders who express high levels of spirituality demonstrate a more positive self-concept, better attitude toward parenting and perception of family climate, more active coping style, and greater satisfaction with their social support than women who are in recovery but expressed lower levels of spirituality (Brome et al. 2000). Notably, treatment providers need to understand how African-American women relate to traditional religion and spirituality and how that relates to positive mental health outcomes. For an overview of spirituality and religion and its implications for psychotherapy with African-American families, refer to Boyd-Franklin and Lockwood 2009.

Role of an Afrocentric perspective

Though it is important not to make the assumption that all African-American women want to identify with a particular African tradition, acknowledgment of the richness of the African-American heritage or adoption of an Afrocentric perspective is another crucial component of a culturally and gender-responsive treatment program for many African-American women. As an example, The Iwo San Program, located in Cleveland, Ohio, incorporated an Afrocentric component in treatment, along with cognitive–behavioral therapy and an Afrocentric approach to the 12-Step program, with a primary goal of increasing the women's understanding of what it means to be African American and of promoting self-pride through embracing African ancestry, history, and culture (CSAT 2003b). Women learned and used the "Seven Principles" from the Swahili tradition and community as a guide for daily living. (For review, see text box below.)

The concepts of empowerment, the positive role of African-American women in the family and larger community, and the ability to build on their inherent strengths in the face of adversity are important to culturally responsive treatment (Rhodes and Johnson 1997). By incorporating an Afrocentric worldview in substance abuse treatment, African-American women will likely benefit from this critical protective factor in enhancing self-image, self-esteem, and centeredness in recovery (Roberts et al. 2000).

Role of group, cognitive–behavioral, and family therapy

Group therapy and adapted cognitive–behavioral therapy (CBT) show promise when grounded in the African-American worldview (Brown et al. 1995; Holcomb-McCoy 2004; Washington and Moxley 2003). By placing emphasis on the importance of community, group therapy can be a powerful and culturally appropriate approach that provides a supportive recovery environment and acts as a buffer to stressors associated with recovery. In essence, it is an opportunity to reinforce or rebuild a community connection that supports health. (Refer to Figure 6-1 for a review of promising practices and strategies.)

CBT may be a noteworthy substance abuse treatment approach if adapted to fit the African-American worldview. Yet, minimal research has been carried out on the effectiveness of CBT and substance use disorders. Between 1950 and 2006, only 12 studies have examined CBT among ethnically diverse populations, with only one study focused on substance abuse and CBT (Horrell 2008). While this one study suggests effectiveness with CBT (as measured by reduction in frequency and amount of drug

---

Nguzo Saba: The Seven Principles

Umoja (Unity)

Kujichagulia (Self-Determination)

Ujima (Collective Work and Responsibility)

Ujamaa (Cooperative Economics)

Nia (Purpose)

Kuumba (Creativity)

Imani (Faith)

Source: Karenga 1998. Note: These seven principles are associated with each day of celebration of Kwanzaa.

use among African-American clients), the results need to be cautiously interpreted due to a high participant dropout rate. To date, more research is needed to examine the effectiveness of CBT with ethnically diverse adult populations with substance use disorders. While research is limited, there is emerging evidence that CBT can be a helpful approach among African-American clients. Kelly (2006) states that CBT may offer African-American women an opportunity of empowerment, supported by a nonjudgmental and collaborative therapeutic relationship, and centered on skill and support system development. It can be easily adapted to match a strength-based approach rather than a deficit model. To help decrease the Eurocentric bias in CBT, clinicians should avoid projecting or overemphasizing the value of cognition without incorporating the relevance of emotional expression and spirituality. As important, CBT should recognize and emphasize the importance of family and community support as an integral part of recovery.

Regardless of approach, treatment should evolve around the premise that family and community are essential elements to healing and recovery. Treatment programs and counselors can endorse these values within the program by using mentors from the community for women in early stages of recovery (Stahler et al. 2005). Overall, more attention is needed to involve and incorporate a multisystems framework including a family systems approach in treatment. Family therapy is characteristically a more pertinent mode of therapy for African-American women (Boyd-Franklin 1989).

Resiliency factors

Consistent with earlier work (Hill 1972), Gary and Littlefield (1998, p. 99) identified the following resiliency factors in their study of African-American families:

- A high degree of religious or spiritual orientation (as evidenced by church membership, church attendance, a sense of right and wrong, teaching moral values, and a shared religious core)
- A sense of racial pride (telling their children about Black history, discussing racism in one's family, telling children what it is like to be African American, preference for being identified as an African American)

Advice to Clinicians and Administrators:
Substance Abuse Treatment and African-American Women

Clinical:

- Incorporate a strengths-based approach versus reliance on a traditional deficit model.
- Use an Afrocentric perspective, when appropriate and welcomed, to provide a framework for recovery.
- Involve family members and community to build a network of safety and support.
- Recognize the relevance of spirituality with the client, and encourage involvement to enhance or secure recovery.

Program Development:

- Use elements of the African-American heritage or adopt an Afrocentric perspective to provide a more culturally responsive treatment program.
- Create program policies and procedures that support rather than limit family and community involvement.
- Develop treatment strategies that strengthen a sense of community within the treatment program, and create avenues to broaden this sense of community beyond the program; i.e., providing outreach activities or inviting community members to treatment graduation exercises.
- Invest in workforce development for African-American staff.

Staff Training:

- Provide culturally competent staff trainings promoting an understanding of—
  - African-American history and heritage.
  - The role of racism and discrimination in stress-related health issues and substance abuse.
  - The potential role and importance of spirituality in recovery.
  - Various African traditions and beliefs, and the knowledge of resources to support an Afrocentric perspective with the client.
  - The value and necessity of outreach services to the African-American community.

- A strong achievement orientation (high expectations for achievement and attainment, goal directedness, etc.)
- Resourcefulness (possessing personal talents and skills, self-reliance, self-sufficiency, independence, and the ability to cope with crises)
- Family unity (possessing a sense of cohesiveness, family pride, family togetherness, and commitment; i.e., the family comes first)
- Display of love and acceptance (the ability to affirm one another and to respect, appreciate, and trust one another)
- An adaptability of family roles (having role flexibility, sharing responsibility, and communicating with one another)
- A strong kinship bond (e.g., a high degree of commitment to the family, a feeling of mutual obligation, kin interaction, and support)
- Community involvement (service to others and membership and active involvement in community organizations)

Asian- and Pacific-American Women

Demographics

Asian origins can be traced to many countries, including Cambodia, China, India, Japan, Korea, Laos, the Philippines, Vietnam, and others. By some counts, the number of national and ethnic groups is nearly 50, representing more than 60 primary languages (Barnes and Bennett 2002; Grieco 2001; New York State Education Department 1997). The three largest groups of Pacific Islanders are Hawaiians, Guamanians or Chamorros, and Samoans (from the Mariana Islands, of which Guam is the largest). In all, 24 different groups are considered Pacific Islander, and individuals from many of these groups have migrated to the United States. More than half of U.S. residents who are Pacific Islanders live in California and Hawaii (Grieco 2001). Yet, over the past few decades, the Asian-American and Pacific-Island populations have become increasingly dispersed across the United States (U.S. Census Bureau 2001*f*).

Asian and Pacific Americans are a rapidly growing group, increasing by more than 7 million over the last 20 years (U.S. Census Bureau 2001*c*). According to the 2002 Census, Asian and Pacific Americans constitute about 4.4 percent of the total U.S. population (12.5 million individuals), of whom slightly more than half (51.6 percent) are women (U.S. Census Bureau 2001*d*). Asian- and Pacific-American women represent 13 percent of all women of color (U.S. Census Bureau 2001*d*). They are a relatively young group with 25 percent under age 18. Asian and Pacific Americans are both more likely to occupy one or the other end of the continuum in educational and income levels—either obtaining the highest educational and income levels or experiencing considerable poverty and a lack of education in comparison to non-Hispanic whites (Reeves and Bennett 2003).

Substance abuse among Asian and Pacific Americans

Although Asian and Pacific Americans constitute about 4 percent of the population, they represent less than 1 percent of admissions to substance abuse treatment facilities in 1999. However, this represents an increase in treatment admissions of 37 percent from 1994 to 1999 among this population (SAMHSA 2004).

Alcohol

In comparison to other ethnic groups, this population has the lowest percentage of current drinking history and of past year alcohol dependence or abuse (SAMHSA 2006). According to the results from SAMHSA's 2006 National Survey on Drug Use and Health (NSDUH; SAMHSA 2007), the rate of binge alcohol use was also the lowest among Asian Americans. Of the 3,951 Asian- and Pacific-American women admitted for substance abuse treatment in 1999, 27 percent of admissions were for alcohol abuse, a relatively low proportion (SAMHSA 2004).

Lower percentages of alcohol intake may be, in part, a result of the genetic disposition of the "flushing" response among Asians (Collins and McNair 2002). More than 25 percent of Asians possess a gene that causes a slower metabolism of normal oxidation of acetaldehyde. With elevated levels of acetaldehyde in the blood, individuals may experience a range of physical reactions including perspiration, heart palpitations and tachycardia, nausea, headaches, and facial flushing. Individual reactions can vary in intensity and time of onset, which also contributes to the amount of alcohol consumed (Weatherspoon et al. 2001).

Alcohol patterns are largely influenced by the norms established within Asian communities in the United States, or by the cultural norms established in the country of origin. The low drinking rates among women of all Asian- and Pacific-American groups seem to derive in part from the large numbers of abstainers among the foreign-born population. Those born in the United States are more likely to use alcohol and tobacco. Various studies have shown that educated, young, middle-aged Asian-American women, with higher levels of acculturation, are more likely to drink than other subpopulations of Asian-American women (Gilbert and Collins 1997; Towle 1988). Among Asian-American groups of recent immigrant status, it is more difficult to determine specific substance abuse and dependence patterns. In addition, recent immigrants are less likely to seek treatment and less able to access treatment services; therefore, they are not as likely to be represented when assessing prevalence.

Regarding cultural norms, solitary drinking practices generally are discouraged and often carry significant consequences. Among recent and other first-generation immigrants, the importance of maintaining face, coupled with insufficient understanding of substance use–related problems, can result in denial of substance abuse problems, family sanctioning, or collusion in substance abuse–related behaviors if drinking practices exceed cultural practices and expectations (Chang 2000). According to the TEDS (SAMHSA 2006), 26 percent of Asian and Pacific Americans identify alcohol as their primary drug of choice upon treatment admission.

Illicit drug use

The rates of illicit drug use are relatively low among Asian- and Pacific-American women compared with other racial and ethnic groups. Currently, methamphetamine (33 percent) bypasses alcohol as the primary drug

---

Advice to Clinicians and Administrators:
Substance Abuse Treatment and Asian- and Pacific-American Women

Note: Minimal treatment research is available pertaining to substance abuse treatment among Asian- and Pacific-American women. Therefore, information was gathered using literature across various modalities in behavioral health to help support the following recommendations.

Clinical:

- Address the importance of ethnic heritage and assess the level of acculturation in the beginning of treatment in order to avoid making assumptions regarding cultural values, family structure, gender roles, and styles of communication.
- Incorporate drug and alcohol education in order to reduce the stigma attached to substance abuse and dependence.
- Approach treatment from the vantage point of promoting overall health rather than focusing solely on substance abuse; include a holistic connection between body, mind, and spirit. There is value in reframing the presenting problem by placing emphasis on the positive aspects for change.
- Provide a nurturing environment that does not encourage cultural and gender-related tendencies toward self-blame (Kitano and Louie 2002).
- Develop trust and build a therapeutic alliance to help decrease internalized feelings of guilt and shame.
- Honor the importance of family as the focal point, and that maintaining family honor, obligations, and responsibilities are central to women.
- Focus on problemsolving, goal-oriented, and symptom-reduction strategies to circumvent the likely shame associated with delving into past alcohol or drug use behavior.
- Explore the history of trauma and the potential for posttraumatic stress symptoms and disorder. Many older immigrant Asian-American women have been exposed to losses, torture, and other types of war-related trauma.

Advice to Clinicians and Administrators: Substance Abuse Treatment and Asian- and Pacific-American Women (continued)

Program Development:

- Use a psychoeducational model as an integral ingredient in treatment.
- Consider the appropriateness of home visits to engage families from the outset prior to individual treatment services.
- Incorporate native language services or community resources, e.g., interpreter services.
- Provide separate treatment groups for women to reduce restrictions imposed by gender role expectations.
- Develop a psychoeducational family treatment program to support the individual in relation to her family and to provide education regarding addiction.
- Implement a lecture series that addresses both Western and traditional concepts of disease and treatment.
- Consider the adaptation of a peer-to-peer support group to establish or support culturally appropriate individual and community supports for recovery.

Staff Training:

- Provide culturally competent staff training to promote an understanding:
- Of the diversity of Asian- and Pacific-American women and of the relevance of cultural, language, and socioeconomic barriers.
  - Of the role of acculturation in alcohol and drug use practices.
  - That reporting substance abuse problems can be a significant source of shame for women and her family, and can be perceived as hurtful toward family.
  - Of the importance of "otherness" and the relevance of community and family in the perception of self-identity as a women.
  - That family is central, along with the maintenance of family obligations.
  - That individuals with socially stigmatized behaviors, such as drug abuse, may experience significant consequences from their family and community.
  - That traditional gender roles are often restrictive and influenced by generational and acculturation levels.
  - That communication is more likely to follow a hierarchy pattern whereby elders are respected.

Sources: Chang 2000; Kitano and Louie 2002; McGoldrick et al. 1996; Torsch and Xuequin 2000.

of abuse upon treatment admission. After methamphetamine, the most frequent cause of admission for illicit drug use among Asian-American women is marijuana (16 percent), followed by opioids (11 percent), and cocaine/crack (11 percent) (HHS 2008a). Yet, variations exist across subpopulations in drug and alcohol patterns.

Clinical treatment issues

Foremost, treatment providers need to understand, acknowledge, and incorporate cultural values within the treatment process. The family is the center of most Asian and Pacific Island cultures and is an important consideration for effective treatment for women. The definition of family is expansive

> "Acculturation... refers to the manner in which individuals negotiate two or more cultures where one culture is considered dominant while the other culture is perceived to have less cultural value" (Leong et al. 2007, p. 424).

and includes not only immediate and extended family members determined by blood and marriage, but also other members of the community. Among women, family ties, loyalties, cultural expectations, and beliefs can serve as a protective factor against substance abuse (Joe 1996). Moreover, the concept and value of interrelatedness among family, community, environment, and the spiritual world is essential in many Asian and Pacific Island cultures, and these tenets should be woven throughout the treatment program and clinical services (for an overview of treating Asian- and Pacific-American clients and their families, refer to Chang 2000).

More than 65 percent of the Asian-American population is foreign-born (U.S. Census Bureau 2004). Thus, stress specific to immigration and acculturation is more likely. This has significant implications for treatment planning and services in a variety of ways, particularly in accessing and addressing acculturation stress and its relationship to substance use and other psychological symptoms, specifically depression (Chen et al. 2003).

A complex set of barriers to care can discourage Asian- and Pacific-American women from availing themselves of substance abuse treatment and other health care. Asian-American women who do not speak English or whose cultural traditions include a sense of shame for ill health often do not seek medical care (Leigh 2006). The problem is compounded by the unsurprising denial of substance abuse in a climate that favors family ties, a reverence for authority, and the dearth of culturally responsive substance abuse treatment services (Kitano and Louie 2002, p. 352). In addition, women typically

assume the role of primary caretaker, holding the essential responsibility of nurturing and supporting the family, even at the expense of individual health concerns.

The development of empirically supported methods is evolving, yet research relevant to specific treatment needs among Asian- and Pacific-American women is sparse. Borrowing from the field of cross-cultural psychotherapy (Chang 2000; Leong and Lee 2006), treatment requires thorough assessment that includes such factors as circumstances of immigration, degree of assimilation, ethnic background, and health beliefs. The Asian American Multidimensional Acculturation Scale shows considerable promise in assessing women's multidimensional levels of acculturation (Chung et al. 2004). It provides a more comprehensive assessment of acculturation and its effect on psychological functioning. Although outcome research specific to Asian- and Pacific-American women in substance abuse treatment is lacking, preliminary research with Asian Americans in community-based substance abuse treatment found no overall group differences in treatment retention and outcomes (Niv et al. 2007).

Resiliency factors

As mentioned above, Asian and Pacific Americans share an ethic of hard work and family orientation, as well as a cultural concept of interrelatedness among family, community, environment, and spiritual world. In addition, the following observations have been noted in the literature:

- If incorporated thoughtfully into the treatment process, the family can have a significant influence on treatment outcome. At the very least, consideration should be given to the family's role in substance abuse as well as to members' participation in treatment and influence on recovery (Chang 2000).
- Some clients might find incorporation of indigenous treatment modalities—such as healing ceremonies, acupuncture, meditation, massage, tai-chi, and herbal medicines—helpful (Kitano and Louie 2002).

American-Indian and Alaska-Native Women

Demographics

In the 2000 census, those who reported Alaska Native or American Indian as their only race/ethnic group totaled nearly 2.5 million, while the number reporting Alaska Native or American Indian in combination with another race/ethnic group numbered 4.1 million (U.S. Census Bureau 2001e), or 1.5 percent of the U.S. population. Alaska Native/American Indian is the smallest of the four major racial/ethnic groups currently recognized in the United States. Their small numbers, however, mask significant diversity.

The largest concentrations of Native people reside in three States: Arizona, California, and Oklahoma (U.S. Census Bureau 2001f). However, American Indians and Alaska Natives may live anywhere in North America on and off reservations or other forms of tribal land, in rural or urban areas, and within villages (Coyhis 2000). Today, American-Indian and Alaska-Native nations (e.g., Navajo, Iroquois) encompass more than 560 federally recognized Tribes, including more than 220 Alaskan villages, in addition to numerous Tribes that are not yet federally recognized. Historically, this diversity, as well as the separation of this group into many small segments scattered throughout the United States, has complicated efforts to identify commonalities through classification (NIH; ORWH 1999). Nevertheless, some experiences shared by many Tribes have been noted (NIH; ORWH 1999):

- Rapid change from a cooperative, self-sufficient, clan-based society to a family-based community dependent on trade
- Prior government criminalization of the use of native language and spiritual practices
- Deaths of members of the older generations to infectious diseases and war
- Loss of the ancestral lands

The rates of unemployment, poverty, and education; poor health status; and alcohol and drug use vary by Tribe and by region. The current poverty level is 27 percent among Native Americans (U.S. Census Bureau 2006). Unemployment hovers at about 13 percent for females older than age 16 (Indian Health Service [IHS] 2002). The proportion of family households maintained by women with no spouse is approximately 21 percent (U.S. Census Bureau 2000).

Substance use among American Indians and Alaska Natives

Although representing only 1.5 percent of the U.S. population, American Indians/Alaska Natives represented 2.1 percent of all admissions to publicly funded substance abuse treatment facilities. Of these, 36 percent were female (SAMHSA 2004). Based on the NSDUH, including alcohol and illicit drugs, Native American women were more likely than any other ethnic group to have met criteria for past year need for substance abuse treatment (OAS 2006a). For more comprehensive information on substance abuse treatment, see the planned TIP *Substance Abuse Treatment with American Indians and Alaska Natives* (CSAT in development e).

Alcohol

Nearly 14 percent of Native-American women were dependent on or abused alcohol between 2004 and 2005 (SAMHSA 2007). Compared with other substances, alcohol was by far the most frequently reported reason (52 percent) for admission to a treatment facility among women (OAS 2006a). The data also show that this group initiates alcohol use at an earlier age than other racial/ethnic groups (SAMHSA 2004). Among women of all races aged 35 to 44, 4.9 per 100,000 died of alcohol-related disease. However, the alcohol-related death rate among American-Indian and Alaska-Native women in this age range is 67.2 per 100,000 (IHS 2002). According to the CDC (2001), American-Indian women have higher rates of alcohol abuse, chronic liver disease, and cirrhosis than any other racial/ethnic group in the United States.

Illicit drug use

Among Native Americans, the rate of current illicit drug use (12.6 percent) is higher than any other race or ethnicity in United States according to the NSDUH (SAMHSA 2006). After alcohol abuse, the most common cause for Alaska Native and American Indian admission to treatment is methamphetamine (15 percent; SAMHSA 2006), followed by marijuana (13 percent), and cocaine/crack (7 percent; SAMHSA 2006). According to one study investigating gender differences among Alaska Natives in inpatient treatment (Malcolm et al. 2006), women reported higher rates of cocaine dependence in addition to alcohol dependence while men had higher rates of marijuana and alcohol dependence. Although the trend for inhalant abuse is declining among American Indians, studies have shown that American-Indian females are using inhalants more than American-Indian males (Beauvais et al. 2002). Among urban American-Indian women who abuse drugs, Stevens (2001) found that most lived below the poverty level, were unemployed and homeless, experienced a particularly high number of pregnancies and stillbirths, and had children remanded to the custody of State and tribal child protective services.

Clinical treatment issues

Substance use patterns and treatment issues among many groups of American Indians and Alaska Natives have not been studied adequately; as a result, many issues specific to these groups are not well known. Overall, wide variations in alcohol and drug use patterns—along with access to treatment and other needed health services—exist across American-Indian and Alaska-Native communities (Berkowitz et al. 1998; Vernon 2007). While similar barriers exist for Native-American women in comparison to other women with substance use disorders, Native-American women often encounter more barriers that impede access to treatment; i.e., economic hardships, treatment accessibility, lack of screening and assessment, and gender-responsive programming (Berkowitz et al. 1998; Parks et al. 2003).

Comprehensive attention to health care and health status is crucial for treatment of American-Indian and Alaska-Native women. Stevens (2001) suggests that medical and substance abuse treatment providers need to work hand-in-hand to meet the needs of Native-American women, and that primary care providers should routinely screen for alcohol and drug abuse and discuss the negative health consequences of substance use in a culturally responsive manner during regular examinations.

Unfortunately, few American-Indian and Alaska-Native women who abuse alcohol and illicit drugs are referred or enrolled in treatment programs of any type. For Native-American women living in rural areas, available treatment programs usually are neither woman-centered nor culturally specific. Moreover, many Native-American women are reluctant to attend treatment programs with non-Native Americans (Hussong et al. 1994). Some prefer participating in reservation-based programs, while others may be reluctant to participate in small community programs or urban health centers due to concerns surrounding confidentiality (Jumper Thurman and Plested 1998). Others may seek treatment elsewhere but express concerns surrounding available support upon reentering the reservation after treatment (Berkowitz et al. 1998). Subsequently, Native-American women are more likely to need help deciding on the location of their treatment program.

Trauma-informed services

American-Indian women are disproportionately affected by violent crimes, childhood sexual abuse, and physical abuse. Nearly three-fourths (73.3 percent) of Alaska-Native women in one program reported sexual abuse histories (Brems 1996). Beyond specific traumas among Native Americans, treatment programs need to incorporate a culturally responsive framework that understands and addresses the legacy of historical and cumulative trauma (Robin et al. 1997), including forced acculturation and deculturalization (e.g., loss of cultural, community, individual identity) of American-Indian and Alaska-Native communities. These losses have sometimes been expressed in higher suicide and homicide rates among Native-American community members. As part of recovery, women will likely need to address the loss of family members or friends. Likewise,

Advice to Clinicians and Administrators:
Substance Abuse Treatment and Native-American Women

Clinical:

- Assess for the history of traumatic events, including sexual and physical abuse, and the diagnosis of PTSD.
- Provide trauma-informed services that encompass the impact of cumulative stress from historical trauma to specific trauma.
- Recognize that the role of "helper" may extend beyond substance abuse counseling to seeking advice for other health concerns, for other family members, or for other life circumstances or stressors.
- Acknowledge the importance of family history and extended family members, and as deemed appropriate, involve family members during the course of treatment.
- Explore the woman's beliefs regarding healing and knowledge of cultural practices. Don't assume that a Native-American woman follows traditional practices.
- Understand and acknowledge the specific Tribe's cultural values, beliefs, and practices, including customs, habits, sex roles, rituals, and communication styles.

Program Development:

- Take time to invest in the individual Native community and learn the perceptions toward non-Native counselors.
- Use treatment as a prevention opportunity for FASD. Provide an interactive program that not only educates women on the cause and prevalence of FAS and Fetal Alcohol Effects (FAE), but provides an understanding of the behavioral effects that are often associated with this syndrome.
- Incorporate comprehensive HIV/AIDS prevention and intervention services into treatment.
- Adopt trauma-informed services and consider an integrated model of specific services for substance-use disorders and trauma.
- Combine contemporary approaches with traditional/spiritual practices; i.e., medicine wheel, "Red Road to Wellbriety" (White Bison), smudging, sweat lodge ceremony, and talking circle.
- Implement a skills training program to help Native-American clients learn how to successfully negotiate both traditional and majority cultures after treatment (Hawkins and Walker 2005).

Staff Training:

- Promote an understanding of the role of historical and intergenerational trauma as well as cultural oppression along with its impact on Native-American clients and its role in substance abuse.
- Provide learning opportunities that highlight the nature, history, and diversity of American-Indian and Alaska-Native communities.
- Address biases and myths associated with Native-American clients; e.g., firewater myth.
- Invest in learning the various and specific cultural patterns in coping with stress that may be unique to the specific community or Tribe.

**Advice to Clinicians and Administrators:Substance Abuse
Treatment and Native-American Women (continued)**

Staff Training (continued):

- Review and discuss the prevalence of HIV/AIDS, FASD, suicide and violence, and other health related risks among Native-American communities.
- Use local tribal members as resource people in training and as staff members in treatment programs.

Source: Coyhis 2000; Evans-Campbell 2008; and Trimble and Jumper Thurman 2002.

screening for traumatic events, posttraumatic stress disorder (PTSD), grief, and depressive symptoms should be routine. Treatment programs for Native-American women need to incorporate culturally congruent trauma-informed and integrated trauma services to build a stronger bridge to recovery (Saylors and Daliparthy 2006).

HIV/AIDS prevention and intervention comprehensive services

In 2005, Native Americans ranked third in HIV/AIDS rates, with Native-American women accounting for 29 percent of the diagnoses. While rates vary from community to community (Vernon and Jumper Thurman 2005), the rise in HIV/AIDS cases among Native-American communities reflects the need for attention in program development and treatment services for substance use disorders among women. Simoni and colleagues (2004) coined the term "Triangle of Risk" in reference to the HIV risk factors: history of sexual trauma, injection drug use, and HIV sexual risk behaviors. Each risk factor is highly interrelated to the other factors and strongly associated with substance use disorders. While risk factors are not limited only to the "triangle of risk" (Vernon 2007), the prevalence of these risk factors clearly represents the necessity of comprehensive HIV/AIDS prevention and intervention services among Native-American women seeking treatment for substance abuse.

Fetal alcohol prevention services

Fetal Alcohol Spectrum disorders (FASD) are very serious problems in some Native communities. A four-State study showed that fetal alcohol syndrome (FAS) among American Indians and Alaska Natives occurred at the rate of 3.2 per 1,000 population over a 2-year period, compared with 0.4 per 1,000 in the total population of the same four States (Hymbaugh et al. 2002). As a means of prevention, gender-responsive treatment services have an opportunity to educate Native-American women on the impact of alcohol and drugs on fetal development. By adding prevention approaches for FASD in treatment, women can make better and more informed decisions regarding alcohol use during pregnancy.

Culturally congruent substance abuse services

Treatment professionals must approach health and well-being through the complementary lenses of culture, history, and the beliefs of Native-American people (LaFromboise et al. 1998; Stevens 2001). For many Native-American women, the journey to reclaim their identities and culture is central to recovery (Brems 1996). The most critical feature for

> "The work we do today will provide for the freedom of our future generations (Mohawk)."
>
> *Source:* The Freedom Way: The Native American Program at the Margaret A. Stutzman Addiction Treatment Center, NY

treatment of American-Indian and Alaska-Native women is that programs be culturally responsive, gender-responsive, and community-based, and that they "reaffirm cultural values and consider the individual in the context of the community" (LaFromboise et al. 1998, p. 150). A series of IHS-funded focus groups for women in treatment found that an emphasis on cultural activities was important to the women (Berkowitz et al. 1998), including sweat lodges, powwows, talking circles, tribal music and crafts, traditional foods, and meetings with medicine people and tribal elders. For many women, participating in tribal activities gave them a sense of belonging—some for the first time (Berkowitz et al. 1998). This is important because the reasons that some Native-American women have given for alcohol and drug use include low self-esteem and "not fitting in with the white world" (Hussong et al. 1994). While it should not be assumed that every Native-American woman *is* traditional; traditional healing should be made available as a treatment option or as an adjunct to treatment.

Family and community involvement

Strong ties to family and community make community-based approaches appropriate because substance abuse is considered a family and community problem (Berkowitz et al. 1998). In some Native-American communities, alcohol consumption is the norm; abstainers may be ostracized. When drinking together is a major family activity, the woman who abstains may, in effect, lose her family. With such high rates of alcohol and drug use, a woman's family and friends are unlikely to offer strong support for recovery. By acknowledging the role and the importance of family and community in either perpetuating the substance use or in providing a nurturing recovery environment, treatment providers must involve family and community members from the outset. As highlighted in the IHS-funded research on substance abuse treatment for Native Americans, comprehensive treatment must embrace and encourage community involvement and commitment to support long-term recovery (Berkowitz et al. 1998). Literature suggests that the key factor in

maintaining abstinence among Native-American women is the presence of tangible support (Oetzel et al. 2007).

Resiliency factors

In recent years, American-Indian communities have organized to promote their economies and cultures. In the mid-1990s, an Executive Order mandated the establishment of tribal colleges on or near reservations, and at least 50 percent of the registered student population of these colleges must, by definition, be American Indians or Alaska Natives. Currently, American Indians are developing economic enterprises in the casino, recreation, and computer industries. Along with these advances, American-Indian and Alaska-Native peoples are revitalizing their native languages and cultures. Recent trends include movement back to the reservation. In addition, many American-Indian communities are very proactive about substance abuse issues.

On reservations, many women have gone back to talking circles and are promoting the need to do things within cultural, family, and community contexts, including the creation of communities that are alcohol free (Berkowitz et al. 1998). The Williams Lake Band in Canada, for example, has become entirely alcohol and drug free. Another success story involves the Alkali Lake Band in British Columbia, which achieved a communitywide sobriety rate of 95 percent over a 15-year period (Berkowitz et al. 1998).

Sexual Orientation and Women

Demographics

Several factors prevent an accurate measure of the number of women who identify as lesbian or bisexual, among them the absence of standardized terms and definitions of sexual orientation and gender identity (Dean et al. 2000). However, general estimates of sexual orientation as lesbian or bisexual range from 1 to 10 percent of the female population (Laumann et al. 1994; Michaels 1996).

Hughes and Eliason (2002) present definitions that are inclusive and highlight the differences between sexual orientation and gender identity. Their definition of "lesbian" or "gay" is "a woman or man whose primary sexual and emotional attachments are to persons of the same sex" (p. 266). "Bisexual" refers to "men or women who have sexual and/or emotional attachments to both men and women" (p. 266), although typically not at the same time.

Substance Use Among Lesbian and Bisexual Women

Limited research on alcohol and drug abuse has focused on issues related to sexual orientation (Hughes and Eliason 2002). What is known, however, is that within-group differences are significant. Early research attempts, specifically methods of data collection, may have reinforced misconceptions and stereotypical interpretations of substance use within these groups. Studies in the 1970s and 1980s revealed high rates of alcohol use and abuse among lesbians,, yet most surveys were conducted at bars. Other methodological limitations that remain consistent to the present time are sample size and absence of control groups (Hughes and Eliason 2002). In addition, studies that evaluate drug patterns are often focused on gay men. Little is known about illicit and prescription drug abuse patterns among lesbian and bisexual women. In two population-based studies, researchers found more drug use and heavy drinking among bisexual and lesbian women than among heterosexual women (Diamant et al. 2000).

Alcohol

Later research (Cochran et al. 2000; Hughes et al. 2000) supports the idea that earlier estimates of the relationship between sexual orientation and alcoholism are inflated. Nonetheless, these and other studies (Case et al. 2004; Cochran et al. 2000, 2001; Cochran and Mays 2000; Gilman et al. 2001; Parks and Hughes 2005; Sandfort et al. 2001) suggest that lesbian women—in comparison to heterosexual women—are more likely to use and abuse alcohol, less likely to decrease their use of alcohol with age, and

more likely to report alcohol-related problems. Literature suggests that this greater prevalence of substance use and abuse may be related to more opportunities to drink, fewer traditional sex role expectations, and different social conventions about drinking (Hughes and Wilsnack 1997).

Illicit drugs

While little is known about drug patterns among lesbian and bisexual women, research suggests that they are at a heightened risk for drug use, with specific subpopulations showing more prevalence, such as young adult lesbian women (Hughes and Eliason 2002). In two studies (Cochran et al. 2004; Corliss et al. 2006), researchers report that women with female sexual partners had at least one symptom of dysfunctional drug use and were more likely to display impairment and meet criteria for any drug dependence in comparison to heterosexual women. Lesbians report greater problems associated with marijuana, cocaine, and hallucinogens. In a study conducted in urban primary care sites, bisexual women were about twice as likely as heterosexual women to report having used illicit drugs in the past month (Koh 2000).

Clinical Treatment Issues

Few studies of substance use disorders have included sufficient numbers of lesbian women to permit separate analyses, and no studies have focused exclusively on bisexual women. In the few studies that are available, findings are inconclusive regarding the efficacy of separate treatment groups. Only 6 percent of substance abuse treatment services offer special programs or group therapy for gay men and women (SAMHSA 2005). For a comprehensive overview of treatment issues among lesbian and bisexual women, review SAMHSA's Center for Substance Abuse Treatment (CSAT) manual, *A Provider's Introduction to Substance Abuse Treatment for Lesbian, Gay, Bisexual, and Transgender Individuals* (CSAT 2001b). This manual provides information to administrators and clinicians about appropriate diagnosis and treatment approaches that will help ensure

Advice to Clinicians and Administrators:
Substance Abuse Treatment and Lesbian and Bisexual Women

Clinical:

- Explore coping style and enhance coping skills needed to manage stress associated with self-disclosure and the habitual "coming out" process, to deal with attitudes from others regarding sexual orientation, and to address feelings of alienation from family members who are rejecting of sexual orientation.
- In addition to appropriate family members, consider friends as a vital component of treatment and support structure. Studies (Kurdek and Schmitt 1986; Mays et al. 1994) report that lesbians generally receive greater support from friends than from family. By using social support from family and friends, counselors will likely enhance psychological well-being.
- Assess for interpersonal violence. Rates pertaining to partner violence or abuse among lesbian women are similar to those of heterosexual women (see, e.g., Coleman 1994; Renzetti 1994) and partner abuse often is accompanied by alcohol use (Schilit et al. 1990). Assess for the history of traumatic events, including sexual and physical abuse, and the diagnosis of PTSD.

Program Development:

- Consider a specialized group that addresses issues unique to lesbians in recovery.
- Implement policies that address the potential woman-to-woman sexual relationships that can develop in residential treatment (similar to man-to-woman relationship policies in treatment).
- Incorporate educational components in treatment that address relevant legal issues and the inherent issues that may arise in addressing medical, child custody, and financial needs.

Staff Training:

- Provide education on the multiple risk and protective factors that may either increase or buffer risk for substance use disorders.
- Impart knowledge about legal issues, including living wills, powers of attorney, advance directives, restrictions imposed by HIPAA, as well as a referral base to assist lesbians in securing these services.
- Address myths and stereotypes associated with gender roles and sexual behaviors, including the possible assumption that lesbians in relationships play either male or female roles or they are hypersexual or promiscuous. It is important for staff to recognize that lesbian relationships maintain the same patterns of stability and sexual behavior as heterosexual relationships.
- Review supportive strategies in assisting clients in determining whether or not to self-disclose sexual orientation in treatment.
- Assist staff to understand the impact of stigma associated with lesbian and bisexual women.
- Review the "coming out" process and the stages of identity.

Source: Ayala and Coleman 2000; CSAT 2001b; Jordan and Deluty 1998; Oetjen and Rothblum 2000; Wayment and Peplau 1995.

the development or enhancement of effective lesbian, gay, bisexual, and transgender (LGBT)-sensitive programs.

Sexual Orientation and Women of Color

Prevalence studies of substance use and abuse in lesbian, gay, and bisexual populations rarely have included sufficient numbers of racial and ethnic minority persons to permit separate analyses. However, limited available data suggest that patterns of substance use among lesbian women of color are more similar to those of their Caucasian lesbian counterparts than to those of their heterosexual racial and ethnic counterparts (Hughes and Eliason 2002). All racially and ethnically diverse group members face similar responses to their sexual orientation that can be stressful to psychological well-being, and reluctance to seek professional help can increase further their risk for negative psychological outcomes (Greene 1997).

Social support for treatment is known to be important in helping women stay in treatment and avoid relapse. Although African-American lesbian and bisexual women may receive support from fewer sources than African-American heterosexual women when they are in treatment for alcohol dependence, the quality of that support appears the same for the two groups (Mays et al. 1994). African-American gay women may prefer counselors of the same race who identified themselves as lesbians (Matthews and Hughes 2001).

Relatively little is known about alcohol abuse among Hispanic/Latina lesbian and bisexual women, although some researchers (Nicoloff and Stiglitz 1987; Peluso and Peluso 1988) believe it is more prevalent among Hispanic/Latina lesbian women than heterosexual Hispanic/Latina women (Reyes 1998).

For Asian Americans, cultural issues play a major role in sexual identity and culturally normative behavior. Asian-American lesbian women pose a cultural dilemma by virtue of their individual and sexual identification. If sexuality is expressed without jeopardizing family integrity and the individual's role in the family, then it may be tolerated (Chan 1997). Many Asians find it difficult to conceive of losing that familial connection and are therefore uncomfortable with assuming a minority sexual identity. Given this context, it is likely that Asian Americans who are openly lesbian probably are relatively acculturated. Chan (1989) found that, although they identify both with their Asian-American and lesbian identities, most of these women identify more strongly as lesbian. The implications of this with regard to substance abuse remain unexplored.

American Indians and Alaska Natives traditionally uphold a worldview that all things are interrelated and dependent upon one another. Identity formation, specifically sexual identity, is conceptualized through this broader lens. Therefore, sexual identity is typically not defined using definitive terms, such as lesbian or bisexual, but rather through more expansive concepts that embrace roles within the culture and community. Native Americans are more likely to use the term "two-spirit" to capture both male and female sexuality and gender expression (Evans-Campbell et al. 2005). Research focused on substance use disorders among two-spirited Native Americans is limited, and empirical literature highlighting two-spirit women is non-existent. In a study comparing two-spirited men and women with Native heterosexual peers, two-spirit individuals had significantly higher rates of lifetime illicit drug use; greater sustained drinking among urban Natives; and greater likelihood to use alcohol to increase sociability, regulate mood, and decrease anxiety and feelings of inferiority (Balsam et al. 2004).

Resiliency Factors

In general, lesbian women are more likely to have long-term relationships and friendships similar to heterosexual women. The stability in relationships may provide a strong platform in recovery provided the environment does not support or encourage continued alcohol abuse or drug use. Moreover, the woman's fortitude

Substance Abuse Among Specific Population Groups and Settings in managing prejudice and discrimination as a direct result of sexual orientation may provide a powerful example and symbol of personal strength in working toward recovery.

Women in Later Life

Demographics

Approximately 21 million women aged 65 and older reside in the United States. In 2003, women accounted for 58 percent of the population aged 65 and older (Federal Interagency Forum on Aging-Related Statistics [FIFARS] 2004); women older than age 65 constitute 7.3 percent of the total population. The oldest of the population (persons 85 years and older) are among the most rapidly growing age cohort in the Nation. The increasing number of older women corresponds to a growing incidence of health-related problems that were once considered solely men's diseases.

A Hidden Disease

Older years are filled with many adjustments and challenges, often including loss of spouse and close friends, retirement, and reduced income. Some women turn to alcohol or drugs to help meet these life changes. Because many older women live alone (40 percent of those aged 65 and older [FIFARS 2004]), their substance use is difficult to measure (Moore et al. 1989). Older women tend to hide their substance use because they attach greater stigma to it than men do (CSAT 1998d). Older women are less likely than older men to drink or use drugs in public, so they are less likely to drive while intoxicated or engage in other behavior that might reveal a substance use disorder (SAMHSA 2008).

Substance use disorders in older women often go undetected by primary care professionals because of a lack of appropriate diagnostic criteria and because many signs of abuse can be mistaken for other conditions more prevalent in later life (e.g., cognitive impairment, anemia, physiological consequences from falls). It is not unusual for older patients to show poor compliance with the recommended use of their medications (Menninger 2002). TIP 26

Substance Abuse Among Older Adults (CSAT 1998d), recommends best practices to identify, screen, assess, and treat alcohol, prescription medication, and other drug abuse among people aged 60 and older.

Risk Factors

Alcohol dependence and prescription drug abuse are the top two substance use issues for older women (CSAT 1998d). Numerous risk factors are associated with substance-related problems among older women including losses or deaths, financial problems, health problems, age-related changes in metabolism, synergistic effects in combining alcohol and other drugs, and changing roles (Epstein et al. 2007). Researchers found that when women were deprived of their usual roles as wife, mother, or employee, their problem drinking increased. Older women with fewer role demands have fewer competing activities (Wilsnack and Cheloha 1987).

Timing of Onset

Alcohol- and drug-related problems in older women can be longstanding or can begin in later life. Women with early-onset alcohol dependence have a high incidence of major depression, anxiety, and bipolar disorder and simply continue their drinking habits as they age (CSAT 1998d). Women with late-onset use appear both physically and psychologically healthier. They are more likely than those with early-onset use to have begun or increased drinking in response to a recent loss such as death or divorce. Both groups appear to use alcohol almost daily outside the home and at home alone and are likely to use alcohol to respond to hurts and losses (CSAT 1998d).

Substance use among women in later life

Alcohol

In comparing trends from 1992 to 2002 in alcohol abuse and dependence among women as they age, the National Epidemiologic Survey on Alcohol and Related Conditions showed a significant inverse relationship between rates of dependence and successive age groups—that as

Signs of Alcohol-Dependence and/or Drug Abuse in an Older Woman

- Neglected appearance and poor hygiene
- Frequent car accidents
- Numerous physicians and prescriptions
- Neglect of home, bills, pets, etc.
- Malnutrition and anemia, and empty food cupboards
- Withdrawal from social activities and self-isolation from family and friends
- Mood swings or erratic behavior
- Repeated falls or evidence of falls (leg bruises)
- Urinary incontinence
- Cigarette burns
- Attempts or thoughts of suicide
- Depression
- Unexplained chronic pain or other health complaints
- Confusion and/or memory impairment
- Blurred vision or blackouts
- Seizures or tremors

Source: Cohen 2000; CSAT 1998*d*

women age, prevalence of alcohol dependence decreases (Grant et al. 2006). While there is earlier empirical evidence to support that late-middle-age to older women have fewer drinking problems (known as "maturing-out"; Brennan et al. 1993), this trend has to be approached with a conservative lens since older women tend to hide their use and not seek alcohol treatment. In addition, the prevalence and risk of alcohol abuse and dependence among women appears to vary among subgroups. For example, widowed women were found to be three times more likely than married women to drink heavily (The National Center on Addiction and Substance Abuse at Columbia University [CASA] 1996). The most consistent predictors of alcohol-related problems among women were friends' approval of alcohol use, financial stressors, and avoidance coping (Moos et al. 2004).

Prescription Drugs

Prescribed medications are the most common drugs of abuse, outside of alcohol, among older adults (National Institute on Drug Abuse [NIDA] 2001). Approximately 30 percent of all prescriptions and 40 percent of all benzodiazepine prescriptions are prescribed to elderly individuals. An older woman is more likely than an older man to visit a physician and to be prescribed a psychoactive drug. Problems can result if prescriptions are written by several physicians who do not know the full range of prescribed and over-the-counter medications being taken. Older women often are prescribed medications highly susceptible to abuse (NIDA 2001). Medications frequently prescribed for and used by older women include anxiolytics and sedative-hypnotics. Alcohol–drug interactions are more likely to occur among older adults simply because they take more medications than younger adults and may continue to drink at levels consistent with earlier patterns. These interactions can cause problems in older adults because of slowed metabolism in later life and greater reliance on medications for chronic medical conditions (CSAT 1998*d*). With

Advice to Clinicians and Administrators:
Substance Abuse Treatment and Older Women

Review TIP 26 Substance Abuse Among Older Adults (CSAT 1998d), for further guidance in providing substance abuse treatment to older women.

Clinical:
- Introduce coping strategies, including relaxation methods, to enhance feelings of self-efficacy in handling life stressors.
- Incorporate counseling services that address issues of grief along with substance abuse treatment as needed.
- Use additional resources to reinforce the need for and support of treatment including, but not limited to, extended family members, healthcare providers, faith-based services, etc.
- Incorporate behavioral activation therapy to help address depressive symptoms among older women who have substance use disorders. This behavioral approach helps clients to recognize the connection between life stressors, mood, and less effective coping behaviors. It encourages and provides strategies to help the client to monitor mood and daily activities with an emphasis on strategies to increase the number of enjoyable activities (Cuijpers et al. 2007).
- Recognize and address the potential losses associated with changes in caregiver roles.

Program Development:
- Create access to treatment through nontraditional delivery; e.g., home-based or mobile community services.
- Provide educational programs on metabolism and interaction of alcohol and drugs, particularly prescription medications, at senior citizen centers.
- Create addiction treatment services or programs designed for older adults only.
- Provide home services or develop a one-stop multidisciplinary program that provides needed healthcare and nutritional services, psychoeducational groups, financial services, transportation, counseling, etc.

Staff Training:
- Review the more common signs of drug misuse among older women, including mental and physical symptoms as well as suspicious requests for refills.
- Provide an introduction to prescription drugs with emphasis on the physiological effects of anxiolytics and sedative hypnotics.
- Provide education on the physiological impact of alcohol and drug intake among older women.
- Emphasize the heightened alcohol sensitivity among women and the increased vulnerability among older women.
- Explore the relationship between alcohol problems and higher rates of depression and prescription drug use.
- Address the need and roles of a multidisciplinary treatment to ensure quality of care for older women in substance abuse treatment.

Source: Eliason and Skinstad 2001; Satre et al. 2004; Scogin et al. 2007.

age-related changes, prescription medications are more potent, less predictable in effects, and more likely to increase negative outcomes (Allen et al. 2006).

Clinical Treatment Issues

Screening and brief interventions, particularly cognitive–behavioral and case management approaches, may be especially useful in limiting alcohol abuse in older women; although research with older women has been limited, results are promising (Blow and Barry 2002). Alcohol dependence in an older woman may be observed first when she presents at an acute-care medical setting with complaints such as depression, memory loss, frequent falls, or chronic pain that may have been exacerbated by alcohol. These are not and should not be presumed to be normal consequences of aging. This is an appropriate time to intervene and discuss the benefits of sobriety as well as treatment options.

Treatment should be supportive, respectful, and non-confrontational. If possible, providers should gather personal information about the client from family members, neighbors, clergy, or others with the client's permission. Labels such as "alcoholic" or "addict" should be avoided and replaced with words such as "drinking" and "drinking problem" (Cohen 2000). It is important to be direct and honest, to explain that assistance is available, and to provide instructions on where help can be secured. A substance abuse treatment professional can help the older woman develop a support system. Some women may respond better if approached about their drinking in the safety of their homes or at a familiar medical facility where they feel comfortable. Programs such as Alcoholics Anonymous can be an important resource, particularly if the group meets during the day and is composed of older women.

A well-coordinated approach to substance abuse treatment for older women should include an interdisciplinary treatment team with family or significant others involved in a plan of individualized support services. Since it may be difficult to address the needs of older women in residential treatment programs (where the majority of clients are much younger), treatment may be more effective when delivered at senior centers, congregate meal sites, outpatient geriatric medical programs, nursing homes, home care programs, or peer outreach (Cohen 2000). Recent studies are providing promising results. In an outcome study comparing men's and women's abstinence rates in an outpatient group, 79 percent of women reported abstinence from alcohol at the 6-month followup, compared to 54 percent of the men (Satre et al. 2004).

Resiliency Factors

Using a strengths-based narrative approach can help capitalize on each woman's life experiences and give meaning to her recovery. By providing an opportunity to explore her life events, history, personal attributes, and triumphs in spite of adversity, counselors can use this history to help reinforce the woman's resilience and abilities to support recovery.

Women in Rural America

Demographics

Rural America contains 17 percent of the U.S. population (Economic Research Services 2007). In many rural areas, the population is aging steadily. Rural areas have a higher proportion of older persons and higher poverty rates among the elderly than urban areas, and women constitute 65 percent of the rural poor age 65 and older. In addition, poverty rates in rural settings are three times higher for widows than for married women (USDA 2007).

In reviewing specific hardships that may not be independent of the effects of either chronic or acute alcohol and drug use, a welfare study identified common material hardships experienced by women. More than 56 percent of rural women respondents report unmet medical needs and telephone disconnection as the most prevalent hardships, followed by food insufficiency, housing problems, improper winter clothing, and utility disconnection (USDA 2007). With added burdens generated by age, substance abuse, and poverty, local communities are faced with many challenges in meeting the diverse needs of women in rural settings.

Substance Use Among Women in Rural Settings

Substance abuse is a major rural health concern. While alcohol and drug patterns vary little across most age groups in urban and rural settings, emerging patterns among rural youth show a rise in use—thus providing a forecast of potential patterns of abuse and dependence. While rural and urban areas experience similar drug-use problems, the consequences may be greater in rural areas because of limited access to health care and substance abuse treatment. For example, only 10.7 percent of hospitals in rural areas offer substance abuse treatment services compared to 26.5 percent of metropolitan hospitals (Dempsey et al. 1999). Currently, there are minimal studies focused on substance use disorders among rural women (Boyd 2003).

Risk factors for substance use disorders among women living in rural areas of the United States are significant. Many rural families are impoverished, and women often experience stress associated with limited resources (Boyd 1998). A history of childhood victimization is another risk factor for substance use disorders among rural women, as for all women. A qualitative study described rural women's perspectives on becoming alcohol dependent, and many reported some form of sexual abuse. This study reported that some rural women began drinking in adolescence as a means of self-medication to ease the pain of their problems (Boyd and Mackey 2000a, b).

Alcohol

Beliefs and expectations about alcohol strongly predict potential alcohol abuse. Women in some rural communities hold more positive beliefs about alcohol than those in other communities or in comparison to urban women. The beliefs involve the notion that alcohol enhances sexual, physical, and social pleasure; reduces tension; and increases arousal, power, and control over life circumstances (Boyd 1998; Marlatt et al. 1988).

Clinical Treatment Issues

Poverty is a significant barrier in obtaining health services, and this barrier is more common for women than for men, especially in rural areas. Women in some segments of rural America perceive financial barriers to health care significantly more than men in rural areas and, consequently, experience poorer health than men (Beck et al. 1996b). Women with substance use disorders who live in rural areas may face a unique set of clinical issues that may challenge substance abuse professionals. These issues can include greater geographic and personal isolation, limited access to substance abuse treatment and mental health services (Ryland and Lucas 1996), poverty, and issues of confidentiality. While rural women often face the same obstacles in obtaining substance abuse treatment services that challenge women anywhere, rural women are more likely to encounter a lack of child care, available treatment slots, transportation, and phone service, and possess a reluctance to address and disclose to staff (Tatum 1995).

Treatment programs need to be culturally and ethnically appropriate for the community. Clinicians and other staff members may need to consider issues such as distance (e.g., how many miles from home to clinic), time and season

> Beyond the traditional therapy method used in many urban areas, the Appalachian tradition of storytelling has been used to help rural clients engage in treatment, gain insight into their problems, and learn new coping skills to address problems associated with substance use (Leukefeld et al. 2000).

Advice to Clinicians and Administrators:
Substance Abuse Treatment and Women in Rural Areas

Clinical:

- Screen for co-occurring disorders, and refer as needed.
- Obtain a history of traumatic events, including sexual abuse.
- Incorporate screening procedures to aid in appropriate referral to other health and social services.
- Explore potential reluctance in seeking help outside of immediate community.
- Assess for a history of interpersonal violence, and recognize that rural women have often reported learning that violence toward women is acceptable.
- Explore beliefs and attitudes toward alcohol and drug use.

Program Development:

- Develop partnerships among other local agencies and neighboring communities to share resources to aid in the delivery of services in remote areas.
- Develop a center that houses a network of services including health, mental health, substance abuse, and other social services.
- Develop a screening, assessment, and referral service for substance use disorders within the Temporary Assistance to Needy Families (TANF) program.
- Provide services that support substance abuse treatment attendance including child care, transportation, and mobile treatment.
- House support groups in the treatment facility, and consider providing or subsidizing transportation as a means of continuing care support.
- Create professional training, network activities, and opportunities for staff to decrease feelings of isolation and staff turnover and to invest in workforce development.
- Develop psychoeducational community programs to help reduce alcohol and nicotine use during pregnancy.
- Consider the use of telecounseling services in rural areas for assessment, pre-treatment, counseling, and/or follow-up services.
- Develop outreach services to address substance use and abuse issues among the aging population of rural women.

Staff Training:

- Emphasize the prevalence of social shame among rural women who have substance use disorders.
- Discuss the cultural issues that may support a reluctance to seeking treatment outside of the immediate community.
- Review the challenges of anonymity in small communities, the strategies that can enhance privacy, and the need to address and ensure confidentiality in treatment.
- Examine the potential hidden attitudinal barriers among women seeking substance abuse treatment including distrust of the "system," expectation of failure, and positive beliefs regarding the benefits of alcohol and/or drug use.

Source: Baca et al. 2007; Boyd 1998; 2003; CSAT 2003b; Howland 1995; Wilkins 2003.

(e.g., the demands of planting and harvesting, coordinating appointments with other trips to town), and even weather conditions to provide culturally acceptable services to rural clients (Bushy 1997). Another aspect of rural life is that communities are smaller and more close-knit so that everyone is familiar with the personal affairs of his or her neighbors. If, for example, a woman is arrested for driving under the influence, the chances are significant that the person in authority knows her or her family (Boyd 1998). Similarly, women in rural areas may know the law enforcement authority and, perhaps, know the substance abuse treatment provider as well. For rural women entering treatment who have been abused, their abusers may also be well known to the community. Prior reports of abuse may or may not be believed, and may set off counter-reactions against her.

Women may wish to seek treatment outside the community, even if they have to travel long distances. They may choose not to be seen going to the counselor's office or may have a preexisting relationship with the counselor. Conversely, women from rural communities may be reluctant to seek treatment outside of their communities, viewing treatment providers as "outsiders." As to other identified clinical issues among rural women with substance use disorders, the incidence of co-occurring disorders is suspiciously lower than among women from major metropolitan areas, perhaps because it is underdiagnosed and, as a result, undertreated (Kessler et al. 1994).

Several treatment programs have been developed for use with rural residents. Among these is Structured Behavioral Outpatient Rural Therapy (SBORT), a cognitive–behavioral intensive outpatient approach consisting of two phases: pretreatment and treatment. The three-session pretreatment phase consists of individual counseling to increase readiness for change. The treatment phase involves 12 sessions in 6 weeks and consists of storytelling and "thought mapping" to develop recovery skills (Clark et al. 2002). Storytelling is used to encourage clients to share their experiences and to help them relate to the presenting material in treatment. During thought mapping, the group examines important

incidents before and after prior use of alcohol or drugs. Treatment focuses on problemsolving strategies and other cognitive strategies, relaxation techniques, coping skills to deal with cravings, and encourages the utilization of self-help (Hall 1999). Specific outcome studies on SBORT for rural women in substance abuse treatment are lacking.

Resiliency Factors

In rural communities, there is typically a pattern of stability in residence, interpersonal relationships, and community. This stability can be a protective factor in recovery by providing sustained support. Likewise, large extended families, involvement in religious activities, and faith are attributes that are not only common in rural America but can serve as a conduit for treatment (Van Gundy 2006). From prevention to continuing care, counselors and administrators need to take advantage of these qualities in programming and clinical practice.

Resources for Other Special Populations and Settings

Women With Physical and Cognitive Disabilities

> Review TIP 29 *Substance Use Disorder Treatment for People with Physical and Cognitive Disabilities*. This is a practical resource for information on addressing treatment issues in this population (CSAT 1998e).

The 2000 Census reported that about 44 million noninstitutionalized adults have disabilities, including approximately 20 percent of adults younger than age 65 and 40 percent of those older than 65 (U.S. Census Bureau 2002). These individuals span all ages and racial, ethnic, and cultural backgrounds. One study (Larson et al.

2005) found that women with trauma histories and co-occurring substance use and mental disorders had high rates of physical disabilities, with the greatest number (15 percent) of disabilities being injury/musculoskeletal/ connective tissues problems. Although little research exists regarding the extent of combined disability and substance abuse, people with disabilities generally use substances at the same or higher rates than those without disabilities (CSAT 1994e). In some cases, the disability can exacerbate the risk factors for substance use disorders.

Women with disabilities are affected by several factors that can increase the likelihood of substance abuse and dependence (Ferreyra 2005):

- Increased dependence on others for basic needs
- Potential use of prescription medication for chronic pain
- Facilitation of substance use by family and friends to help cope with the disability
- Social isolation (lack of social support, unemployment, etc.)
- Insufficient referral for substance abuse treatment by primary physician or caregiver caused by lack of recognition
- Inaccessible substance abuse treatment programs

Women in the Criminal Justice System

Women in criminal justice facilities face numerous challenges including, but not limited to, greater health issues and higher prevalence of co-occurring disorders; increased likelihood of pregnancy and need for prenatal care; history of sexual violence and other forms of abuse; and childcare, custody, and parenting issues. The number of female inmates in all criminal justice facilities has been increasing at a faster rate than the number of male inmates. Between 1995 and 2002, the average annual growth rate of incarcerated females was 5.4 percent, compared with 3.6 percent for males (Harrison and Karberg 2003). Among the prison population, from 1990 to mid-2001, the number of female inmates jumped 114 percent; the male population grew by 80 percent in the same period (Beck et al. 2002). African Americans and Hispanics/Latinas account for nearly two-thirds of incarcerated women. Their median age is in the 30s. Nearly half of those in State prisons and other correctional facilities have never been married (Greenfeld and Snell 1999).

Among State prisoners, females were more likely than males to be sentenced for drug offenses (29 percent versus 19 percent; Sabol et al. 2007). Among Federal defendants in 2004, the leading drug arrests and sentences among women were related to methamphetamine (Bureau of Justice Statistics 2004). Women were more likely than men to have used methamphetamines in the month before their offense (Bureau of Justice Statistics 2006). According to U.S. Department of Justice, an estimated 52 percent of females in comparison to 44 percent of males incarcerated in local jails were dependent on or abusing drugs. In the last decade, more than half of all female prisoners reported being under the influence of alcohol or drugs at the time they committed the crime, with drug use being more prevalent (Greenfield and Snell 1999). In addition to TIP 44 *Substance Abuse Treatment for Adults in the Criminal Justice System* (CSAT 2005c), refer to *Gender-Responsive Strategies: Research, Practice, and Guiding Principles for Women Offenders* (Bloom, Owen, and Covington 2003) for more information.

Review TIP 44 Substance Abuse Treatment for Adults in the Criminal Justice System. This is a practical resource for information on addressing treatment issues in this setting (CSAT 2005c)

Women Who Are Homeless

Review the planned TIP *Substance Abuse Treatment for People Who Are Homeless*. This TIP is a practical resource for information on addressing treatment issues in this setting (CSAT in development g).

According to the Annual Homeless Assessment Report to Congress (2008), nearly 3 percent of Americans experience homelessness at any one time. Approximately 23 percent are chronically homeless with homelessness disproportionately affecting African Americans (44 percent of the total homeless population). Less is known about homeless women. Data collections often have missing personal identifiers, leading to less than reliable estimates of homeless women and homeless women and their children.

In exploring factors associated with women who are homeless (literal definition of homelessness: sleeping in shelters, public places, abandoned buildings, etc.), literature suggests significantly higher prevalence rates of domestic violence and serious health problems including HIV. Most women who are homeless do not have a criminal record. Nearly half never lived independently prior to losing their housing arrangement, and that housing arrangement mainly disintegrated between the woman and extended family members, spouse, or significant other. More than 25 percent reported loss of employment as the immediate cause of homelessness, while another 25 percent of women reported domestic violence as the cause (Levin et al. 2004). Other factors that contribute to homelessness include illness, recent relocation (Lehmann et al. 2007), hospitalization, severe mental illness, substance use disorders, high-risk pregnancy, increased rents, or fire (SAMHSA 2003b; Levin et al. 2004). The majority of women who are homeless using shelters have children (83 percent; HUD 2008). It is estimated that 84 percent of homeless adults with families are women (AHAR 2007).

Substance abuse among women who are homeless

Alcohol abuse and drug use has increased among homeless women in the past 20 years (North et al. 2004). Numerous studies (Koegel et al. 1999; North et al. 2004a; Robertson et al. 1997) provide estimates on lifetime and current substance use disorders among homeless women with lifetime estimates ranging from 56 to 63 percent and current estimates spanning 38 to 58 percent. Twenty percent of homeless admissions to substance abuse treatment are women, with admission rates higher among African-American women. Upon admission, prevalence rates of alcohol-related admissions were similar to all female admissions, while prevalence of cocaine/crack and heroin were more likely reported among homeless women (OAS 2004a).

SAMHSA offers a Homelessness Resource Center, a virtual community located at www.homeless.samhsa.gov. For providers who serve the homeless, this site offers information on a wide range of programmatic and clinical topics, provides access to related resources, including a one-stop site for all Federal Government materials on homelessness, and provides a place to share ideas and to gain support.

7 Substance Abuse Treatment for Women

Overview

While women are as likely to stay and engage in treatment as men, substance abuse counselors need to attend to individual, counselor, and environmental variables to secure the best retention rates based on level of care and presenting problems. This chapter begins with gender-specific factors that significantly influence treatment retention of women. Other highlights include women's treatment issues and needs (beginning with the role of relationships—including family and partners), parenting issues and treatment needs (including pregnancy and children), and several co-occurring disorders (including anxiety, mood, and eating disorders) that are most prevalent among women and are likely to require attention during the course of treatment. Significant consideration is also given to trauma, trauma-informed services, and integrated treatment for women with trauma-related symptoms and substance use disorders.

Treatment Retention

The many factors that influence clients to enter treatment are often the same ones that keep them in treatment. Treatment retention refers to the quantity or amount of treatment received by a client. Today, retention is more likely defined using the term "length of stay," and is measured by months or a timeframe rather than by the number of sessions (Comfort and Kaltenbach 2000; Greenfield et al. 2007a). Historically, literature has reflected that treatment duration (retention) has served as one of the most consistent predictors of posttreatment outcome, yet literature remains limited regarding the specific relationship between retention and outcome among women with substance use disorders. (For literature reviews on retention and outcome factors for women with substance use disorders, see Sun 2006; Greenfield et al. 2007a.)

Gender is not likely to predict retention in substance abuse treatment. For some time, it has been assumed that women are more likely to leave treatment, but some literature counters this view (Joe et al. 1999). Do women have lower retention rates than men? This is a difficult question to answer because treatment retention often involves the contribution and interaction of numerous variables. Studies have begun to identify these variables and how they relate to each other to influence treatment retention rates among women (see Ashley et al. 2004), but further research is needed to understand the complexity and interactions of these variables.

Psychiatric symptoms, drugs of choice, motivation levels, class, race, ethnicity, criminal justice history, addiction severity, and patterns of use are common factors that typically influence or predict retention among clients in general (see Simpson 1997). Among women, several factors have been identified that influence or predict retention. The following section highlights these factors. Nonetheless, this is not an exhaustive list of retention conditions or issues, but one that is limited to factors that are evident across several studies or that provide some insight into women's issues that need further empirical exploration.

Factors That Influence Retention Among Women

Sociodemographics

Relationships: Support from a partner during treatment and recovery can contribute significantly to long-term maintenance of abstinence. Some treatment studies suggest that including a partner or significant other in a client's treatment also contributes significantly to successful short-term outcomes (Price and Simmel 2002). For example, couples therapy for women in alcohol and drug abuse treatment contributed to favorable outcomes in one study (Trepper et al. 2000), and a study by Fals-Stewart and colleagues (2005) indicates that behavioral couples therapy was associated with abstinence and sustained recovery. Zlotnick

and colleagues (1996) also found family therapy to be an effective component for women in an outpatient substance abuse treatment program.

It appears that women who develop relationships in treatment are less likely to successfully complete treatment if their new partner discontinues treatment. In one qualitative study, all of the women who did not successfully complete treatment established a sexual relationship during the early phase of outpatient treatment (Ravndal and Vaglum 1994).

Age: Age appears to be a factor that influences retention. According to the Drug Abuse Treatment Outcome Study (DATOS), age has a significant positive effect on retention in residential treatment (Grella et al. 2000). In a study examining variables associated with retention in outpatient services, women younger than 21 were not as likely to successfully complete outpatient treatment (Scott-Lennox et al. 2000). Likewise, criminal justice research found that women who are older at their first arrest were more likely to complete treatment (Pelissier 2004).

Education: Women with a high school education are more likely to stay in treatment. According to two studies (Ashley et al. 2004; Knight et al. 2001), women who have a high school degree or equivalent are more likely to stay in treatment longer and complete treatment than women with less than a high school education. While education level is influential, it may be a reflection of other client characteristics or socioeconomic conditions.

Women of color: Research typically reflects lower retention rates among women of color. While more research is needed to pinpoint the specific factors that lead to lower retention rates among ethnically diverse women, a key variable appears to be economic resources. According to Jacobson, Robinson, and Bluthenthal (2007), limited economic resources may play a more significant role in retention than specific demographics or severity of substance use disorder.

Criminal justice and child protective services referral and involvement

It appears that either referral or involvement with the criminal justice system or child protective services is associated with longer lengths of treatment (Brady and Ashley 2005; Chen et al. 2004; Green et al. 2002). Specifically, Nishimoto and Roberts (2001) concluded that women who were mandated by the criminal justice system to enter treatment and who also had custody of their children were more likely to stay in treatment longer. While some studies reflect mixed results on the effect of women being mandated to treatment by the court, another study (generated from the sample of participants in the Substance Abuse and Mental Health Services Administration's [SAMHSA's] Women, Co-Occurring Disorders, and Violence Study) found that retention was higher among women who had been mandated to treatment (Amaro et al. 2007).

Pregnancy

Pregnancy status can significantly influence treatment engagement and retention. Grella (1999) concluded that pregnant women were more likely to spend less time in treatment, and that pregnancy interrupted treatment. Yet, the length of stay may be more related to the stage of pregnancy. In another retention study among women, women who entered treatment late in their pregnancies had good retention whereas women who entered treatment in their first trimester tended to leave treatment early (Chen et al. 2004).

Pregnancy and co-occurring disorders: Pregnancy often adds to the challenge of retaining clients who have severe psychiatric disorders in treatment. In one study (Haller et al. 2002) that compared retention rates across three groups of women, the group characterized by severe addiction, psychiatric (DSM Axis 1 diagnosis) and personality (DSM Axis 2 diagnosis) disorders had rapid attrition (a 36 percent dropout rate), whereas the groups described as clinically benign or with less severity but with externalizing personality deficits were more likely to complete treatment. In a similar study conducted by Haller and Miles (2004), women with more severe pathology were twice as likely to leave treatment against medical advice. While these studies have limitations, they do shed light on the role of psychiatric issues in retention among women, particularly pregnant women, and the need to provide appropriate intervention earlier in the treatment process. The findings of a study examining the effects of trauma-integrated services suggest that women who receive these mental health services may engage in treatment longer (Amaro et al. 2008).

Treatment environment and theoretical approach

Supportive therapy: The consensus panel's clinical experience has shown that women who abuse substances benefit more from supportive therapies than from other types of therapeutic approaches. Review of the literature indicates that positive treatment outcomes for women are associated with variables related to the characteristics of the therapist (e.g., warmth, empathy, the ability to stay connected during treatment crises, and the ability to manage countertransference during therapy; Beutler et al. 1994; Cramer 2002; Crits-Christoph et al. 1991). Women need a treatment environment that is supportive, safe, and nurturing (Cohen 2000; Grosenick and Hatmaker 2000; Finkelstein et al. 1997); the therapeutic relationship should be one of mutual respect, empathy, and compassion (Covington 2002b).

The type of confrontation used in traditional programs tends to be ineffective for women unless a trusting, therapeutic relationship has been developed (Drabble 1996). Early research on women in treatment demonstrated that women entered treatment with lower self-esteem than their male counterparts (Beckman 1994). Hence, the traditional practice during recovery of "breaking down" a person who abuses substances and rebuilding her as a person is considered unduly harsh and not conducive to effecting change among women who abuse substances (Covington 2008a rev., 1999a; Drabble 1996; Kasl 1992). Although designed to break through a client's denial, these approaches can diminish a woman's self-esteem further and, in some cases, retraumatize her. Approaches based on awareness, understanding, and trust are less aggressive and more likely to effect change (Miller and Rollnick 2002). An atmosphere of acceptance, hope, and support creates the foundation women need to work through challenges productively.

Collaborative approach: Leading practitioners in the field of substance abuse treatment for women suggest that effective therapeutic styles are best characterized as active, constructive, collaboratively and productively challenging, supportive, and optimistic (Covington and Surrey 1997; Finkelstein 1993, 1996; Miller and Rollnick 1991). Effective therapeutic styles focus on treatment goals that are important to the client. This may mean addressing issues of food, housing, or transportation first. Having her primary needs met builds a woman's trust and allows her to address her substance use. A collaborative, supportive approach builds on the client's strengths, encourages her to use her strengths, and increases her confidence in her ability to identify and resolve problems.

Effective therapeutic styles facilitate the client's awareness of the difference between the way her life is now and the way she wants it to be. The client and counselor agree to work together to identify the client's distortions in thinking—discrepancies between what is important to her and how her behavior and coping mechanisms prevent her from reaching her goals. Approaching treatment as a collaboration between equal partners—where the therapist is the expert on what has helped other people and the client is the expert on what will work for herself—may reduce the client's resistance to change.

Type of treatment services

Same-sex versus mix-gender groups: While literature (Grella 1999; Gutierres and Todd 1997; Niv and Hser 2007; Roberts and Nishimoto 1996; Zilberman et al. 2003) generally supports same-sex groups as being more beneficial than mix-gender groups for women, most research surrounding this issue is either too small to generalize, fails to control for other factors that may influence results, or falls short in matching and evaluating same-sex and mix-gender groups using comparable services and program lengths. Inconsistent results are evident when comparing retention and outcome rates between both groups (Kaskutas et al. 2005). Historically, research has not controlled for the confounding variable that female-only groups provide more gender-responsive services than mix-gender groups. These enhanced services may be more responsible for retention and outcome than the gender constellation of treatment. In one study comparing women in a female-only program to a mix-gender group, the author concluded that just placing women in a same-sex group without women-specific treatment services is not effective in improving retention or outcome (Bride 2001).

More rigorous studies are needed to clarify factors. Several qualitative studies (Grosenick and Hatmaker 2000; Nelson-Zlupko et al. 1996; Ravndal and Vaglum 1994) have highlighted that women perceive same-sex or female-only groups as more beneficial than mix-gender groups

Note to Clinicians

While women may perceive female-only groups as beneficial, it is important for clinicians to prepare for and recognize that some women may express hostility toward other women in the group or treatment program. Women are as likely to impose the same societal gender stereotypes that they experience onto other women in the group (Cowan and Ullman 2006). Some women may see other women as a threat to their relationships and engage in competitive behavior in the group process, and other women may impose and project their internalized negative stereotypes onto other group members; e.g., blaming a woman who was victimized by violence or making assumptions about, calling attention to, or labeling another woman's sexual behavior.

because they provide the women more freedom to talk about difficult topics such as abuse and relationship issues and to focus on themselves rather than on the men in the group. TIP 41 *Substance Abuse Treatment: Group Therapy* (CSAT 2005d), provides more information on treatment issues and process using group therapy.

Service delivery: Women who have access to various services in one location appear to have higher retention rates (McMurtrie et al. 1999; Volpicelli et al. 2000). In addition, studies support that women who are involved in or initially receive greater intensive care, specifically residential treatment, are more likely to remain in treatment and in continuing care (Coughey et al. 1998; Strantz and Welch 1995). Retention is also heightened when treatment services also include individual counseling for women (Nelson-Zlupko et al. 1996).

Onsite child care and child services: In two randomized studies (Hughes et al. 1995; Stevens and Patton 1998) comparing women in residential programs whose children stayed with them versus women whose children did not stay with them, women whose children stayed with them had a longer length of stay (retention). Other less rigorous studies provide similar results (Ashley et al. 2004; Metsch et al. 2001; Nelson-Zlupko et al. 1996; Wobie et al. 1997). For more information on children in residential treatment programs, see chapter 5, "Treatment Engagement, Placement, and Planning."

Therapeutic alliance and counselor characteristics

Although the relationship with the counselor is important to both men and women, each gender defines this connection differently. When women and men were asked what was important about the quality of their therapeutic relationships and their recovery from substance abuse, most women answered trust and warmth, and most men answered a utilitarian problemsolving approach (Fiorentine and Anglin 1997). Across studies, women have identified several counselor characteristics they believe contribute to treatment success: non-authoritarian attitudes and approach, confidence and faith in their abilities, and projection of acceptance and care (Sun 2006). Overall, the therapeutic alliance appears to play a paramount role in predicting posttreatment outcome (Gehart and Lyle 2001; Joe et al. 2001; Miller et al. 1997).

Staff gender: Research on the impact of gender differences in client–counselor relationships is limited across mental health professions and is nearly non-existent in the substance abuse field. Although women show greater preference for female staff in addiction treatment, further research is needed in examining the role of gender in treatment retention and outcome among women in individual versus group counseling, same-sex versus mix-gender groups and treatment programs, and women at different levels of substance abuse treatment. In a study that examined how clients in inpatient substance abuse treatment would view their ideal male and female counselor, gender was not considered an important variable even

Implications for the Male Counselor

"Men may need to pay particular attention to certain issues when counseling women. The issues of anger, autonomy, power, and stereotypical roles have great impact on women clients and are extremely important issues for women in therapy. For some women, because of previous dependence on men, their emotional responses to anger are more likely to be repressed and viewed as unacceptable. For other women, autonomy and power are often seen as masculine traits and inappropriate for women. Men's greater, or perhaps different, familiarity with anger, autonomy, and power can potentially provide therapeutic benefit for their women clients" (DeVoe 1990, p. 33).

Improving Transitions and Retention Rates for Women

Programs that maintain relationships or connections with women throughout their treatment and during step-down transitions from more intensive to less intensive treatment appear paramount in maintaining high levels of retention. Using supportive telephone calls between residential and outpatient addiction treatment is an effective strategy for women. Women are more likely than men to attend continuing care if a telephone intervention is implemented (Carter et al. 2008). In addition, women are more likely to stay in treatment during transitions to less intensive levels of care if it is the same treatment agency (Scott-Lennox et al. 2000).

though the majority of clients preferred a female therapist (Jonker et al. 2000). Prior research on therapist preference in counseling highlighted that nearly 95 percent of women who expressed a preference specified a female counselor (Stamler et al. 1991). Grosenick and Hatmaker (2000) reported that 82 percent of the women and treatment staff in a residential program treating pregnant women and women with children believed it was important to have female staff, while 38 percent of the clients and 46 percent of the staff sample asserted that male staff were important. For those who endorsed the importance of male staff, they indicated that men serve as male role models for children and provide a male perspective on various clinical issues, such as relationships.

In a study that examined the influence of both client–counselor race and gender composition in treatment retention among African-American clients in intensive outpatient groups (Sterling et al. 1998), no significant gender differences were found. Nonetheless, several trends were evident. Female clients treated by female counselors stayed in treatment 5 days longer than mix-matched gender groups (mix-matched refers to clients being matched to counselors of the opposite sex), and women in gender-matched groups at discharge were more likely to continue outpatient care. The authors suggested that different results may have transpired if they had examined the role of gender and race in client–counselor relationships in individual substance abuse counseling versus group therapy. Research focused specifically on client–counselor race and gender composition in women's treatment is lacking.

Client's confidence in the process

A woman's successful experience in other life areas and her level of confidence in the treatment process appear important to staying in treatment. Kelly, Blacksin, and Mason (2001) compared two groups of women—a group that completed treatment and another group that did not—to ascertain factors affecting substance abuse treatment completion. They found that women who had prior successes were more apt to complete treatment. While self-efficacy may play an important role, methodological issues and other factors may be as responsible for the study's results, namely the limited economic resources in the group of non-completers. In addition, other general retention studies have highlighted the importance of the therapist's prognosis of client retention; thus the counselor's confidence may be as significant to retention as the client's confidence (Cournoyer et al. 2007). Further gender-specific retention research is needed to address the role of self-confidence and confidence in the treatment process.

Theoretical Approaches for Women

In a meta-analysis of studies on treatment approaches, Wampold (2001) attributed more than half of the effect of therapies to therapeutic alliance—a key element of all the theoretical approaches. Some approaches have significant clinical and empirical support in substance abuse treatment research literature (including motivational interviewing, cognitive–behavioral therapies, and some psychodynamic approaches), however, research highlighting the role of gender differences is in its infancy, and limited research is available that delineates gender-specific factors that contribute to the effectiveness of these therapies. Data available at the time of publication is referenced throughout this TIP. For general information on counseling theories, refer to TIP 34 *Brief Interventions and Brief Therapies for Substance Abuse* (CSAT 1999*a*); TIP 35 *Enhancing Motivation for Change in Substance Abuse Treatment* (CSAT 1999*b*); and TIP 47 *Substance Abuse: Clinical Issues in Intensive Outpatient Treatment* (provides an overview of counseling theories; CSAT 2006*c*).

Women's Treatment Issues and Needs

Relationships and the Need for Connection

Relationships are central in women's lives—as part of their identities, as sources of self-esteem, as the context for decisionmaking and choices, and as support for day-to-day living and growth (Covington and Surrey 1997; Finkelstein 1993, 1996; Miller 1984). Connections are relationships that are healthy and supportive—mutual, empowering, and emotional resources. "Disconnections" involve relationships that are not mutual and empowering: one member is dominant, there is imbalance in the give and take, or a disparity exists in emotional supportiveness. Disconnections range from feeling "unheard" or "unknown" to extreme forms of disconnection, such as sexual abuse and violence. Disconnections create major difficulties for most women, such as lowered self-esteem, feelings of powerlessness, and lack of assertiveness. The experience of relationships as connections and disconnections is a central issue in personality development, with repeated severe disconnections potentially having serious psychological and behavioral consequences.

The Influence of Family

Treatment providers should be sensitive to the relational history women bring into treatment, both positive and negative. For instance, the extended family often functions as a safety net that provides women with child care, financial support, and emotional and spiritual guidance (Balcazar and Qian 2000). However, few studies have examined the role of the extended family in the development of substance abuse and recovery. While research on the extended family tends to define its role as primarily protective, drinking and drug use in the family can contribute to the development of abuse. Many women who abuse substances were raised in families where there was chemical abuse, sexual abuse, violence, and other relational disconnections. These family relationships form a basic model for the relationships women later develop with others.

Women with a substance-using family background may develop adult relationships that mimic these broken family dynamics. Thus many women who have family members who used substances also may have a partner or friend who abuses substances. Relationships that center on substance use, or include emotionally or physically negative, harmful behavior (whether past or present), can play a significant role in enabling a woman's continuing substance use.

To assess the impact of a client's family relationships, treatment providers should explore the role of the extended family in her life and try to determine how her substance abuse has affected her relationships with family members. Counselors should also help a client to explore her current relationships outside her family in the light of her substance use. Counselors may need to work with some clients to help them understand the negative effects these relationships can have.

In addition, skills related to improving the quality of relationships—such as communication, stress management, assertiveness, problemsolving, and parenting—can be an important part of treatment. To help clients learn these skills, treatment providers can model connection with clients, provide support, help clients repair or replace hurtful or damaging relationships, and help clients "redefine" their families (Knight et al. 2001b). Family therapy is a more essential approach in substance abuse treatment for women. For more guidance in employing family therapy, refer to TIP 39 *Substance Abuse Treatment and Family Therapy* (CSAT 2004b).

If maintaining or reconnecting with extended family members is not an option, plans should be made to find alternatives in developing a support system or a "family of choice." However, the grief associated with the loss of the original family needs to be addressed. Treatment programs can help women connect with natural supports in the community—friends, work colleagues, and significant others (Knight and Simpson 1996). Developing or maintaining

---

Advice to Clinicians: Relational Model Approach

Beginning in the 1970s, a number of theorists started to examine the importance of gender differences in psychological development. Jean Baker Miller's Toward a New Psychology of Women (1976) offered a new perspective on the psychology of women that challenged the basic assumptions of traditional theories. Carol Gilligan, a developmental psychologist, gathered empirical data on fundamental gender differences in the psychological and moral development of women and men (Gilligan 1982).

Drawing on Miller's and Gilligan's work, theorists have been developing a relational model of women's psychology. The three major themes in relational theory are:

- *Cultural context.* Recognizes the powerful effect of the cultural context on women's lives.
- *Relationships.* Stresses relationships as the central organizing feature in women's development. Traditional developmental models of growth emphasize independence and autonomy. This model focuses on women's connection with others.
- *Pathways to growth.* Acknowledges women's relational qualities and activities as potential strengths that provide pathways to healthy growth and development.

The relational-cultural theory affirms the power of connection and the pain of disconnection for women, with repeated disconnections having adverse consequences for mental health (Covington and Surrey 1997; Jordon and Hartling 2002). As a result, the approach requires a paradigm shift that has led to a reframing of key concepts in psychological development, theory, and practice. For example, instead of using the "self" as the sole focus, the model focuses on relational development.

According to Miller, "Women's sense of self becomes very much organized around being able to make and then to maintain affiliations and relationships" (Miller 1984, p. 83). More than men, women find an activity more satisfying and more pleasurable when others are involved. Therefore, for women, relationships directly affect their feelings of empowerment, self-worth, and self-esteem.

Substance abuse treatment often provides a woman her first opportunity to establish new, healthy relationships—especially relationships with other women. Accordingly, counselors should help women to "examine past relationships, including issues of loss, violence, and incest; to validate and build upon [their] relational skills and needs; to learn how to parent successfully; …to let go of problematic, abusive relationships" (Finkelstein 1996, p. 28); and to confront the loss of a primary relationship with their drug of abuse (Cramer 2002).

positive relationships can improve women's self-esteem and increase their feelings of self-efficacy (Finkelstein et al. 1997). Further, a high degree of social support is positively related to better treatment outcomes (Laudet et al. 1999).

Partner Relationships

Many women drink and use substances to maintain relationships and cope with the pain and trauma of lost relationships. Some women feel they are expected to maintain relationships at all costs, even if those relationships are undermining, abusive, or otherwise detrimental. Women may stay in harmful relationships because of economic or social dependence. Treatment providers sometimes unknowingly reinforce this expectation by focusing on the importance of relationships to the exclusion of helping their clients increase their feelings of autonomy, healthy solitude, and individuality—also important needs for women.

Once a woman's significant relationships have been examined relative to her substance use, the counselor and client can work together on a plan for reconnecting with significant others during recovery (if possible). Yet, engaging a partner in a woman's treatment can be challenging, especially in balancing issues of the woman's and her partner's needs, safety concerns, and lack of funding for partner and family services. Few models within women's treatment programs exist that include partners and other family members, and even fewer address lesbian partners. Price and Simmel (2002) provide an overview of the issues surrounding a partner's influence on a woman's addiction and recovery and examples of model programs. They recommend starting with a thorough assessment after a woman has identified her partner(s) and given permission to involve the partner in treatment.

As women become healthy through participating in treatment and developing appropriate relationships, and as other supports (e.g., financial, housing) are put in place, it is hoped they will choose to reevaluate relationships that are detrimental to their well-being and recovery. When women decide to end significant relationships, counselors should realize that ending these significant relationships is a real loss that must be mourned while new attachments are being created. However, some women often choose to continue to participate in, or may be unable to escape, destructive relationships.

Tolerating or accepting a client's relationships that the counselor finds objectionable is complicated because a woman's substance abuse frequently is maintained in connection with her partner (Amaro and Hardy-Fanta 1995), and maintaining this relationship can increase her risk of relapse. Thus, any relationship that enables a woman to continue to abuse substances or threatens her safety becomes a therapeutic issue between a counselor and a female client. The counselor should acknowledge a woman's feelings about that relationship, regardless of the counselor's opinion about what is best for the client. However, if a client is in danger of being victimized, the counselor should primarily be focused on ensuring her safety. Initially, staff should take immediate measures to increase physical safety in the treatment environment—in both outpatient and inpatient settings. In addition to validating her experience, it is important to help facilitate a safety plan that may necessitate additional referrals to domestic violence hotlines and shelters. To review a sample personalized safety plan for domestic violence, refer to Appendix D in TIP 25 *Substance Abuse Treatment and Domestic Violence* (CSAT 1997b).

Safety issues for the client or her children may preclude the partner's involvement. If the client does not feel safe involving her partner, the emphasis should change to safety planning.

Several curricula focus on a woman's relationships in recovery and help her identify, assess, and evaluate both destructive and empowering relationships and support systems. Covington's curriculum, *Helping Women Recover* (2008a, 1999a), allows women to examine their relationships and support systems. Najavits' *Seeking Safety* (2002a) and *Woman's Addiction Workbook* (2002) include information that assists women in understanding healthy and unhealthy boundaries, strategies

Advice to Clinicians:
Considerations in Involving the Partner in Treatment

In deciding whether or not to involve a woman's partner in treatment, primary consideration should be given to her safety and to the partner's willingness to participate in treatment. The following important issues should also be assessed to determine participation and level of treatment involvement and to establish an appropriate treatment plan:

- **History of violence:** Has there been a history of violence in the relationship, including threats and other emotional, physical, and/or sexual abuse; protection orders; police reports; or citations for domestic violence or assaults? Is there a history of impulsivity with client or partner? Has there been a history of violence outside the relationship, in previous relationships, or with children? Is there a recognizable progression of violence in the relationship?

- **History of substance use in the relationship:** How influential has this partner been regarding the client's continued drug and alcohol use? Does the partner see the woman's alcohol and/or drug use as a problem needing treatment? Has the history of the relationship been centered upon using or providing drugs and alcohol? How often are alcohol and other drugs used when engaged in activities with each other or during sexual intimacy? Is the client or partner worried about having sex without being under the influence of substances? Has the client left prior treatment experiences prematurely due to this relationship? Is the client worried that her partner is going to leave either as a result of her use or of her treatment? Does the client acknowledge that her use has impacted the relationship? Is she able to describe how her substance use has affected the relationship?

- **Partner's history of substance use:** What is the partner's attitude toward alcohol and drug use? Does he/she use as well? Is he/she in recovery? Has the partner been arrested, charged, or convicted of alcohol or drug related offenses? Does the client minimize the influence of her partner's current drug and alcohol use?

- **Accessibility:** Does the partner have the financial resources and transportation to attend treatment? Are there potential barriers that limit physical attendance, such as distance from program, transportation, work schedule, financial resources, childcare responsibilities?

- **History of mental illness:** Are there any known mental health issues with the partner or client that have or will impact the relationship?

- **Relationship support of the partner:** Has the partner been emotionally supportive throughout the history of the relationship? Currently, how emotionally supportive is the partner regarding the client's treatment and recovery? Does the partner play an essential role in childcare? Does the partner provide financial support? Has the partner ever threatened to leave, withdraw financial support, or threaten the custody of the children?

- **Commitment to relationship:** Is there a current commitment to maintaining the relationship?

for identifying persons who can be positive (supportive) or negative (destructive) influences on their recovery, tactics for enhancing or minimizing those influences, and activities to enhance support from other women. Cohen's *Counseling Addicted Women: A Practical Guide* (2000) provides client and staff activities surrounding relationship issues.

Sexuality

Healthy sexuality is integral to one's sense of self-worth. Sexuality represents the integration of biological, emotional, social, and spiritual aspects of who one is and how one relates to others. If healthy sexuality is defined as the integration of all these aspects of the self, it is apparent how substance abuse can have an impact on every area of a woman's sexuality. In addition, sexuality is one of the primary areas that women say change the most between substance abuse or dependence and recovery and is a major trigger for relapse (Covington 2008a, 1999a, 2007).

Women and men are socialized into different gender roles. For example, many men are taught to seem knowledgeable about sex and be comfortable with their bodies. In contrast, women struggle more with body image and are socialized to be less assertive sexually or risk being labeled as promiscuous. This polarization of sex roles is mirrored in society's belief about male and female substance use. Women who use substances are perceived as being more eager for sex and more vulnerable to seduction (George et al. 1988). This is reflected in the stronger stigma against women with substance use disorders, which is often expressed in sexual terms and labels women as promiscuous or sexually loose. Sexual terms are rarely used to describe men with substance use disorders.

Recovery and healing goes beyond abstinence from alcohol or drugs to developing relationships with others. Many women will need to explore the connections between substance abuse and sexuality, body image, sexual identity, sexual abuse, and the fear of sex when they are alcohol and drug free. Therefore, the consensus panel believes that discussion of women's sexual issues is an important part of substance abuse treatment. The following are some of the sexual concerns that women report during early recovery:

- *Sexual identity*. Counselors may need to help a woman determine her sexual identity as a heterosexual, lesbian, or bisexual person. Substance abuse during adolescence can interrupt the healthy development of sexual identity. Circumstances such as prostitution or incarceration may lead women to participate in sexual activity with other women. Some women use drugs to suppress their sexual feelings toward other women. Others use drugs to act on their erotic attachment to other women and may feel confused about their sexual identity when in recovery. Once the substance of abuse has been removed from a woman's life, the counselor can help her discover whether her identity is heterosexual, lesbian, or bisexual (Covington 1997). For review of sexual identity stages of development and its relationship to substance abuse, see *A Provider's Introduction to Substance Abuse Treatment for Lesbian, Gay, Bisexual, and Transgender Individuals* (CSAT 2001b, pp. 61–67).
- *Fear of sex while abstinent*. Many women enter treatment with little or no experience of sexual relationships without being under the influence of substances. For women with a history of sexual trauma, using alcohol and drugs to manage emotions while having sex may have served as an important coping mechanism. Subsequently, women may become fearful of having sex without the assistance of substances (Covington 2000,

Clinical Activity:
Exploring the History and Influence of Relationships: Sociogram

Using a simple diagram (referred to as a sociogram) that was pioneered by J. L. Moreno in the 1940s, clients can highlight their most influential female and/or male relationships (including positive and negative attributes). Starting with this diagram, counselors can use this activity as a foundation to help women explore how these relationships influence current relationship patterns, preference for male or female friends, attitudes toward other women and/or men, and the development of support systems.

Depending on your goal, you can have the client focus only on the men or women who have been most influential in their lives. Generally, the exercise provides more clarity for the client if you focus on only one gender at a time. Yet, your selection depends on your treatment goal, the client's current struggles, and previous relationship history. If the woman is having a difficult time connecting with other women in treatment, it may be helpful to start with a history of her female relationships. Even though there are other ingredients that influence how a woman relates to and views other women (namely gender socialization), a sociogram that begins with the history of female relationships may enhance awareness of the issues that impede her ability to relate to other women. At other times, it may be more fruitful to focus on the history of male relationships with women due to clinical issues that involve men. Here are directions and a sample of a sociogram on female relationships:

Provide the client with a piece of paper and a pencil, and ask her to list the most influential females throughout her life. The list should include women who have had the most significant impact—both positive and negative. It should not be limited to family members, but instead include women throughout her lifespan up to the present day. The list should consist of women who have had a powerful influence even if the encounter was brief. You could ask her to limit the list to six to eight women for this exercise. She can always go back and add individuals later on.

After compiling this list (it takes about 3 to 5 minutes), have the client turn the page over and draw a circle (about the size of a quarter) in the middle of the page and have her place her own name within the circle. Referring back to her list of influential women, ask the client to draw a circle for each influential woman on the piece of paper and to place the circles in reference to how influential they have been in her life—placing the most influential women closer to her circle and other women with less influence farther away on the page. The circle can be placed anywhere on the paper. For example, if you have a client with a physically abusive mother and the client feels that this history prevented her from trusting other women, she may place the circle, labeled "Mother" quite close to her circle.

After instructing the client to draw and place the circles on the page so that the placement represents how influential or how much she believes this relationship affected her, ask the client to go back and list three things in each circle that she learned about other women based on each specific relationship. For example, you may say to the client, "What did you learn about women based on your relationship with your mother and how your mother was with you? Select three things and write them in the circle that is labeled 'Mother.'"

Upon completion, have the client present her sociogram. This exercise works quite well in a women's group and in individual counseling. In group, it promotes a dynamic discussion on how women learn to relate to each other, and it creates an opportunity to understand how each client's history of female relationships can influence current relationships in treatment and recovery. As a counselor, you can promote further discussion by asking the following questions:

Substance Abuse Treatment for Women

Are there any themes or recurrent patterns in this sociogram?

1. How does this history influence your relationship with other women in treatment, in therapy groups, and in support groups?

2. Can you provide a specific and recent example of how your history of relationships affected or contributed to a specific situation in treatment?

Sample Sociogram Exercise: "What have I learned from each relationship about other women?"

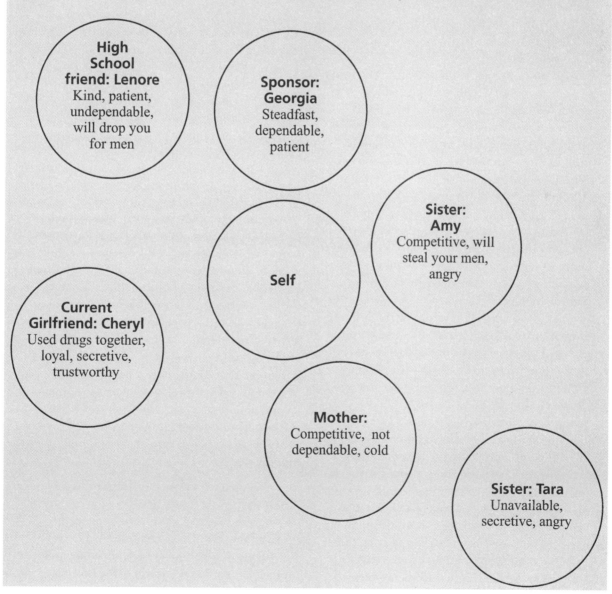

1997). Trauma survivors may view sex as taboo or hurtful and their sexual responses as bad. In addition, sexual relationships sometimes can trigger painful memories of past abuse that can create difficulties for women, particularly in early recovery (Covington 1997; Finkelstein 1996).

- *Sexual dysfunctions.* Alcohol and drugs interfere with sexual sensitivity and enjoyment in many ways. They disrupt the delicate balance of a woman's hormonal system, interfering with her body's emotional, reproductive, and physiological functions (Greenfield and O'Leary 2002). Women with substance use disorders have the same kinds of sexual dysfunctions as those without the disorder (lack of orgasm, lack of lubrication, lack of sexual interest, etc.), but they have more problems more often (Covington 2000).

- *Sexual and interpersonal violence.* Sexuality often is associated with violence and abuse for female clients with histories of trauma. Consequently, they may be fearful, angry, and distrustful, and have difficulty functioning sexually. Given the association between substance abuse and sexual abuse (Ullman et al. 2005), women who have been abused may use alcohol or drugs to numb the emotional pain of the abusive experience. This can create a spiraling relationship where many women use substances to alleviate the sexual difficulties they are experiencing. But the alcohol or drugs only exacerbate the problem. Women who are under the influence of drugs are at greater risk for sexual and physical aggression (Blume 1991; Testa et al. 2003), and this remains true with pregnant women who have substance use disorders (Velez et al. 2006).

- *Sexually transmitted diseases (STDs).* The use of alcohol and drugs increases the likelihood of contracting STDs, including HIV/AIDS. There are three primary reasons for this increased risk. When drunk or high, many women neglect to protect themselves against STDs or to make sure they do not use contaminated needles (Evans et al. 2003; Pugatch et al. 2000). Often women with substance use disorders find themselves in relationships with men who are also chemically dependent, thereby increasing the risk that their partner may have STDs or are HIV positive. In addition, rates of other infectious diseases among women with substance use disorders tend to be higher than among other female populations (CSAT 1993c; Grella et al. 1995). Notably, preliminary findings suggest that women who inject illicit drugs and have sex with other women exhibit increased HIV infection and risk behaviors in comparison to other people who use injection drugs (Young et al. 2005).

In addition to research pertaining to prevalence, counselors need to address clinical issues associated with infectious diseases. Specifically, shame and stigma are highly associated with sexually transmitted diseases and HIV infection (Fortenberry et al. 2002), and, as a result, women who are addicted and infected with a sexually transmitted disease are likely to perceive and experience a more profound sense of shame and higher levels of stigma—potentially serving as a barrier to engaging in help-seeking behavior.

Pregnancy

Pregnancy creates stress for many women. Literature suggests that this stress can come from the woman's physical discomfort; her anxiety about the health of her fetus and how she will care for her baby; or her shame from the social stigma of using drugs, alcohol, or tobacco while she is pregnant (Daley et al. 1998). Providers can create an atmosphere that supports talking freely about pregnancy and recognize that ambivalence toward pregnancy is a normal reaction. Counselors should make a careful assessment of the woman's existing parenting and other family responsibilities and of the social services and economic resources the mother needs.

Some women experience feelings of ambivalence about their pregnancy that become apparent during treatment. Educational programs, particularly for young women, that review the effects of alcohol, drug, and tobacco use on pregnant women and their fetuses may provide motivation to enter treatment, but this information will probably also generate concern over the status of their fetus. Counselors should be supportive of the client as she processes this emotionally difficult information. Counselors must understand a woman's guilt, shame, and unspoken feelings about the effects of substance use on fetal health and development. Counselors can advocate for fetal well-being but must also give the mother information that is nonjudgmental. It is important for counselors to stress that "it is never too late to stop," and that whenever pregnant women reduce or stop drug and alcohol use, benefits are obtained!

Women should be encouraged to consult with an obstetrician or geneticist regarding their concerns of prenatal exposure on the fetus. However, caution should be exercised in evaluating pregnancy outcomes based on use of alcohol, drugs, or tobacco during pregnancy and their possible effects on the newborn. It is almost impossible to make accurate predictions on neonatal outcomes. Nevertheless, a woman should have support from her substance abuse counselor to meet with her prenatal care provider to discuss these issues.

After detoxification and stabilization, counselors should offer the important message that abstinence, staying in substance abuse treatment, and prenatal care can reduce the impact of substance use on the fetus (Bolnick and Rayburn 2003). Research indicates that a positive environment is as enriching to a child's early growth and development as prenatal exposure to substances is detrimental (Frank et al. 2001; Hurt et al. 2001). After the child is born, a mother can work to create a positive environment for her child's healthy development. This approach emphasizes the recovering woman's control and self-efficacy; it is another element of empowerment for recovering women (Covington 2002a).

Parenting

A woman's relationship with her children and her identity as a mother play a vital role in her sense of self. These relationships are important in recovery from substance use disorders. The consensus panel believes that substance abuse treatment programs should offer treatment that addresses the critical component of parenting connections to children, as well as a full range of children's physical and mental health care, along with other services, whether within a treatment program itself, or by referral to a collaborating agency. Refer to chapter 5 for more specific information on programming across each level of care for women who are pregnant and/or have children.

Most mothers who are in substance abuse treatment feel a strong connection with their children and want to be good mothers. Most want to maintain or regain custody of their children and become "caring and competent parents" (Brudenell 2000, p. 86). Women who believe they have not cared for their children adequately or who believe that they are perceived as having neglected their children carry enormous guilt (Sun 2000). Therefore, for many women, maintaining caring relationships with their children is sufficient motivation to keep them in treatment. Unfortunately they often have inadequate role models in their own lives or lack the information, skills, or economic resources that could make motherhood less difficult (Camp and Finkelstein 1997; Moore and Finkelstein 2001). They also have the challenge of balancing the work necessary for recovery with their tasks as mothers. Another challenge treatment providers may face is the mother who is developmentally disabled to the extent that her mothering is inadequate. Ensuring the safety of her children while respecting the mother's choice to care for them requires careful case management to provide support for the mother.

People take from their family relationships a basic sense of their own identity and an equally basic model for the relationships they later develop with others. Mother–child relationships are understood to be the model for the child's future relationships. At the same time, because women tend to develop their sense of self through relationships, a woman's identity is also deepened when she becomes a mother. Society places a high value on a woman's ability to mother, and her own perceived success or failure in this endeavor forms an important aspect of her self-concept. For a mother with a substance use disorder, this concept can be paramount (Feinberg 1995).

Parenting programs

Research findings are inconsistent in demonstrating the effectiveness of behavioral parenting programs for improving the parent–child relationship and children's psychological adjustment among mothers who have substance use disorders (for review, see Suchman et al. 2004; Suchman et al. 2007; Velez et al. 2004). More research is needed to evaluate the most effective parenting approaches and to address research methodological issues surrounding parenting program evaluations. In general, literature appears to support combining behavioral training with attachment-based parenting interventions (relational model).

A strengths-based relational approach to parenting assumes maternal assets already exist that can be identified and built on, and that the emotional quality of the parent–child relationship is equally important in improving the parent–child relationship and psychological adjustment of the child. In essence, parenting is a relationship—not solely a set of skills. Some topics for parenting skills and relationship building include:

- Age- and developmentally appropriate behavioral expectations for children.
- Children's emotional, physical, and developmental needs.
- Parenting styles and other childrearing practices, including attachment-oriented approaches (defined as enhancing the parent's ability to accurately perceive and sensitively respond to the emotional needs reflected in their child's behavior) (Slade and Cohen 1996; Suchman et al. 2006).
- Strategies to improve nurturing that begin with helping mothers find a way to nurture themselves as an important step in learning how to nurture their children.
- Constructive discipline strategies without corporal punishment.

- Anger management strategies to assist parents in learning how they can appropriately manage their strong feelings.
- Appropriate parent–child roles including modeling opportunities.
- Integration of culturally congruent parenting practices and expectations.

Clients need time to practice these new parenting skills and change patterns of behavior to improve interactions with their children (CSAT 2000b). It is helpful to match parenting, coaching, or other support groups to the woman's ability to cope with her children and the other problems she is facing. Substance abuse counselors must simultaneously help mothers address their other ongoing challenges while teaching them to be better parents (Camp and Finkelstein 1997). Programs that provide support and parent training to mothers can also help children by building their self-esteem, supporting them educationally and emotionally, and assisting them to achieve developmental milestones.

Children affected by maternal alcohol and drug dependence have increased vulnerability for physical, social-emotional, and academic problems (Conners et al. 2004; VanDeMark et al. 2005). Moreover, analysis from SAMHSA's Women, Co-Occurring Disorders and Violence Study (WCDVS) suggests that children are also at an increased risk for physical child abuse when the mother has a current history of mental health symptoms, alcohol and drug use severity, and trauma (Rinehart et al. 2005). Thus, children need more than just adequate child care.

The consensus panel recommends that an onsite child specialist or one available by referral should be a standard element of programs that include children. Assessment and screening for developmental and learning delays and social problems is necessary, as are play and expressive therapies that help children acknowledge and express feelings about their parents' problems. Children should be provided with information regarding their mother's substance use disorder in an age-appropriate manner. Counselors can help the mother and children frankly discuss issues surrounding substance use and recovery. A staff member providing therapeutic services for children should conduct substance abuse prevention activities for children of all ages.

While a woman is learning to parent, her children need assistance to overcome the effects of her substance abuse. It is likely their mother has been emotionally and physically unavailable at times. Counselors can help children realize that their mother's behavior was unintentional and, as she regains control of her life, she will likely become more available. In addition, Alateen; psychoeducational curricula, such as the National Association for Children of Alcoholics "Celebrating Families™;" and onsite individual and group therapy can provide further support to children.

Parenting issues for women with trauma histories

A history of trauma can affect both how a woman experiences parenting and how effective she is as a parent. Factors that affect a woman's parenting include the extent of trauma history, who the abuser was, and a woman's parenting role models, as well as whether she has been involved with trauma work or has developed the skills to manage trauma memories and feelings (Melnick and Bassuk 2000). Several major parenting issues for trauma survivors can be identified:

- Many women feel shame, guilt, and self-blame, which can interfere with their emotional availability to their children. This includes a mother's self-criticism or depression when evaluating current parenting as well as her belief that she deserves blame for inadequate parenting, or feeling that her children's behavior is an attack because they had inadequate parenting.
- Interaction with a child can trigger a mother's traumatic past. This includes experiencing a child's misbehavior as a traumatic trigger, children's distress or need for bonding reminding a mother of her own vulnerabilities, and having posttraumatic

stress disorder (PTSD) symptoms triggered by normal developmental events such as breastfeeding, bathing a child, and providing sexual education to a child. Likewise, a mother may experience heightened anxiety and vigilance when one of her children reaches the same age that her own prior sexual abuse or trauma began or occurred. For example, if a client witnessed her younger brother getting shot when she was 12, she may encounter more traumatic stress symptoms as her oldest child reaches the same age as her brother.

- A mother may internalize and reenact the role of both victim and perpetrator in response to trauma. This may cause her to worry that her children will be mistreated and lead to either overprotectiveness or helplessness, a reluctance to set limits out of fear of identifying with a perpetrator.
- Female clients will need to come to terms with having been inadequately nurturing parents at times and with the complexities of providing a better relationship with their children (Melnick and Bassuk 2000).

Trauma-informed parent training assists mothers in identifying their triggers, learning appropriate boundaries and discipline, and learning nurturing behaviors so they can care for their children in healthy ways. As the mother becomes more stable, she will need to be prepared for the possibility that her children will feel safer in acting out their previous distress. Programs can prepare women in early recovery for this predictable event with information, coaching for effective parenting, and reframing the children's behavior as a signal that they feel safer and can afford to express themselves.

Children who are not in a mother's care

Regaining custody or re-establishing their role of primary caregiver can be a major motivating factor for women in treatment. Professionals at all levels of care are encouraged to support the relationship between mothers and children and to support and facilitate ongoing connections with their children in foster care or with relative caregivers. Since parent–child visiting is an essential ingredient toward reunification, substance abuse treatment providers may be able to provide supervised visits, offering an opportunity for therapeutic intervention and the mother's attention to her relationship with children not in her custody. Yet, numerous factors inhibit visitation, including the mother's health status, transportation needs, and support from others (Kovalesky 2001), and staff should be aware of these variables. Ultimately, counselors will need to help women recognize how their recovery needs can complicate meeting their children's needs and determine the pacing of reunification efforts.

Occasionally, a mother in substance abuse treatment expresses a desire not to keep her children. The woman may feel unable to be a mother or has no support in doing so, or her children have been cared for by others for a long time. In other cases, it is possible that these children were the result of rape or prostitution. Sometimes it is in the best interest of both the mother and the child(ren) for the mother to relinquish care. Counselors must be careful to allow the decision to belong to the woman, to listen to her ambivalence, and to support her regardless of her decision (CSAT 2001b).

Children with special needs

Some mothers with substance use disorders have children with special needs, possibly as a result of alcohol or drug use during pregnancy, inadequate prenatal care, poor nutrition during pregnancy, or other factors. In addition to coping with the personal guilt, mothers will find that these children demand extra care and attention and create additional stresses during recovery. Careful assessment of these children by trained professionals is essential. An educational and/or treatment plan should result from an assessment that is integrated with the mother's treatment plan. Because so many of the children who are included in treatment with their mothers have emotional or developmental problems, there is a real need for child specialists on staff (Conners et al. 2004; CSAT 2000b). A linkage to programs for children

with special needs and children with disabilities would be an asset in providing the services these children need.

History of Trauma

Trauma can result from numerous experiences, including emotional, physical, and sexual abuse, as well as assault, war, natural disasters, terrorism, and interpersonal violence that occurs between family members or with intimate partners. Women who experience or witness violence, particularly actions that threaten their lives and safety, can become traumatized by these events (Herman 1997). The *Diagnostic and Statistical Manual of Mental Disorders, 4th Edition, Text Revision* (DSM-IV-TR) defines trauma as "involving direct personal experience of an event that involves actual or threatened death or serious injury, or other threat to one's physical integrity; or witnessing an event that involves death, injury, or a threat to the physical integrity of another person; or learning about unexpected or violent death, serious harm, or threat of death or injury experienced by a family member or other close associate" (American Psychiatric Association [APA] 2000a, p. 463).

Women respond to and are affected by trauma in a variety of ways. Based on their histories, circumstances, and other factors, some women experience traumatic stress symptoms that dissipate over time, while other women are resilient to the effects of trauma and recover from it quickly (Foa and Rothbaum 1998). Some women develop psychological disorders including PTSD and other anxiety and mood disorders, and other women may use alcohol, tobacco, and drugs to cope with the trauma and its symptoms. Still others may replicate their trauma by engaging in problematic parent–child interactions, including abuse and neglect (McMahon and Luthar 1998). A family history of anxiety, early traumatic violence, and repeated exposure to trauma can predispose an individual to develop severe problems. The Adverse Childhood Experiences Study (Felitti et al. 1998) reflected a strong association between health risk behavior and disease for both adult men and women to exposure to emotional, physical, or sexual abuse, and household dysfunction during childhood.

The relationship between trauma and substance abuse

Substance abuse and victimization appear to be highly correlated; drug abuse increases the risk of violent assault, and victimization appears to increase the risk of substance abuse (El-Bassel et al. 2005; Kendler et al. 2000; Kilpatrick et al. 1997). Nevertheless, the connection between substance use and abuse and interpersonal violence often is complex, especially for women. Men who abuse substances are at high risk of committing violence against women and children. Women who use substances are more at risk for being abused because of relationships with others who abuse substances, impaired judgment while using alcohol or drugs, and being in risky and violence-prone situations (Testa et al. 2003). Survivors of abuse may become dependent on alcohol and drugs to manage trauma symptoms and reduce tension and stress from living in violent situations. Thus begins a cycle of "victimization, chemical use, retardation of emotional development, limited stress resolution, more chemical use, and heightened vulnerability to further victimization" (Dayton 2000; Steele 2000, p. 72).

A history of trauma is common in the lives of women with substance use disorders. Female survivors of sexual trauma were found, in one study, to be dependent on more substances, to have had more hospital stays and emergency department visits, and to be less able to care for their children than women who had not been sexually abused (Young and Boyd 2000). Girls who suffer physical and sexual abuse by dating partners are more likely to engage in risky behaviors such as smoking, binge drinking, and cocaine use (Silverman et al. 2001). In another study, adverse childhood circumstances predicted binge drinking among adult women (Timko 2008).

Alcohol and drug use by trauma survivors can be adaptive at first. Some victims use substances to numb psychological effects of the trauma.

Some substances help survivors dissociate the trauma from their consciousness (Herman 1997). Women who have histories of violence and trauma have a higher propensity for substance use disorders and are more likely to encounter a difficult recovery from substance use disorders. Their treatment is typically complicated because of the interrelationship between trauma and substance use, the role that substances play in managing traumatic stress symptoms, and sequelae from the experience of trauma such as depression and other psychological disorders. To obtain more specific information on the impact of trauma, traumatic stress disorders, symptoms of PTSD and associated symptoms, and treatment approaches, refer to TIP 42 *Substance Abuse Treatment for Persons With Co-Occurring Disorders* (CSAT 2005e) and the planned TIP *Substance Abuse and Trauma* (CSAT in development *h*).

Interpersonal violence

Violence dramatically affects the physical and emotional health of victims and witnesses. The United Nations defines violence against women as "any act of gender-based violence that results in, or is likely to result in, physical, sexual or psychological harm or suffering to women, including threats of such acts, coercion or arbitrary deprivation of liberty, whether occurring in public or in private life" (United Nations General Assembly 1993, p. 2). The National Violence Against Women Survey (Tjaden and Thoennes 1998; 2000; 2006), conducted in 1996, estimated that in the year before the survey, almost 2 million women were physically assaulted and more than 300,000 women experienced a completed or attempted rape. Estimates of lifetime incidence increased to more than 50 million women who were physically assaulted and almost 20 million who experienced rape or attempted rape. Moreover, sociologists have commented that this level of violence has created a culture of fear for many women, observing that women feel they need to be alert and aware of their surroundings to protect themselves against assault and rape (Gordon and Riger 1989).

Women are more likely to become victims of intimate partner abuse (Catalano 2007), and men and women become victims of interpersonal violence under different circumstances. Women often experience violence in the privacy of their home (Catalano 2007; Covington 2002a; Tjaden and Thoennes 2006). Both boys and girls are at risk for physical and sexual abuse by parents and people they know, but this risk changes over the course of life. As girls move into adolescence and adulthood, they continue to be at risk for interpersonal violence. Often their abuser is someone with whom they have a relationship. For example, about one in five high school girls reportedly has suffered sexual or physical abuse from a boyfriend (Ackard and Neumark-Sztainer 2003; Silverman et al. 2001, 2004). For an overview of violence and women, see Figure 7-1.

Violence and abuse also occur in lesbian relationships. While research is limited, studies reviewed by Renzetti (1993) have indicated that lesbians experience partner violence at about the same rate as heterosexual women. As is the case with violence in heterosexual relationships, alcohol consumption often is part of the battering (Schilit et al. 1990). In comparing the prevalence of domestic violence between homosexual males and females, the National Coalition of Anti-Violence Programs (2007) reports there are no overall differences.

Childhood sexual and physical abuse

A history of childhood sexual or physical abuse (or both) is a significant risk factor for the development of a substance use disorder (Evans and Sullivan 1995). Two models help explain this—the distress coping model and the emotion regulation model. It is likely that substances not only serve as means of coping with negative emotions generated by childhood abuse, but

Figure 7-1
Violence and Women

- The strongest risk factor for being a victim of intimate partner violence is being female.
- One of every six women has been forcibly raped at some time in her life, and women are as likely to be raped as adults as they are as minors.
- While women are at a significantly greater risk in comparison to men of being raped by all types of offenders, 43 percent of all female victims were raped by either a current or former intimate partner.
- Between 25 and 50 percent of women will be abused by male partners during their lifetime.
- Women are injured as a result of domestic violence about 13 times more frequently than men.
- Women with fewer resources or greater perceived vulnerability—girls and those experiencing physical or psychiatric disabilities or living below the poverty line—are at even greater risk for domestic violence and lifetime abuse.
- Interpersonal violence is characterized by a pattern of physical, sexual, or psychological abuse. The most common pattern in domestic violence is escalation in frequency and severity over time.
- When women are violent toward family members, it often is in self-defense.
- A history of intrafamilial violence may be the most influential risk factor for a woman's abuse of substances.
- Violence in the media significantly affects attitudes and behaviors related to violence. It increases fear and mistrust, desensitizes people to violence, and glamorizes risk-taking behaviors and violence.

Source: American Psychological Association 1996; Brownridge 2006; Tjaden and Thoennes 2006

in regulating emotions by enhancing positive feelings (Grayson and Nolen-Hoeksema 2005; Simpson 2003; Ullman et al. 2005).

A study of 1,411 women born between 1934 and 1974 found that women who experienced any type of sexual abuse in childhood were more likely than those who were not abused to report drug or alcohol dependence as adults. In fact, childhood sexual abuse was associated more strongly with drug or alcohol dependence than with any other psychiatric disorder. This study is based on data from women in the general population, as opposed to clinical studies of women in treatment (Kendler et al. 2000).

Clinical studies have documented that up to 75 percent of women in substance abuse treatment have a history of physical and/or sexual abuse (Ouimette et al. 2000; Teusch 1997). Earlier studies have shown that women who abuse substances are estimated to have a 30- to 59-percent rate of current PTSD (Najavits et al. 1998), which is higher than the rate in men who abuse substances (CSAT 2005a). A history of sexual and/or physical abuse puts women at risk for psychiatric hospitalization (Carmen 1995), depression (Herman 1997; Ross-Durow and Boyd 2000), eating disorders (Curtis et al. 2005; Janes 1994; Miller 1994; Smolak and Murnen 2001), and self-inflicted injury (Dallam 1997; Haswell and Graham 1996; Miller and Guidry 2001). See also TIP 36 *Substance Abuse Treatment for Persons With Child Abuse and Neglect Issues* (CSAT 2000b).

Co-Occurring Disorders

When working with women with co-occurring mental and substance use disorders, substance abuse treatment counselors need to apply the tools of the mental health professional, especially in knowing when and where to refer clients with co-occurring disorders. Substance abuse treatment providers do not necessarily have to be trained as mental health professionals, but making appropriate referrals and coordinating the services needed by these clients requires a solid grasp of the differences in treatments, role of medications, and available resources. The following section provides an overview of co-occurring issues and highlights

three disorders that are prevalent in substance abuse treatment among women. For more in-depth coverage of treatment for those with co-occurring substance use and mental disorders, review TIP 42 *Substance Abuse Treatment for Persons With Co-Occurring Disorders* (CSAT 2005e).

An overview of issues

Both the substance abuse and mental health care fields understand that clients can enter treatment with issues they perceive as interwoven, whether or not the services themselves are. To address the dilemmas facing the people they serve, mental health, substance abuse, and trauma services are opening a dialog with one another, paving the way toward providing an appropriate, integrated system of care for each client in every system.

An integrated care framework provides assessment and treatment wherever the woman enters the treatment system, ensures necessary consultation for her issues when a given individual or program does not have the necessary expertise, and encourages all counselors and programs to develop competence in addressing co-occurring disorders. When women are assessed at a facility that does not have all the services they need, staff members at that facility are responsible for ensuring that the women are assessed at other appropriate facilities. Too often, services may over- or under-treat one of the disorders (Miller 1994a). Staff members also are responsible for following up with the cooperating facility to ensure that clients receive proper care.

The need for ongoing evaluation of co-occurring disorders is critical because both substance abuse and substance withdrawal can mimic or mask co-occurring psychiatric disorders. The client's internal turmoil can result in overwhelming affect and chaotic behavior that creates heavy demands for providers. Women with co-occurring substance use and mental disorders are likely to have PTSD, other anxiety disorders, depression, or eating disorders (particularly bulimia). While women are also more willing to identify social and psychiatric problems, they appear to have more difficulty in acknowledging problems with substance use (Mangrum et al. 2006). Treatment services that provide an integrated system of care can naturally assist women in exploring the interaction and impact of substances and mental health without supporting or reinforcing the polarization of each disorder that can arise when one disorder is easier to acknowledge by the client.

Co-occurring mental and substance use disorders often result in poor psychosocial functioning, health problems, medication noncompliance, relapse, hospitalizations, homelessness, and suicidal behavior (Reed and Mowbray 1999). Co-occurring disorders are associated with poorer treatment outcomes for women with substance use disorders and contribute to high rates of treatment dropout (Bernstein 2000). Among women in the child welfare system, the prevalence of co-occurring disorders is high and the need for services is paramount. More often than not, mothers' co-occurring disorders interfere with the likelihood of family reunification—especially if there are numerous needs, such as vocational, housing, and mental health services (Choi and Ryan 2007). Thus, appropriate referrals and case management are needed to retain these clients in substance abuse treatment and to afford the best possible outcome for women and their children.

Pregnant women and co-occurring mental illness

Pregnancy can aggravate the symptoms of co-occurring mental illness. This can be a result of the hormonal changes and stresses that occur during pregnancy, some medications given during pregnancy or delivery, the stresses of labor and delivery, the challenges and hormonal changes with lactation, and adjusting to and bonding with a newborn (Grella 1997). Women with co-occurring disorders sometimes avoid early prenatal care, have difficulty complying with healthcare providers' instructions, and are unable to plan for their babies or care for them when they arrive. According to the literature, women with anxiety disorders or personality disorders have a greater risk of postpartum depression (Grella 1997), and mood disorders affect treatment outcome among pregnant women who are drug dependent (Fitzsimons et al. 2007). More outcome research is needed to evaluate the role of co-occurring disorders among pregnant women and the impact of treatment for co-occurring disorders on prenatal and postnatal care.

It is important to remember that women can become depressed not only after childbirth but during pregnancy. According to the National Women's Health Information Center (HHS

Advice to Clinicians:
Women With Co-Occurring Disorders

- Provide women who have co-occurring disorders with comprehensive coordinated services using an integrated treatment model.
- Screen and assess for trauma as a standard practice for women in treatment for substance use disorders.
- View services as long term, suggesting a range of continuing care services and peer support, such as 12-Step programs, group therapy, or women's support groups.
- Maintain regular contact with clients and advocate for them; adapt case management models that promote regular contact with clients.
- Attend to a client's reaction to medication and compliance, particularly when a woman is treated for psychiatric illnesses. Learn about medications effective for anxiety, depression, and other mental disorders; their safety profile, side effects, and possibilities for cross-addiction; and length of time needed for symptoms to decrease.
- Offer encouragement to women with co-occurring disorders and reward them for gains made in treatment to help them establish a stronger sense of self-worth.

Source: DiNitto and Crisp 2002.

Postpartum Depression: An Under-Diagnosed Disorder

According to the DSM-IV-TR (APA 2000*a*), postpartum depression begins within 4 weeks after delivery. Episodes occurring after this period are considered "ordinary" depression. Risk factors for postpartum depression include a history of depression, psychological distress or psychiatric diagnosis before or during pregnancy, or a family history of psychiatric disorders (Nielsen Forman et al. 2000; Steiner 2002; Webster et al. 2000). Prospects for recovery from postpartum depression are good with supportive psychological counseling accompanied as needed by pharmacological therapy (Chabrol et al. 2002; Cohen et al. 2001; O'Hara et al. 2000). Antidepressants, anxiolytic medications, and even electroconvulsive therapy have all been successful in treating postpartum depression (Griffiths et al. 1989; Oates 1989; Varan et al. 1985). (Note that some medications pass into breast milk and can cause infant sedation.) Patients with postpartum depression need to be monitored for thoughts of suicide, infanticide, and progression of psychosis in addition to their response to treatment.

The term "postpartum depression" encompasses at least three different entities:

- Postpartum or maternity "blues," which affects up to 85 percent of new mothers
- Postpartum depression, which affects between 10 and 15 percent of new mothers
- Postpartum psychosis, which develops following about one per 500–1,000 births, according to some studies (Steiner 1998)

Postpartum blues is temporary depression occurring most commonly within 3–10 days after delivery and may be caused by progesterone withdrawal (Harris et al. 1994), a woman's emotional letdown that follows the excitement and fears of pregnancy and delivery, the discomforts of the period immediately after giving birth, fatigue from loss of sleep during labor and while hospitalized, energy expenditure at labor, anxieties about her ability to care for her child at home, and fears that she may be unattractive to her partner. Anticipation and preventive reassurance throughout pregnancy can prevent postpartum blues from becoming a problem. Women with sleep deprivation should be assisted in getting proper rest. Symptoms include weepiness, insomnia, depression, anxiety, poor concentration, moodiness, and irritability. These symptoms tend to be mild and fleeting, and women usually recover completely with rest and reassurance. Followup care should ensure that the woman is making sufficient progress and not heading toward a relapse to substance abuse.

Postpartum depression is a more severe case of the postpartum blues that does not go away after a few days. Beyond the temporary weepiness, irritability, and emotional letdown that follows delivery, postpartum depression involves a longer-term experience of despair, discouragement, guilt, self-reproach, and withdrawal from social contact. In many ways, postpartum depression resembles the grief and mourning that follows bereavement. Women may also lose their appetite and thus also lose weight, experience insomnia and severe mood swings, and have trouble coping with simple daily tasks, including the care of their newborns.

Postpartum psychosis is a severe mental disorder. Women with this disorder lose touch with reality and may have delusions, hallucinations, and/or disorganized speech or behavior. Women most likely to be diagnosed with postpartum psychosis are those with previous diagnoses of bipolar disorder, schizophrenia, or schizoaffective disorder, or women who had a major depression in the year preceding birth (Kumar et al. 2003). Other studies reviewed by Marks and colleagues (1991) indicate that other risk factors for postpartum psychosis include previous depressive illness or postpartum psychosis, first pregnancy, and family history of mental illness. Recurrence of postpartum psychosis in the next pregnancy occurs in 30–50 percent of women (APA 2000*a*). Peak onset is 10–14 days after delivery but can occur any time within 6 months. In most cases, the severity of the symptoms mandates pharmacological treatment and sometimes hospitalization. The risk of self-harm and/or infanticide is widely reported and monitoring of mother–infant by trained personnel can limit these occurrences.

2009), several factors increase a woman's chance of depression prior to delivery: minimal support from family and friends, a history of depression or substance abuse, a family history of mental illness; anxiety about the condition of the fetus, problems with previous pregnancies or birth(s), relational or financial problems, and age of mother (younger women).

Many pregnant women with co-occurring disorders are distrustful of substance abuse and mental health treatment providers, yet they are in need of multiple services (Grella 1997). One concern is whether the mother can care adequately for her newborn. For her to do so requires family-centered, coordinated efforts from such caregivers as social workers, child welfare professionals, and the foster care system. It is particularly important to make careful treatment plans for women with mental health problems that include planning for childbirth and infant care. Women are often concerned about the effect of their medications on their fetuses. The consensus panel believes that treatment programs should work to maintain a client's medical and psychological stability during her pregnancy and collaborate with other healthcare providers to ensure that treatment is coordinated. Providers also need to allow for evaluation over time for women with co-occurring disorders. Re-assessments should occur as they progress through treatment.

Anxiety Disorders

Anxiety disorders encompass physiological sensations of nervousness and tension, psychological worry characterized often by apprehension and rumination, and behavioral patterns of avoidance linked to the perceived source of anxiety. Some anxiety disorders have stronger familial ties than others. Anxiety disorders can develop without an identified stressor or event or by exposure to acute or prolonged stress, (such as a traumatic event or a chronic condition such as living with poverty, in a dysfunctional family system, or as a result of migration and acculturation). PTSD, panic disorders, agoraphobia without panic, simple phobia, and generalized anxiety disorder are more common among women than among men (APA 2000a; Kessler et al. 1994; NIMH 2007). Among individuals with substance use disorders, traumatic stress reactions and PTSD are quite prevalent among women. As a result, this section will primarily focus on PTSD starting with a brief overview of treatment considerations for women with anxiety disorders. For more detailed information regarding anxiety disorders and trauma, refer to TIP 42 *Substance Abuse Treatment for Persons With Co-Occurring Disorders* (CSAT 2005e) and the planned TIP *Substance Abuse and Trauma* (CSAT in development h).

General treatment considerations for anxiety disorders

Women with anxiety disorders often seek medical help for physical (somatic) complaints such as fatigue, trembling, palpitations, sweating, irritability, sleeping problems, eating problems, irritable bowel syndrome, chronic pain, or dizziness. The symptoms of substance use and anxiety disorders are easily confused; therefore, abstinence must be established before a woman in substance abuse treatment is diagnosed with anxiety disorder. However, this does not preclude providers from working with

Note to Clinicians

It is important to remember that women can become depressed not only after childbirth but during pregnancy. According to the National Women's Health Information Center (HHS 2009), several factors increase a woman's chance of depression prior to delivery: minimal support from family and friends, a history of depression or substance abuse, a family history of mental illness; anxiety about the condition of the fetus, problems with previous pregnancies or birth(s), relational or financial problems, and age of mother (younger women).

Substance Abuse Treatment for Women

women to develop coping skills and strategies to manage the symptoms of anxiety.

Cognitive–behavioral therapies (CBT) are effective treatments for anxiety disorders (Hofmann and Smits 2008) including, but not limited to, stress inoculation and other anxiety management strategies, desensitization processes, and imaginal and in-vivo (live reenactments) exposure therapies. Nonetheless, other types of therapy that address the underlying stress-producing events may be required (Frank et al. 1998). Clinical experience indicates that women with anxiety disorders and substance use problems may benefit from alternative therapies as an adjunct to CBT, including acupuncture, exercise, and mindfulness meditation. One study indicated that socially phobic female outpatients being treated for alcohol dependence had better outcomes with CBT than with 12-Step facilitation therapy (Thevos et al. 2000).

Benzodiazepines, which are commonly prescribed for anxiety disorders, can also be addictive and thus present a major problem for women with a substance use disorder. Providers may prescribe sedating antidepressants or selective serotonin reuptake inhibitors (SSRIs; Zweben 1996) instead. Newer nonaddicting medications, both SSRIs and non-SSRIs, are being prescribed as anti-anxiety agents (NIMH 2007). Other options include anticonvulsants, antihypertensive agents, and newer neuroleptic medications.

PTSD

Although some type of trauma has been experienced by many women who use substances, not all women who have been traumatized will develop PTSD. An anxiety disorder, PTSD may involve other anxiety symptoms including panic attacks and avoidance (Brady et al. 2000). Refer to Appendix E for DSM-IV-TR criteria for PTSD. For those women who have PTSD, their symptoms will involve persistent re-experiencing of trauma-related events, avoidance of trauma-related material, and arousal (APA 2000a; Refer to Figure 7-2, p. 162, for PTSD symptom clusters). In addition, they will present other associated symptoms, such as depression and sleep disturbance. Subsequent to a heightened state of arousal, many women report significant sleep difficulties characterized by nightmares, trouble falling sleep, frequent awakenings or problems in staying asleep, and apprehension in going to sleep. Among women with a history of sexual assault and PTSD, sleep difficulties have been noted as a significant motive to drink (Nishith et al. 2001).

Along with the physiological and psychological symptoms that so often characterize PTSD, the experience of trauma can impact core assumptions and beliefs about self, others, and life (for review, see Janoff-Bulman 1992). One study (Hall 2000) demonstrated that the severity of the effects of trauma is evident in two core beliefs identified by survivors of childhood abuse who are in recovery: "I am nothing" (feeling inconsequential) and "I am bad or wrong." In addition to the abuse or trauma itself, experiences that lead to feeling inconsequential include being unprotected from danger, telling someone about the abuse but not being believed, being told lies to conceal the abuse, and being unprepared for life transitions. This can lead to shutting down emotions and social isolation (Boyd and Mackey 2000a; Hall 2000). The perpetrator may have put the blame on them ("you asked for it").

Treatment of PTSD

Unlike other memories, memories of traumatic events may seem to have vague cognitive content. Rather, they often are sensory fragments such as

---

Note to Clinicians

Anxiety in a client can increase a counselor's anxiety. A tip for staff working with women who abuse substances with anxiety disorders is to "slow down," that is, start with general and non-provocative topics and proceed gradually as clients become more comfortable talking about issues.

Figure 7-2
PTSD Symptoms

Symptoms	Client Experience	Clinical Suggestions
Reexperiencing • Flashbacks • Intrusive memories • Nightmares	• Feelings of being tossed from present and thrown into the nightmare of the past • Feeling of being out-of-control • Feeling of incompetence in managing symptoms or triggers	• Grounding techniques • Develop support system • Education about trauma and the symptoms of PTSD • Create sense of safety • Sleep hygiene strategies • Imaginal rehearsal of dreams • Cognitive and coping skills to help separate past experiences from present moment
Hyperarousal • Heightened startle response • Irritability or heightened aggression • Hypervigilance of environment • Sleep disturbance	• All-or-none thinking • Fatigue • Feeling overwhelmed and terror of being overwhelmed by feelings • Difficulty in managing anxiety and engaging in self-soothing skills	• Normalize the symptoms • Ability to reassure • Containment strategies • Increasing coping and self-soothing capacities • Anxiety management training • Cognitive restructuring
Numbing and Avoidance • Staying away from persons, places, and things that remind client of trauma	• Disconnection from others' and own feelings • Mechanical experience of life; possible discussion of painful events with limited affect • Dissociation (not knowing or remembering events or periods or experiencing oneself as separate from what one was experiencing) • Repeated use of substances or engagement in behaviors to avoid distress • Isolation; profound loneliness • Ineffective defense against overwhelming feelings	• Affect regulation skills • Cognitive–behavioral strategies to build coping skills • Education regarding substance use disorders and opportunities to draw connections between substance use and distress • When appropriate and with adequate training, use exposure strategies including desensitization, eye movement desensitization and reprocessing, prolonged exposure therapies

Sources: APA 2000*a*; Cramer 2000; Melnick and Bassuk 2000; and Najavits 2002*b*.

sights, sounds, smells, or kinesthetic sensations and emotional states (van der Kolk 1996). Developing the ability to organize the traumatic events into coherent thoughts and narrative that can be expressed in some way can significantly lessen somatic symptoms (see Figure 7-3; van der Kolk 1996). Some treatment methods support the premise that the trauma must be made conscious, effectively experienced, and integrated into present life (Volkman 1993). Some treatments suggest that coping strategies are the effective path in addressing PTSD, while other approaches heavily rely on the premise that repeated and prolonged exposure to anxiety-evoking material will gradually reduce PTSD symptoms through the process of extinction/habituation (Foa et al. 2007). A review of psychological treatments for PTSD is beyond the scope of this TIP. For a review of treatments, refer to the article, *Psychosocial treatment of posttraumatic stress disorder: A practice-friendly review of outcome research* (Solomon and Johnson 2002), along with the TIPs highlighted in the introduction to the Anxiety Disorders section earlier in this chapter.

Women with substance use disorders and PTSD

Substance abuse and the effects of trauma interact in complex ways in an individual. A treatment provider cannot assume that one is a primary problem and the other secondary. Nor is it always beneficial to delay working on trauma symptoms until the client has been abstinent for a predetermined minimum amount of time. The counselor should focus on the client's current crisis and stabilizing her affect.

Substance abuse can prevent full recovery from PTSD, and continuing PTSD symptoms may perpetuate use of substances and the development of substance use disorders. Two studies report double the lifetime prevalence of PTSD in women than in men: 11.3 percent versus 6 percent and 10.4 percent versus 5 percent (Breslau et al. 1991; Kessler et al. 1995, respectively). These studies found that women were twice as likely as men to develop PTSD after exposure to a trauma, suggesting that women are particularly vulnerable to PTSD or that the particular type of trauma experienced by women is more likely to result in PTSD. In a study that sampled 558 cocaine-dependent outpatient clients on current rates and symptoms of PTSD, women were three times more likely to meet diagnostic criteria for PTSD (Najavits et al. 2003).

Najavits and colleagues (1997) cite studies demonstrating that women with substance use disorders have higher rates of PTSD (30 to 60 percent) in comparison to men, most often as the result of physical or sexual assault. Women with substance use disorders have also been found to

---

Figure 7-3
Helpful Skills for Trauma Victims

- Self-knowledge, including attention to bodily cues
- Self-regulation, including recognizing triggers and expressing emotions appropriately
- Self-soothing; for example, using relaxation or guided imagery and keeping a journal
- Self-esteem and recognizing which behaviors to change
- Self-trust, including learning when to trust one's own judgment and how to make decisions
- Limit setting and assertiveness, including recognizing personal limits and defending them
- Clear expression of needs and desires; for example, identifying a need, evaluating the need, and planning how to fill it
- Realization that the healthiest relationships have mutuality and reciprocity and learning to create them

Source: Adapted from Harris and Fallot 2001*a*.

have higher rates of repeated trauma by family perpetrators than men who abuse substances (Grice et al. 1995). Rape has been found to be the most likely form of violence to lead to PTSD for both women and men, and female rape victims may be particularly vulnerable to developing substance use disorders because of the traumatic nature of rape (Kessler et al. 1997).

More research is needed in evaluating outcome and the role of PTSD and relapse. Women who relapse often are labeled as "resistant" when, in fact, victimizations that have not been addressed could account for the difficulty in stopping substance abuse (Root 1989). Trauma survivors sometimes use alcohol and drugs to medicate the pain of trauma and consequently are perceived as "treatment failures" because their trauma experience is misunderstood or not identified (Covington 2008a rev., 1999a). In an outcome study comparing women with and without PTSD in treatment for substance use disorders, the authors found that individuals with both PTSD and substance use disorders relapsed more quickly and that PTSD was a predictor of relapse (Brown et al. 1996).

While women with PTSD appear to possess more psychological risk factors associated with relapse than men, another outcome study comparing men and women in an outpatient treatment setting highlighted that women are more likely to engage in treatment, thereby offsetting the higher risks for relapse (Gil-Rivas et al. 1996). Women with PTSD may benefit from relapse prevention therapy as an effective short-term treatment for substance use disorders and PTSD. In a study evaluating the efficacy of cognitive–behavioral relapse prevention therapy for substance use disorders (only), the "Seeking Safety" program (manual-based treatment for substance abuse and PTSD), versus "standard" community care, women who were engaged in either relapse prevention therapy or the "Seeking Safety" program showed sustained improvement in substance use and PTSD symptoms at 6- and 9-month followups in comparison to women in standard care (Hien et al. 2004).

Substance abuse treatment: Trauma-informed treatment approach

When providing treatment, clinicians need to be aware that most female clients are trauma survivors, even if they do not meet criteria for PTSD. During the past 20 years, the treatment community responded to this treatment need in varying ways. Several years ago, most providers first treated the substance use disorder then addressed trauma-related issues later. As knowledge in the field grew, collateral services were offered that treated substance abuse and trauma issues concurrently. A "trauma-informed" program has an awareness of the pervasiveness of traumatic events and translates that awareness into integrated services that support the coping capacity of clients. This capacity enables a woman to stay and participate in treatment, to engage in a positive therapeutic alliance, and to learn to cope with the aftermath or consequences of trauma. The text box below provides an example of a trauma-informed approach to treatment.

A trauma-informed approach adjusts services to meet the needs of women who have a history of trauma. In 6- and 12-month outcome studies evaluating program and person-level effects among women with co-occurring disorders and trauma (Morrissey et al. 2005; Morrissey et al. 2005a), programs that provided integrated services (mental health, substance abuse, and trauma) displayed increased positive effects on mental health and substance use outcomes. Programs can use Appendix F, Integration Self-Assessment for Providers, to determine the extent to which their agency integrates treatment for substance abuse, mental illness, and trauma.

To be trauma-informed means to know of past and current abuse in the life of a woman. But more importantly, it means to understand the roles that violence and victimization play in the lives of women seeking substance abuse and mental health services, to design integrated service systems that accommodate the vulnerabilities of a trauma survivor, and to deliver services that facilitate participation in treatment (Harris and Fallott 2001b). Being trauma-informed does not mean that the program forces clients to reveal their trauma unwillingly. Nor does it mean that substance abuse treatment counselors need the level of expertise that is required to help women resolve all their problems related to trauma. However, knowledge about violence against women and the effects of trauma helps counselors to:

- Consider trauma when making assessments and treatment plans.
- Avoid triggering trauma reactions or retraumatizing women.
- Adjust staff behavior with clients and other staff members, and modify the organizational climate to support clients' coping capacities and safety concerns.

- Allow survivors to manage their trauma symptoms successfully so that they can access and continue to benefit from treatment services.
- Emphasize skills and strengths, interactive education, growth, and change beyond stabilization.

Clinical considerations in trauma-informed services

A history of trauma should alert counselors to the potential for co-occurring mental disorders, such as PTSD, depression, anxiety disorder, or personality disorders that can impede treatment unless addressed early. Once the trauma has been identified either during the assessment process or in early treatment, the

The Women Embracing Life and Living (WELL) Project

The aim of the SAMHSA-funded Women Enhancing Life and Living (WELL) Project was both to integrate treatment services and to encourage trauma-informed services for women with co-occurring substance use and mental disorders who have histories of violence. The project used relational strategies to facilitate systems change across three systems levels: local treatment providers, community or regional agencies, and the State government.

Substance abuse treatment clinicians in the study reported they tended to be insensitive to trauma/violence issues because they were unaware of the overlap between these two issues (there were notable exceptions among staff at programs that were gender-specific and evidence-based). Clinicians who were cross-trained or attempted to provide a broader range of services to clients often encountered restrictions embedded in existing procedures, forms, and documentation requirements that made integrated care more difficult.

Clients in the study recounted their frustration at having to slant their histories depending on the agency or practitioner they were addressing, and at having to conceal part of their histories to receive certain services. Rather than promoting wholeness and recovery, the experience in the treatment program recreated the secrecy of abuse and fed the stigma associated with their illnesses.

The WELL project worked within three communities to address this fragmentation and to increase awareness of the importance of integrating an understanding of trauma into services offered to women. It began by convening leadership councils at the State and the local levels. Project activities included cross-training for clinicians, convening a consumer advisory group to provide guidance, submission of recommendations from the local leadership councils to the State level, and visits by consultants to each agency to assist clinicians in putting their training into practice. These activities resulted in greater understanding of trauma-related issues by clinicians, stronger linkages to community services for women with histories of trauma, and more referrals to these services.

Source: Markoff et al. 2005.

Note to Clinicians and Administrators

Preliminary data support that integrated trauma-focused interventions for women in substance abuse treatment programs appear to be safe, thus presenting no differences in adverse psychiatric and substance abuse symptoms or events in comparison to standard care (Killeen et al. 2008). So often, clinicians and administrators fear and hold the misperception that addressing trauma-related issues is counterproductive and produces deleterious effects on women in substance abuse treatment. While the selection of services and the planning on how these services are delivered is important in maintaining the integrity of care for the client, integrated trauma-focused interventions are not only a viable option but an essential component of treatment for women with substance use disorders.

counselor can begin to validate a woman's experience and acknowledge that she is neither unique in her experience nor alone. If women are not questioned directly, the abuse may go unrecognized and untreated. Many women who are dependent on alcohol or drugs experience difficulty in recovery and relapse if violence and abuse issues are not addressed in treatment. Women may need help understanding the serious long-term effects of violence, sexual abuse, and incest on their functioning and on the risk of relapse (Covington 2003; Finkelstein 1996; Najavits 2006).

In many instances, counselors can address trauma and its relevance to substance abuse treatment effectively. In other cases, complex or severe problems related to trauma that exceed the counselor's competence may be present initially or may arise during treatment. Clients with such problems should be referred to a specialist—typically a licensed mental health professional trained in trauma within the treatment program. Trauma-informed counselors can recognize when a therapeutic relationship is stretching their abilities, but the decision to refer a client requires understanding of the situation and supervisory consultation and agreement.

Major trauma-related clinical issues that counselors need to address or attend to during the course of treatment include:

- *Outreach.* Efforts to engage women in treatment include flexible scheduling, ready availability, identification of client interest in and need for treatment, and ongoing evaluation. Outreach includes informing the community of services offered and initiating contact with agencies that should refer women for assessment and counseling (Elliott et al. 2005).

- *Assessment and referral.* A counselor needs to understand the nature of a woman's exposure to trauma—the type of abuse, when it occurred, whether it was a one-time event or repeated over time, the relationship between the client and the perpetrator (family member, acquaintance, stranger), and what occurred if the woman previously disclosed the experience (Bernstein 2000). It requires treatment by a clinician who is trained in treating traumatic stress disorders. Women who score high on a posttraumatic stress assessment should be referred for treatment to address their PTSD concurrently with their substance abuse treatment. Counselors should be candid when they cannot provide the treatment the client needs and may need to make a referral.

- *Psychoeducation.* One of the counselor's major functions in treating a woman in recovery who has a trauma history is to acknowledge the connection between substance abuse and trauma. This acknowledgment validates a woman's experience and helps her feel that she is not alone and that her experience is not shameful. Sharing prevalence data can reduce her sense of isolation and shame (Finkelstein 1996).

- *Normalizing the symptoms.* In addition, it is important to educate and discuss the

Advice to Clinicians:
When Is a Woman Ready for Trauma Processing?

Many counselors and clients assume that "working on trauma" means telling the story of what happened. Although exposure therapy is a widely known treatment method (Foa and Rothbaum 1998), it is controversial in the substance abuse treatment field. Questions remain about whether it is a safe treatment to conduct with clients who are abusing substances or engaged in self-destructive behavior. A study on exposure therapy for people in substance abuse treatment showed that many clients could not tolerate the work, with 61.5 percent not completing the minimum dose of treatment. Those who engaged in the treatment did well in outcomes—including reducing substance use and employment problems—but more research is needed to determine client factors that would identify who would best benefit from this type of treatment (Brady et al. 2001).

Some experts recommend not asking the client to tell her story until she has achieved some abstinence or safe functioning, whereas others assert that this is a case-by-case decision. Staff and clients should not be led to believe that the "real work" is telling the trauma story. CBT is equally effective and may be preferred for some. Najavits (1998) has identified signs to determine when a woman with substance abuse disorder is ready for trauma-exploration work:

- She is able to use some coping skills.
- She has no major current crises or instability (e.g., homelessness, domestic violence).
- She wants to do this type of work.
- She can reach out for help when in danger.
- She is not using substances to such a degree that emotionally upsetting work may increase her use.
- Her suicidality has been evaluated and taken into account.
- She is in a system of care that is stable and consistent, with no immediate planned changes (e.g., discharge from inpatient unit or residential program).

typical symptoms associated with PTSD to help normalize the client's physiological and psychological experience. Similar to other anxiety disorders, clients are often overwhelmed by symptoms leading to the belief that they cannot manage them or that they are not going to survive them. Some relief arrives when a client knows that they are having a normal reaction to an abnormal event or set of circumstances.

- *Safety, support, and collaboration.* Trauma often creates profound disconnection in two areas: interpersonal relationships and internal feelings. Some women who experience traumas become isolated, feeling that the only safety is in solitude; others compulsively reenact dangerous relationships (Najavits 2002b). Alternating between the

experience of feeling overwhelmed and shutting down, women come to treatment profoundly discouraged about the value and safety of relationships. For a client, safety is psychological and physical, internal and external. A major goal of treatment is to develop a therapeutic alliance. Ideally this alliance creates a safe place within which the woman can learn to trust and have new, meaningful experiences. For a substance abuse treatment program, safety is an organizational or system issue that calls for counselor readiness, collaboration with the client, staff training and supervision, and continual self-assessment of strengths and limitations (Markoff et al. 2005).

- *Tracking level of distress.* Counselors need to monitor their own and their clients' level of distress. Counselors must observe the client for signs of discomfort. For example, if a client is hyperventilating, the counselor needs to help the client gain mastery of her breathing before proceeding. Using a scale of 1 to 100 to measure the client's subjective units of distress (SUD scale) can be a helpful tool in assessing the client's perception of current distress and in comparing her levels of distress from one session to the next (Wolpe 1969). It also provides tangible feedback to both the counselor and client.

- *Regulation of level of closeness and distance.* Carefully maintained boundaries between the counselor and the client maximize the effectiveness of the therapeutic relationship and ensure that treatment does not re-create the original trauma. For example, counselors should not physically intrude on a client who is "shut down"—does not want to be touched.

- *Timing and pacing.* The counselor addresses trauma issues when the woman is ready and functioning at a level where it is safe for her to explore the trauma; timing is directed by the client. The counselor helps the client identify when she is beginning to feel overwhelmed and how she can slow the process down. Trauma treatment begins with the start of substance abuse treatment and needs to be conducted in a careful and clinically sensitive manner. It is not always clear when and under what conditions it is helpful to a client to tell her trauma story. Sometimes results of this work are positive, but the telling can be harmful when the client does not yet have coping resources to handle the intense telling. Recalling or talking about her traumatic experience can retraumatize a woman. Even if the client wishes to talk about her trauma, it may be unwise if she is in an unstable situation (Najavits 2002a) and does not have a support system or is in danger of decompensation.

- *Coping skills.* A client's knowledge of coping skills helps her manage symptoms and increases her self-sufficiency and self-efficacy. Counselors and programs need to incorporate skill development components—including problemsolving, assertiveness, anger management, communications, and anxiety management—along with stress inoculation and relaxation techniques. Clients need to focus on both disorders and their interactions. More insight-oriented therapeutic work occurs once clients have attained abstinence and control over PTSD symptoms (Najavits et al. 1996, 2002a). Therapy should help women learn to use more healthful methods of coping with negative feelings, interpersonal conflict, and physical discomfort (Stewart et al. 2000).

- *Affect regulation.* Counselors need to assist clients in learning how to increase their tolerance for affective distress. The feeling of jeopardy feels real for both the client and counselor. It is the challenge for the counselor to remain connected with the client during this crisis, neither becoming overwhelmed by the traumatic reenactment nor emotionally abandoning the client by withdrawing (Cramer 2002). Training to handle strong feelings is essential, as is clinical supervision. Like the client, the counselor may feel shame, incompetence, anxiety, and anger. Emotional support from colleagues and supervisors helps counselors avoid defensiveness, client blaming, detachment, secondary traumatic stress reactions, and burnout.

- *Listening skills.* A critical part of therapy for addressing trauma in substance abuse treatment is to help the client gain support and establish safety. Counselors need to be nonjudgmental, empathetic, and encouraging; creating an environment that validates the client's experience through listening and gentle guidance.

- *Acknowledgment of grief and mourning.* The client needs time to grieve many losses. While this grieving process begins from the outset of treatment, the intensity of grief reactions often rises as anxiety symptoms dissipate.

- *Case management.* Case managers or counselors can assist women with solving problems and crisis intervention, locating peer-support groups and afterhours support, and coordinating linkages with other agencies.

- *Triggering and retraumatization.* During treatment, triggering is unavoidable. A trigger sets off a memory of the trauma. It can be a noise, a television show, another person's presence, or anything that is a reminder of the event. Therapist and client must be prepared for the difficult work of coping with triggers. The client is prepared by learning to identify the triggers and in either developing or enhancing coping and self-soothing skills. The difference between retraumatization and triggering is the therapist's ability to stay connected to the affective experience of the client and the client's knowledge that she will not be totally overwhelmed by her intense feelings (Najavits 2002a; Russell 1998). Triggering is inevitable; retraumatization is not. Reenactments are inevitable, but if they occur under controlled conditions and the client feels supported and safe with her counselor, retraumatization does not have to occur. All programs need to be alert to the risk of triggering and retraumatization.

Models of recovery

Since the late 19th century, a number of experts have conceptualized recovery from trauma in stages, describing it in different terms but referring to the same process (Herman 1997). Most of the conceptualizations followed three stages. The first stage is stabilization, preventing further deterioration and ensuring symptom management. During the second stage trauma is remembered, reenacted, and worked through.

Stage three is a return to normal, the time when the client can live with the memories of the trauma, and problems are controlled. In *Trauma and Recovery*, Herman (1997) describes trauma as a disease of disconnection and provides a three-stage model for recovery: safety, remembrance and mourning, and reconnection. During these stages, clients receive consistent support for recovery from their substance use disorders.

Stage 1: Safety

Female trauma survivors in early treatment for substance abuse typically need to be in an all-women group led by a female facilitator. "Survivors feel unsafe in their bodies. . . . They also feel unsafe in relation to other people" (Herman 1997, p. 160). Counselors can ensure that the environment is free of physical and sexual harassment and assess a woman's risk of domestic violence. Counselors teach women to feel safe internally by using self-soothing techniques to alleviate depression and anxiety rather than turning to drugs (Najavits et al. 1996). Women are helped to feel physically and emotionally safe in their relationships with their counselors. The counselor works to develop the client's trust and to help her make the connection between substance abuse and victimization (Hiebert-Murphy and Woytkiw

---

Advice to Clinicians:
Retraumatization

Some staff and agency issues that can result in retraumatization of the client include the following:

- Violating the client's boundaries
- Breaking trust with the client
- Unclear expectations
- Inconsistent enforcement of rules
- Chaotic treatment environment
- Rigid agency policies that do not allow a woman to have what she needs to feel safe
- Disruption in routines
- Disrespectfully challenging the client's reports of abuse
- Labeling intense rage and other feelings about the trauma as pathological
- Minimizing, discrediting, or ignoring the client's feelings or responses
- Disrupting relationships because of shift changes and reassignments
- Obtaining urine specimens in a nonprivate manner

SAMHSA's Women, Co-Occurring Disorders and Violence Study (WCDVS)

In 1998, SAMHSA funded sites in the United States to develop integrated services for women who were the victims of violence and diagnosed with co-occurring mental and substance abuse disorders; services were also available for these women's children. This 5-year study sought to compare more integrated treatment with non-integrated treatment for more than 2,000 women and yielded information on the effectiveness of the integrated services approach for women. WCDVS also addressed the interplay of substance use disorders, trauma, and mental illness and demonstrated the empowerment and healing that comes when female clients are involved directly in their care and recovery. Outcomes for women in the study improved more than the outcomes for those in the treatment-as-usual group when women had a voice in the planning, implementation, and delivery of their treatment and received counseling for all three conditions together.

The study showed that to improve treatment, an increased recognition is needed of the effects that past and present traumas have on women in treatment. Women should be encouraged and helped to play an active role in their healing processes. Additional key findings include, but are not limited to, the following: the need for comprehensive assessment that incorporates the history of trauma, physical and mental health needs, and the impact of co-occurring disorders on child care; the need for systems change to incorporate services for women and children with co-occurring disorders; and that integrated services for mental health, substance abuse, and violence issues in a trauma-informed context appear to be more effective and not more costly than treatment-as-usual.

For an overview of the study, including contact information regarding the involvement of specific programs, refer to http://www.wcdvs.com/pdfs/ProgramSummary.pdf.

Source: Becker and Gatz 2005; Salasin 2005

2000). The client learns to stop using unsafe coping mechanisms such as substance use and other self-destructive behaviors. An alliance between the counselor and the client, whose level of trust has been damaged by trauma, is the goal of this stage.

Stage 2: Remembrance and mourning
In this stage, women tell their stories of trauma. Women mourn the losses associated with their abuse and substance use (Hiebert-Murphy and Woytkiw 2000). More specifically, they mourn their old selves, which the trauma destroyed. Women stabilized in substance abuse treatment may be ready to begin Stage 2 trauma work. A counselor can address the high risk of relapse that exists in this phase through anticipation,

planning, and self-soothing mechanisms (Najavits 2002b). Considerable clinical judgment is required in determining whether the client has adequate coping skills.

Stage 3: Reconnection
Once the woman has coped with past trauma, she can look to the future. She learns new coping skills, develops healthy relationships, and becomes oriented toward the future. Stage 3 groups, traditionally unstructured, can be comprised of both women and men. This phase corresponds to the ongoing recovery phase of substance abuse treatment. For some women, reconnection can occur only after years of working through trauma issues.

It is important to emphasize that the majority of clinical work surrounding trauma in substance abuse treatment programs and in early stages of recovery from substance use disorders should focus on safety, client skills in establishing safe behaviors, and early trauma recovery skills—specifically coping skills such as grounding, emotional regulation, and stress management strategies.

Treatment programs and curricula for substance use disorders and trauma

The following trauma-specific curricula are designed to address treatment issues with women who have a history of trauma and trauma-related symptoms and substance abuse. These programs are mainly focused on establishing safety and support, providing psychoeducation, and developing coping strategies and skills surrounding the sequelae of trauma and substance use disorders (for review of integrated trauma treatment models see Finkelstein et al. 2004 and Moses et al. 2003).

The Addiction and Trauma Recovery Integration Model (ATRIUM; Miller and Guidry 2001): Based on Miller's Trauma Reenactment Model, ATRIUM is a 12-week program that integrates psychoeducational and expressive activities for individuals with trauma-related and substance use problems. The ATRIUM model assesses and intervenes at the body, mind, and spiritual levels and addresses issues linked to trauma and substance abuse experiences such as anxiety, sexuality/touch, self-harm, depression, anger, physical complaints and ailments, sleep problems, relationship challenges, and spiritual disconnection.

Beyond Trauma: A Healing Journey for Women and A Healing Journey: A Workbook for Women (Covington 2003a, b): The theme of this 11-session integrated program for trauma treatment is the connection between substance abuse and trauma in women's lives. It includes a psychoeducational component for teaching women about trauma and its effects on the inner self (thoughts, feelings, and beliefs) and the outer self (behavior and relationships, including parenting). The program emphasizes coping skills, cognitive–behavioral techniques, and expressive arts, and is based on the principles of relational therapy. It includes a facilitator's manual, participant's workbook, and videos.

Helping Women Recover: A Program for Treating Addiction (Covington 2008a, b rev., 1999a, b): This 17-session step-by-step guide integrates the theoretical perspectives of substance abuse and dependence, women's psychological development, and trauma in four modules (self, relationships, sexuality, and spirituality). The program includes a facilitator's guide to work with such issues as self-esteem, sexism, family-of-origin, support system, mothering, and self-soothing issues. A Woman's Journal provides self-tests and exercises to help clients with substance use disorders create personal guides to recovery. There is a separate version for women in the criminal justice system (Covington, 2008a, b rev., 1999a, b).

Seeking Safety (Najavits 2000, 2002b, 2004, 2007): This manual-based, cognitive, behavioral, and interpersonal therapy model for substance use disorders and PTSD focuses on client safety. It can be conducted in individual or group formats. The manual includes 25 topics and is based on five principles:

1. Safety as the priority of this "first stage" treatment
2. Integrated treatment of PTSD and substance use disorder
3. A focus on ideals
4. Four content areas: cognitive, behavioral, interpersonal, and case management
5. Attention to therapist processes

Several outcome studies have been completed on Seeking Safety, all showing positive results. The studies involve the following populations: women treated in an outpatient setting using a group modality (Najavits et al. 1998); women in prison in a group modality (Zlotnick et al. 2003); low-income and mostly minority women in individual format (Hien et al. 2004); adolescent girls (Najavits et al. 2006); and women in a community mental health setting in group format (Holdcraft and Comtois 2002). In a study that targeted patient and counselor feedback (Brown et al. 2007), results show that clinicians and clients alike were satisfied and felt that the Seeking Safety program was relevant to the treatment program and clients' needs. Seeking Safety has been implemented in a variety of clinical programs in addition to these research studies.

Trauma Adaptive Recovery Group Education and Therapy (TARGET; Ford et al. 2000): TARGET assists clients in replacing their stress responses with a positive approach to personal and relational empowerment. The curriculum includes a one- to three-session orientation, a five- to nine-session core education and skills curriculum, and 26 sessions of applications of recovery principles. TARGET has been adapted for clients who are deaf and for those whose primary language is Spanish or Dutch. TARGET is being evaluated in several treatment settings.

Trauma Recovery and Empowerment Model (TREM; Harris and The Community Connections Trauma Work Group 1998): This 33-session group approach was developed by clinicians with considerable input from clients and includes survivor empowerment, power support, and techniques for self-soothing, boundary maintenance, and solving problems to be covered over 9 months. TREM assists women with the trauma recovery process and includes

social skills training, psychoeducational and psychodynamic techniques, and peer support groups. Each section includes discussion questions, typical responses, and experiential exercises (Harris and The Community Connections Trauma Work Group 1998). TREM is being evaluated in several treatment settings. Preliminary studies showed symptom reduction and client satisfaction (Berley and Miller 2004).

Treating Addicted Survivors of Trauma (Evans and Sullivan 1995): Combining therapeutic approaches with a 12-Step approach to the treatment of substance use disorders, this model for treatment of survivors of childhood abuse who have substance use disorders is based on a medical view of substance abuse as illness. It assumes clients accept the 12-Step approach, uses the principle of safety first to drive all interventions, and has five stages to organize the selection and timing of treatment tactics: crisis, skills building, education, integration, and maintenance (Sullivan and Evans 1994).

Substance Dependent PTSD Therapy (SDPT; Triffleman 2000): This integrated approach showed positive outcomes in a small controlled pilot study that compared it with 12-Step facilitation therapy. SDPT is a 5-month, two-phased, individual CBT method using relapse prevention and coping skills training, psychoeducation, stress inoculation training, and exposure treatment for PTSD. Participants meet twice weekly. The use of the combined approaches for PTSD treatment techniques with clients with substance use disorders is notable. The first phase incorporates understanding and education about PTSD symptoms as part of the overall approach to abstinence. The second phase continues work on substance-related abstinence, while primarily targeting PTSD symptoms. In clinical trials, this model showed equal success rates in women and men.

Mood Disorders

Depression

Major depression is an intense, acute form of depression, often with physiological changes in such areas as sleep, appetite, energy level, and ability to think. Thought content includes feelings of worthlessness and suicidal ideation or plans, although older adults and people from some ethnic groups or cultures sometimes do not express this cognitive component. Major depression has severe, moderate, and mild variants. Even mild major depression is a serious mental disorder.

Major depressive episodes and dysthymia are present in nearly twice as many women as men for both lifetime and 12-month prevalence. Research suggests that women experience more chronicity of depression in comparison to men characterized by earlier onset of symptoms, poorer quality of life, greater social impairment, and greater familial history of mood disorders (Kornstein et al. 2000).

Although rates of depression among women of color in the general population are comparable with those for Caucasian women, the illness is more likely to be undiagnosed and untreated in the former group, according to the literature reviewed (Mazure et al. 2002). Depression may appear through somatic symptoms that are misinterpreted by providers. Of concern is the lack of compliance with treatment regimens using psychotropic medications by women of color, which is possibly related to side effects of the medication. In addition, the sense of loss associated with migration may contribute to high levels of depression among Hispanic/Latina and Asian and Pacific-Islander immigrant women. In a study examining the use of pediatric emergency services with a sample of Mexican- and Central-American immigrants in Los Angeles, the women reported high levels of mental distress (Zambrana et al. 1994). Somatic complaints are common among Hispanic/Latinas and can mask depression or other mental illness.

Women with substance use disorders and depression

Alcohol consumption and alcohol-related problems co-occur with depression more often in women than in men (Graham et al. 2007). Depression usually precedes alcohol abuse in women, whereas alcohol dependence usually comes first among men (Moscato et al. 1997). Two mechanisms have been suggested to explain the pattern among women: (1) alcohol is used to try to relieve the symptoms of depression, and (2) depression renders women less concerned about issues of health and safety, including alcohol consumption (Dixit and Crum 2000). For more in-depth information on depression, refer to the TIP 48 *Managing Depressive Symptoms in Substance Abuse Clients During Early Recovery* (CSAT 2008).

One study indicates that the risk for heavy drinking is higher among women with a history of depressive disorder than among women with no history of depression, and the risk for heavy drinking rises with increasing reports of depressive symptoms (Dixit and Crum 2000). Research suggests that genetic factors contribute to women's susceptibility to both disorders. Among treatment-seeking women, depression is positively correlated with craving (Zilberman et al. 2003). While craving is not consistently associated with relapse, clients who experience cravings express distress in managing and coping with them.

Although it may be difficult to determine whether the depression or substance use disorder is primary, both need to be identified and treated concurrently to minimize relapse and improve a client's quality of life. If a woman's depression is life threatening, the depression must be treated immediately. In general, the disorder with the higher crisis potential needs to be addressed first—but neither should be neglected. Withdrawal symptoms sometimes include depression, and withdrawal symptoms sometimes mask depression. Appropriate treatment requires a thorough history and monitoring of symptoms over time.

Substance abuse treatment and depression

Women with co-occurring substance use disorders and depression can be placed in a variety of treatment settings, depending on the severity of their disorders. Antidepressant and mood-regulating medications are appropriate for women in treatment for both disorders. Clients may require medication to overcome debilitating and incapacitating depressive symptoms so that they can participate in substance abuse treatment. In addition, relief from depression can be significant motivation in recovery. However, it may take time for a client to be stabilized on the appropriate medication and dosage. Women may need education and medication monitoring initially to ensure they are taking their medications as prescribed. Some women may increase their dose thinking that the larger dose provides more help or reduce their dose to prove they are improving. Still other women may have difficulty taking antidepressant medication based upon fear and misinformation that it is addictive.

SSRIs and other new generation antidepressants often are used because their improved side effect profile increases the likelihood of compliance (Zweben 1996). Women with depression may respond to a combination of psychotherapy and medication. CBT and interpersonal therapies (IPT) are evidence-based approaches in treating depression (Butler et al. 2006; deMello et al. 2005; Kuyken et al. 2007), and they can be used as an adjunct to medication or as a principal intervention for mild or moderate depression. For clients who are hesitant to use medications or when the use of medication is contraindicated, CBT and IPT are viable options but appear far less effective when depression is severe (Luty et al. 2007; Markowitz 2003).

Eating Disorders

Between 90 and 95 percent of those diagnosed with eating disorders are women (Hoek 1995), with as many as 5 percent of young women being affected (Frank et al. 1998). Studies have shown that bulimia affects between 2 and 5 percent of women, whereas anorexia is much less common (Frank et al. 1998). About 2 percent of the U.S. population has a binge eating disorder, and it occurs in 10 to 15 percent of mildly obese people (National Institute of Diabetes and Digestive and Kidney Diseases 2001). However, all measures of the prevalence of eating disorders are considered to be estimates by researchers because they represent only cases diagnosed in medical facilities. Women with eating disorders are skilled at concealing their disorders and many remain undiagnosed (Hoek and Van Hseken 2003). Common definitions of eating disorders and behaviors are defined in Figure 7-4.

Substance abuse counselors and mental health professionals have difficulty detecting eating disorders because clients minimize or deny their symptoms and fail to seek treatment out of shame or fear of gaining weight. Counselors should be alert to symptoms of eating disorders that may be serious but do not meet full criteria for an eating disorder diagnosis. Disordered eating behaviors can pose serious health issues and lead to full-blown disorders. In addition, counselors should be aware that eating disorders occur in women from diverse backgrounds.

Note to Clinicians

Women receiving methadone maintenance treatment (MMT) require antidepressant medication that is compatible with methadone, but dosages of both need close monitoring. Although MMT can normalize mood in some women, it is a treatment for opioid dependence, not depression (Zweben 1996). TIP 43 Medication-Assisted Treatment for Opioid Addiction in Opioid Treatment Programs (CSAT 2005b), provides more information.

Although anorexia is seen most often in young heterosexual Caucasian women, girls and women from all ethnic and racial groups have eating disorders and disordered eating at increasing rates. Often these women receive treatment for the accompanying symptoms of an eating disorder, such as depression, rather than for the disorder itself. When they are finally diagnosed, the disorder tends to be more severe (HHS, Office on Women's Health 2000). Overall, studies show that eating disorders are positively associated with all DSM-IV mood, anxiety, impulse-control, and substance use disorders regardless of age, gender, and race-ethnicity (Hudson et al. 2007).

Women with substance use and eating disorders

One study evaluating the role of eating disorder behaviors and its association with substance use (Piran and Robinson 2006) determined that as eating disorder behavior becomes more severe, the number of substance classes used increases as well. Specifically, severe bingeing was consistently associated with alcohol consumption, and dieting and purging was associated with stimulant and sleeping pills/

sedative use. Herzog and colleagues found that 17 percent of women seeking treatment for either anorexia nervosa or bulimia nervosa had a lifetime drug use disorder (Herzog et al. 2006).

Overall, research indicates that substance abuse is accompanied more often by bulimia and bulimic behaviors than by anorexia (Bulik et al. 2004; Holderness et al. 1994; Ross-Durow and Boyd 2000). Nearly one third of women with a history of bulimia also have a history of alcohol abuse, and 13 percent have a history of alcohol dependence. Alcohol abuse and dependence have been found to be related to PTSD and major depressive disorder, which in turn were associated with bulimia. One study demonstrated that alcohol use disorders are highly prevalent among women with bulimia and that the presence of PTSD and depression increases the risk of alcohol abuse occurring (Dansky et al. 2000).

Attitudes toward dieting among young women may be related to increased susceptibility to alcohol and drug use (Zweben 1996). This is both a health issue and a relapse risk because some women may use cocaine or amphetamines (or both) to manage their weight. Additionally, the tendency to overeat affects many women in early recovery. Compulsive or binge eating bears a similarity to abuse of substances other than food and is correlated with depression, thoughts of suicide, and childhood sexual abuse. Women engaging in binge eating sometimes use food as a substitute addiction; others may overeat to compensate for the stress they experience in early abstinence. Elements of the eating disorder take the place of relapsing to the drug of choice (Ross 1993).

Eating disorders need to be viewed in a biopsychosocial context that addresses biological or organic factors, a social component (influence of media and other cultural images enforcing standards of slimness for women), and psychological issues. Eating disorders are correlated with growing up in dysfunctional families where substance abuse occurs (van Wormer and Askew 1997). A strong relationship exists between eating disorders and depression, self-inflicted violence, and suicidal tendencies (APA 2000a; Kuba and Hanchey 1991). Most women with eating disorders meet DSM-IV criteria for at least one personality disorder, such as borderline, histrionic, or obsessive–compulsive personality (Zerbe 1993).

Eating disorders are sometimes present before the onset of alcohol and drug problems and can be obscured by active substance use, or they may be inactive during periods of active drinking or drug abuse. Eating disorders can precede the onset of substance use disorders chronologically, follow them, or develop simultaneously (Bulik and Sullivan 1998). A history of bulimia, anorexia, or compulsive overeating could become a barrier to the successful treatment of a client's substance use disorder if the prior eating disorder goes undetected. Deprived of compulsive involvement with food, a woman may begin to abuse substances. During treatment for substance use, unbeknownst to the therapist, the disordered eating behavior may reappear. Because the eating disorder takes over the function of the substances by helping the client cope, a cycle

can occur that never addresses the common and predisposing factors contributing to both problems. There may be success in that the substance use has stopped; however, this may be a result only of disordered eating or symptom substitution. This disordered use of food masks depression, anxiety, and other symptoms expected to surface during the treatment of substance use, leaving the therapist with no view of the woman's coping abilities without any compulsive and disordered behavior. Eating disorders may coexist with alcohol and drug consumption in other ways (John et al. 2006). Diuretics, laxatives, emetics, stimulants, heroin, tobacco, and thyroid hormone may be attractive to a woman with anorexia or bulimia because of their weight-loss potential or their ability to facilitate vomiting (Bulik and Sullivan 1998).

Substance abuse treatment and eating disorders

Therapeutic modalities include individual, group, and family therapies. A cognitive–behavioral approach is used to address the irrational thoughts that lead to disordered eating behaviors (van Wormer and Askew 1997). CBT has been effective for women with bulimia in reducing the frequency of binge/purge cycles and improving body image, mood, and social functioning. In some instances, the use of tricyclic antidepressants and selective serotonin reuptake inhibitors can improve short-term outcomes, but in all eating disorder cases, medical evaluation should be included (Carr and McNulty 2006; Raeburn 2002).

Interpersonal therapy has been used successfully with women with bulimia, and dialectical behavior therapy recently has begun to be used with this population (Raeburn 2002; Safer et al. 2001). Additional treatment approaches for women with eating disorders that can engage clients include psychoeducation, behavioral contracting, and nutrition monitoring (Frank et al. 1998).

Treating this condition requires specialized training, along with a thorough medical evaluation for problems typically associated with eating disorders. Clients require nutritional counseling to develop healthful eating patterns, medications (usually antidepressants), and discharge planning that addresses both eating and substance use disorders (Marcus and Katz 1990). Eating disorders often surface or are exacerbated when women reduce substance use; in this situation, integrated care and management is the optimal choice.

It is important for counselors to look beyond the earlier profiles of eating disorder cases and consider symptoms among women of color and in various social classes. The HHS Office on Women's Health provides educational materials on eating disorders on its Web site (www.4women.gov/BodyImage).

Addressing Tobacco Use With Women in Treatment

Cigarette smoking is a major cause of lung cancer among women. Approximately 90 percent of all lung cancer deaths are attributable to smoking. Since 1950, lung cancer mortality rates for American women have increased an estimated 600 percent. In 1987, lung cancer surpassed breast cancer to become the leading cause of cancer death among American women. In 2000, about 27,000 more women died of lung cancer (67,600) than breast cancer (40,800; CDC 2001). In 2004, diseases caused by cigarette smoking killed an estimated 178,000 women in the United States. The three leading diseases were lung cancer (45,000), chronic lung disease (42,000), and heart disease (40,000; CDC 2005).

Although it is commonly accepted in the substance abuse treatment field that the use of one addictive drug frequently leads to relapse

---

Advice to Clinicians: Women With Eating Disorders

Substance abuse counselors may want to consider these steps in addressing eating disorders:

- Include an eating history as part of a comprehensive assessment of a client (refer to chapter 4 on Screening and Assessment).
- Refer for medical evaluation.
- Ask the client what happens as a result of the disordered eating behaviors. Does she feel in control, more relaxed, or numb? Approach eating disorders as a response to emotional discomfort.
- Educate the client about eating behaviors as a legitimate health concern.
- Develop integrated services, and coordinate necessary services and referrals (including a referral to a provider that specializes in eating disorder treatment).
- Incorporate nutritional counseling and psychoeducation on eating disorders and disordered eating.
- Institute routine observations at and between meals for disordered eating behaviors.
- Recommend the use of support groups that are designed specifically for the given eating disorder.
- Teach coping skills using cognitive–behavioral therapy and include anxiety management training.

Source: Bulik and Sullivan 1998; Rome 2003

---

to a person's "drug of choice," this has not been clarified in the issue of nicotine use and substance abuse (Burling et al. 2001). Many treatment professionals have thought it too difficult for clients to give up tobacco and still remain abstinent from other substances even after years of being drug or alcohol free. They believed that any attempt to stop smoking could put the recovering person at an increased risk for relapse. It also was assumed that people will quit naturally if they so desire (Bobo et al. 1986).

However, research and experience since the mid-1980s has begun to challenge these assumptions (for review, see Prochaska et al. 2004; Sussman 2002). Research shows that quitting smoking does not jeopardize substance abuse recovery; that nicotine cessation interventions in substance abuse treatment are associated with an increase in long-term abstinence of alcohol and illicit drugs. Prochaska and colleagues (2004) examined outcomes of smoking cessation interventions in 19 randomized controlled trials with individuals both in current addiction treatment and in recovery. The researchers found striking interactions between smoking cessation and success in treatment for other drug abuse. Their first observation was that among both men and women, those who stopped smoking while also quitting other drug use showed higher success rates in abstinence from alcohol and other drugs, even though their rates of relapse to cigarette use was high.

Motivating women to stop smoking involves addressing their concerns about the difficulties and negative consequences of smoking cessation and bolstering their confidence to stop (Miller and Rollnick 2002). Women's motives for stopping smoking include their present health, their future health, and the effect of their smoking on the health of others. Women's concerns about quitting include believing stopping will be difficult, feeling tense and irritable if they quit, enjoying smoking too much to stop, expecting difficulty concentrating after quitting, and anticipating gaining considerable weight after stopping (Lando et al. 1991; Pomerleau et al. 2001). Studies have not

consistently shown differences in relapse rates between men and women, yet women appear to have higher rates of relapse when they fail to adhere to pre-established quit dates (Borrelli et al. 2004). Among women, relapse is significantly related to weight gain, strong negative affect, history of depression, family history of smoking, unemployment, and a history of smoking cigarettes high in nicotine (Cooley et al. 2006; Hoffman et al. 2001; Swan and Denk 1987; Wetter et al. 1999).

Akin to other services, smoking cessation programs should be integrated into substance abuse treatment for women. Providers are encouraged to include smoking cessation in their clients' treatment plans, as this will help send a message to women that treatment providers care about their total health. Further, even temporary cessation from smoking (assisted with nicotine replacement therapy) may give women confidence about remaining abstinent from other substances, and there may be no other opportunity to help them quit smoking. In reviewing the common relapse risks among women, nicotine cessation programs should consider strategies (along with pharmacologic therapies), that address body image, nutritional counseling, and emotional regulation combined with CBTs that target cognitions, establish quit dates, and teach coping strategies to manage anticipated difficulties in maintaining abstinence.

The consensus panel believes that smoking cessation programs should be offered in all substance abuse treatment programs. Clinics can meet a minimum standard of care by adopting some of the following guidelines:

- Require all treatment facilities to be smoke free, and provide nicotine cessation programs for employees as well.
- Provide onsite cessation services and include tobacco and nicotine issues as part of treatment planning.
- Train staff to address nicotine addiction. Substance abuse counseling skills already in place can be applied to help clients achieve and maintain smoking cessation.

- Base counseling sessions on professional guidelines for smoking cessation, such as those supported by the National Cancer Institute and the U.S. Public Health Service.
- Provide all clients access to pharmacotherapy as an aid in quitting tobacco use; for example, nicotine patches and nasal sprays, bupropion (Zyban™), and varenicline (Chantix™), if medically appropriate. Note that few studies have examined the risks associated with nicotine replacement and other pharmacotherapies among pregnant women (for review, see Schnoll et al. 2007; Wise and Correia 2008).
- Identify local resources for referrals for more intensive interventions, such as the American Cancer Society (www.cancer.org) and the American Heart Association (www.americanheart.org).

8 Recovery Management and Administrative Considerations

Overview

The first part of this chapter, aimed at the substance abuse treatment counselor, examines the most critical aspects of recovery management including continuing care services, outcome and relapse variables, and support services. The second part is directed toward substance abuse treatment program administrators and supervisors. This segment looks at the benefits of consumer participation in programming, the characteristics of a healing environment for treatment, and the main components of staff development including staffing, training, and clinical supervision specific to women's programming. Organizational change strategies that focus on how an organization can become gender responsive follow.

Continuing Care

Continuing care services, often referred to as aftercare, are substance abuse services that occur after initial treatment. Continuing care is designed to provide less intensive services as the client progresses in treatment and establishes greater duration of abstinence. The dearth of research on continuing care is particularly evident surrounding gender differences. Several studies are available that show potential patterns, but caution is needed in interpreting the findings due to methodological issues and sample size.

Although women appear more likely to attend aftercare, any transition from one service to the next can be challenging for the client and treatment provider (Carter et al. 2008). In general, clients are more likely to discontinue treatment during these periods. Women often express feelings of disconnection with the new treatment provider and experience additional struggles in managing the added demands and expectations of child care while attending less intensive treatment. Relapse is more prevalent during these periods, especially when there is little compliance or support from family to follow aftercare plans. The initial risk factors that served as a direct or indirect path to substance use often are the same risk factors that reappear in early recovery and sabotage involvement in continuing care, recovery activities, and abstinence. As an example, women who have a history of substance use that involves a significant relationship appear more likely to leave care prematurely due to the influence of a boyfriend, spouse, or significant other.

In one study that gained information from program case managers, it was reported that the women who had prior inadequate drug treatment services were most likely to drop out of continuing services (Coughey et al. 1998). Those women who completed aftercare had two times the amount of prior residential alcohol/drug treatment and longer sobriety time at admission. Equally important, women appear more likely to engage in continuing care if the primary treatment they received involved specialized programming for women (Claus et al. 2007).

Treatment Outcome

Historically, researchers have used posttreatment abstinence rates as the focal point of measuring success. Debate has ensued regarding how to measure treatment outcome and whether or not posttreatment abstinence rates are myopic in that they fail to account for the physical, psychological, and social conditions that improve in the treatment process. Other commentaries have suggested that using abstinence rates as the only benchmark to measure outcome falls short of recognizing the chronic nature of substance dependence disorders—that relapse is not inevitable but a likely event that can

provide a client with a learning opportunity to strengthen recovery skills. Overall, most outcome studies have targeted more immediate responses to treatment, often measuring and following outcome variables no longer than 12 months beyond discharge (Grella et al. 2005). This section examines the many factors that contribute to treatment outcome and includes numerous studies that expand the definition of treatment outcome beyond abstinence rates, including quality of life and other biopsychosocial benefits. The segment ends with a discussion on relapse and prevention for women, and specifically for postpartum women.

Gender is not a significant predictor of treatment outcome. Once in treatment, women are as likely as men to complete treatment and have good treatment outcomes, although outcome differences are noted when evaluating individual and program characteristics (for a comprehensive literature review, see Greenfield et al. 2007a). Women are also as likely to have similar abstinence rates and overall quality of life 1 year after discharge from treatment (Slaymaker and Owen 2006). As shown by previous research (Timko et al. 2002), women show greater increases than men in employment, recovery-oriented social support systems, and participation in self-help groups (Grella et al. 2005). Grella's study found that women have greater reduction in levels of distress, although their levels of distress appear to remain consistently higher than those of their male counterparts at each period of outcome evaluation. For women with posttraumatic stress reactions, literature supports the relationship between the receipt of integrated trauma treatment services and positive treatment outcome (Cohen and Hien 2006; Cocozza et al. 2005). In a posttreatment outcome study measuring factors that predicted 5-year abstinence, 12-Step participation and involvement in social networks that support recovery were among the essential ingredients (Weisner et al. 2003a, b).

Although further evaluation is needed, there appears to be a stronger association between treatment participation and posttreatment outcome among women (Fiorentine et al. 1997;

Hser et al. 2004). Literature suggests that treatment completion and length of stay in residential treatment are important factors in establishing positive posttreatment outcomes among women (Greenfield et al. 2004). Specific posttreatment outcome analysis comparing length of treatment to posttreatment outcome in residential treatment for pregnant and parenting women and their children shows an association between longer lengths of stay and abstinence, improvements in employment and income, decreases in arrests and depressive symptoms, and more positive attitudes toward parenting (Conners et al. 2006). Although studies have begun to shed light on gender differences in posttreatment outcome, future research should continue to examine the specific underlying factors that influence treatment outcomes and how these factors differ between men and women.

Relapse

Gender alone does not predict substance abuse treatment outcomes. Instead, client characteristics are more likely to predict relapse, and these characteristics often influence the risk of relapse differently in men and women (Greenfield et al. 2007b). Women who complete treatment for substance use disorders show no significant differences in relapse rates or only slightly better outcomes compared with men (for review, see Walitzer and Dearing 2006). However, gender differences do emerge across qualitative and quantitative studies that evaluate antecedents or risk factors associated with relapse and the clients' psychological and behavioral reactions to the relapse. Relapse characteristics and reactions specific to women are highlighted in Figure 8-1 (p. 184).

Currently, many relapse prevention programs do not delineate specific strategies and therapeutic approaches for women. Thus, research is needed to develop and evaluate relapse prevention programs and intervention strategies for women. One randomized study is available that evaluates a manual-based, women-only, women-oriented relapse prevention therapy group called Women's Recovery Group (WRG). In this study, WRG produced better outcomes in the 6 months following treatment than a mix-gender group using a standard manual-based program (Greenfield et al. 2007b). A forthcoming book by Greenfield, to be published by Guildford Press,

> Women are as likely as men to experience positive treatment outcomes including similar abstinence rates and overall improvement in quality of life.

Note to Clinicians: Family Reunification

The ability to regain custody of children can significantly motivate mothers to not only enter and pursue treatment but also to maintain motivation for ongoing recovery after treatment. Mothers in early recovery can face numerous challenges and stressors associated with reunification, including time pressures in establishing recovery to avoid termination of parental rights, the maintenance of recovery activities while assuming the parenting role, the management of affect associated with the impact of their past drug and alcohol use on their children's physical and mental health, effective implementation of parenting skills, and others (for review, see Carlson et al. 2006). As a provider, it is important to not only acknowledge the mother's initial enthusiasm and motivation for reunification, but also incorporate preparatory skills, including parenting, stress and anger management, and problemsolving to help fortify personal resources in anticipation of future parenting and childcare issues and challenges.

will provide the protocol for this women-specific relapse prevention group. Figure 8-2 provides examples of topics discussed in WRG.

Postpartum relapse prevention

It is not uncommon for women who abstained from alcohol, drugs, and tobacco during pregnancy to return to use after childbirth (Mullen 2004). The stresses of parenting a newborn and the resumption of activities curtailed during pregnancy can involve a host of triggers. The postpartum period presents numerous triggers for relapse in recovering women who are drug dependent, including:

- Pain and other common discomforts of the postpartum period.
- Fatigue and sleep deprivation.
- Other chronic health problems.
- The stress of role adaptation and caring for a newborn (along with other children for some women).
- Shifts in relationships with partners and family members.
- Interactions with child welfare agencies, courts, and criminal justice agencies.
- Ambivalence about parenting.
- Temporary or permanent loss of custody, whether voluntary or involuntary.
- Reunification after temporary loss of infant custody.
- Guilt and grief related to infant illness or death.
- Other stressors of daily living.

Figure 8-1
Women-Specific Predictors of Relapse and Reactions to Relapse

Relapse Risks Unique to Women
Women are more likely to relapse if they report or display:
- Interpersonal problems and conflicts.
- Low self-worth that is connected to intimate relationships.
- Severe untreated childhood trauma.
- Strong negative affect.
- More symptoms of depression.
- Greater difficulty in severing ties with other people who use.
- Failure to establish a new network of friends.
- Lack of relapse prevention coping skills.

Women's Reactions to Relapse
Women are more likely than men to exhibit the following behaviors during or after relapse:
- Relapsing in the company of others and particularly with female friends or a significant other.
- Escalating use after initial relapse that is positively associated with severity of childhood trauma.
- Seeking help.
- Experiencing slightly shorter relapse episodes.
- Reporting depressed mood.

Women are less likely than men to be affected by the same relapse risks across multiple relapse episodes.

Source: Coyne et al. 2006; Hyman et al. 2007; McKay et al. 1996; Project MATCH 1997; Rubin et al. 1996; Sun 2007; Zywiak et al. 2006.

Figure 8-2
Women's Recovery Group: Manual-Based Relapse Prevention

Group Format: 90-minute sessions
- Brief check-in
- Review of past week's skill practice
- Presentation on session topic
- Open discussion of topic and other recovery-related issues
- Review of session's "take-home message" and upcoming week's skill practice
- Check-out

Content Areas:
- The effect of drugs and alcohol on women's health
- What are the obstacles to seeking treatment and getting into recovery?
- Managing mood, anxiety, and eating problems without using substances
- Violence and abuse: Getting help
- Women and their partners: The effect on the recovery process
- Women as caretakers: Can you care for yourself while taking care of others?
- Women's use of substances through the life cycle
- Substance use and women's reproductive health
- The issue of disclosure: To tell or not to tell
- How to manage triggers and high risk situations
- Using self-help groups to help yourself
- Can I have fun and not use drugs or alcohol?
- Coping with stress
- Achieving balance in your life

Source: Greenfield et al. 2007*b*

Relapse prevention education with emphasis on postpartum triggers will help women anticipate and plan for such triggers. Relapse prevention techniques are often taught in groups using structured curricula that include strategies for maintenance of abstinence and recovery, such as identifying high risk situations; learning refusal skills that can be practiced with peers and staff in advance of "real life" challenges; and recognizing triggers that lead to relapse thinking, drug craving, and eventual use. Although there are multiple new demands placed on recovering postpartum women, using the tools for relapse prevention in the context of a full program of recovery activities is essential for continued abstinence.

During treatment, triggers for drug use should be identified and explored with recovering women prior to program discharge in concert with individualized treatment planning. Many of the services and resources used by the client prenatally should be continued, if not intensified, in the postpartum period. Alumnae groups and in-home visitation programs have assisted women with relapse prevention and family preservation (French et al. 2007; Gruber et al. 2001). Drug-specific research on postpartum women and relapse has primarily examined relapse to smoking after childbirth. In one study, correlates of postpartum relapse to smoking included high maternal weight gain, late or no prenatal care, and stressful life events (Carmichael and Ahluwalia 2000). Other research suggests that postpartum women relapsed to smoking in order to manage emotions, stress, and weight, and because they did not initially quit for themselves (Bottorff et al. 2000; Levine and Marcus 2004). Relapse prevention programs for postpartum women who smoke can decrease future smoking in some of these women (Ratner et al. 2000).

For many perinatal women who are monitored by drug courts, probation, parole, and child welfare agencies, the consequences of relapse can be devastating in terms of the potential for loss of child custody. Perinatal programs, in acknowledgment of the importance of parenting roles and relationships to women, recognize the possibility of relapse and acknowledge that this is the time when assistance to the client and her child should be intensified, not eliminated.

Support Systems for Women

Twelve-Step recovery groups have been a vital resource for over 50 years, and as time has evolved, more women have participated in these recovery support groups. Originally, the Alcoholics Anonymous (AA) program was written by men and primarily for men, and the content and language reflected this bias—a bias that was steeped in the culture of the time period in which it was written. The AA literature has since been revised and updated, yet issues regarding sensitivity to language and the limited focus on cultural and social issues pertinent to women's dependence and recovery remain a

potential roadblock for some women (Covington 1994). Nonetheless, 12-Step support groups have been the most steadfast peer-facilitated program, providing women a viable avenue of support in establishing abstinence, in developing recovery skills, and in maintaining recovery.

Most research on the effectiveness of 12-Step groups has been conducted with men, but some studies have examined gender differences. To date, research results reflect inconsistencies regarding differences in attendance and abstinence rates between men and women. Moos, Moos, and Timko (2006) found that women appeared to gain even greater benefits from AA than men, and women were more likely to attend AA and to attend more frequently. Compared with men, women showed less avoidance coping and greater reduction in depression with continued AA participation. Another study reported no gender differences in 12-Step attendance over a 24-month period, including frequency of participation and drop-out rates (Hillhouse and Fiorentine 2001). For women, availability of support and sponsorship appear to be the main ingredients in perceived social support in 12-Step recovery groups (Rush 2002).

Like men, women have other options for support group involvement. Women for Sobriety is the only self-help program designed specifically for women who are alcohol-dependent. Although women can benefit from participation in groups and from the supporting women-centered literature, availability of support groups is limited. To date, gender-specific outcome research on recovery groups outside of 12-Step programs is minimal.

Administrative Considerations

Consumer Direction, Participation, and Empowerment

The field of substance abuse treatment has a tradition of integrating consumers into service delivery as counselors and case managers, particularly at the direct service level. However, the field is only beginning to learn about and apply the enormous benefits received when these individuals are integrated into the entire fabric of service delivery, from program design to implementation and evaluation. For example, the SAMHSA-funded Women, Co-Occurring Disorders and Violence Study demonstrated a priority on including consumers in all aspects of study design and implementation throughout the 5 years of the study.

Prescott (2001) identifies the important contributions made to service systems and research when consumers are actively involved. When hiring people in recovery as mentors, case managers, counselors, and board members, characteristics to consider include significant time in recovery, ability to handle the expected range of tasks, and considerable training in issues related to recovery in the specific treatment areas (Moses et al. 2004).

Service system benefits include:
- Improving quality of services and systems.
- Contributing to systems knowledge.
- Improving customer orientation.
- Positively affecting policy development.
- Adding diversity.
- Reducing stigma.
- Providing positive role models.
- Promoting increased awareness and education among coworkers.
- Providing knowledge about and linkages to community and alternative resources.
- Increasing client engagement and retention.

Research benefits include:
- Enhancing research design.
- Promoting engagement of research subjects.
- Broadening interpretations and perspectives of research findings.
- Increasing research relevance (Prescott 2001, p. 6).

Active involvement of consumers in all aspects of treatment planning significantly contributes to both recovery and empowerment, and is essential if meaningful, effective services for women and children are to be developed (Schauer et al. 2007). The consensus panel believes consumers should have input into program design as well as management and research evaluation protocols. In addition, training in leadership and advocacy for consumers contributes to their feeling of being part of a group, effecting changes in their lives and communities, learning skills, changing others' perception of their competencies, increasing their positive self-images, and overcoming stigma. These elements are critical components of empowerment (Chamberlin and Schene 1997).

Prescott (2001) lists the benefits to recovering women involved in programs:
- *Positive role model.* Consumers are positive role models when they serve in capacities ranging from chief executive officer to support staff. Women who volunteer at the treatment program or in the community can be positive role models for clients new to treatment.
- *Promotion of specific skills.* As staff members in a treatment program, consumers learn skills to help themselves communicate with community agencies and social service groups and learn how organizations change and ideas are implemented, thereby gaining a sense of control over the environment.
- *Promotion of recovery and well-being.* Being a part of the treatment milieu, having responsibility for an aspect of the program, and working with colleagues whose mission is to promote wellness can help a woman focus her life on maintaining her health and recovery.
- *Increased sense of hope.* The increased security of having employment and perhaps income helps consumers envision their future in a more promising light.

- *Cultivation of self-efficacy.* As consumers acquire the skills they need to make positive contributions to the work of the treatment program, their belief grows in their abilities to handle problems on a broad scale.
- *Decreased stigma.* When consumers play a role in a treatment program, they give evidence that substance abuse is not a character flaw or moral defect but an illness that can be overcome. Their presence sends that message to others and mitigates any internalized stigma of consumers.

Consumer-centered programs incorporate the views of women in recovery in all stages of program design, management, and evaluation. In this way, the quality of services and systems integration improves, coworkers become better educated about the process of recovery, and the stigma of substance abuse is reduced.

Creating a Healing Environment

The primary characteristic of a healing environment is safety. The environment should also be holistic, seamless, and centered on a woman's needs. To promote healing, the therapeutic environment must be inviting and welcoming, with culturally appropriate decorations and pictures. Surroundings should be multicultural, highlighting heroines from many cultures. A connection to women's history and female heroes plays an important role in bolstering women's self-efficacy.

In both residential and outpatient programs, the physical layout must provide privacy and space where women can be quiet and meditative. Private time is needed in their schedules; treatment programs can offer an array of services that pack a daily schedule, but women need time for contemplation and to pursue personal interests. Music and recreational activities should be available. Space dedicated to child care and equipment for children's activities is essential if children are included in the program.

In women's treatment programs, sensitivity to trauma-related issues is critical to a healing environment. A calm atmosphere that respects privacy and maximizes client choices promotes healing. Staff should be trained to recognize the effects of trauma, and women should have a clear understanding of the rules and policies of the residence. A trauma-informed environment must consider:

- Attention to safety.
- Attention to boundaries between staff and participants, among participants, and between participants and visitors (e.g., giving women permission to say no to hugging; hugging can be a common expression of positive emotion for some women, but for those who have been traumatized it could represent an undesired intrusion into their personal space).
- Mutuality in staff–staff and staff–client relationships.
- A nonpunitive atmosphere in which conflict is addressed by negotiation to the extent possible.
- An organizational structure that allows participants access to several layers of staff and administrators.
- Encouragement of assertiveness and leadership.
- Self-care.

Staffing

A woman-centered staff member is an active participant in treatment and considers the specific needs of women in general and of each particular client and how they can be addressed. She weighs the realities and complexities of women's lives and their social and gender roles with a nonjudgmental attitude. Although programs are not always able to hire a woman for each staff position, a program still can adhere to a woman-centered philosophy. A key rationale for having female staff work with female clients is role modeling; people watch more than they listen. A woman-run program shows clients how women can exercise power effectively. Women need to be seen in leadership roles in the program.

This goal does not, however, exclude men as treatment providers for female clients; men who are respectful of women's experiences can help women. They must have a woman-centered perspective and be knowledgeable about women's issues, particularly trauma and domestic violence. In residential programs or other programs with children's services, male staff members can play a valuable role by being healthy male role models for women and their children. Women report that working with a male counselor who is compassionate and respectful can be a healing experience, particularly if they endured negative relationships with men. Ideally, a woman should have the option to choose either a man or a woman as her primary counselor.

Men can serve in a variety of roles in nonresidential programs, including case manager, housing coordinator, couples' or children's counselor, and general equivalency diploma teacher. They can provide a male point of view about parenting and assist in exploring the attitudes and behavior of the clients' partners.

Training

Treatment providers and staff members at all entry points in systems that serve women need to be able to screen, triage, and refer for substance abuse treatment using an approach that supports and encourages women to receive treatment. Because of a lack of knowledge about substance use generally and about women particularly, as well as the tremendous stigma attached to women who abuse substances, it is important that all staff training include a process that identifies, acknowledges, and brings to awareness the biases, judgments, and anger toward women who use and abuse substances. The pervasiveness of substance use and abuse and the negative effect it has on the lives of so many people make it difficult to remain objective as a helping professional. If women are to be identified and referred when in need of treatment for their substance use, those in a position to help must be able to interact in a manner that assists and causes no harm.

Training for point-of-entry providers

Point-of-entry providers see women with a variety of complaints and have the potential to identify and refer women for assessment and treatment. These point-of-entry providers

include those in healthcare, domestic violence, social service, child protection, mental health systems; schools and daycare centers; the criminal justice system; TANF (Temporary Assistance for Needy Families) workers, judges, and clergy. The consensus panel recommends that because these providers are in the position to identify women in need of substance abuse treatment, a minimum standard of cross-training among systems and within interdisciplinary groups is needed. With a heightened focus on cultural and linguistic competency, along with substance abuse education, training can help practitioners avoid creating barriers to treatment when clients are from cultures, ethnicities, or sexual orientations different from their own (Goode et al. 2006). Figure 8-3 defines the attitudes, skills, and knowledge that should be the goals for training an audience of point-of-entry staff.

Training for substance abuse treatment counselors

Although it is widely assumed that clinical staff members who provide substance abuse treatment are prepared to serve both men and women, the training received by clinicians does not always specifically include women-centered treatment. The consensus panel believes that training for clinicians should include information on the psychological growth and development of women, cultural competence, sexual orientation and gender identity issues, the role of relationships in women's development of a sense of self, the importance of children in the treatment process, children's importance in the lives of mothers, and the sense of adequacy in parenting that is vital to self-esteem. Training should include information on the etiology of use and abuse of substances in women and the physiological effects that are unique to women. Counselors also need to be able to disseminate accurate information about the bodily changes and potential effects of substance use on both a pregnant woman and her fetus.

In addition, social roles and status in society strongly influence the patterns, consequences, and context of use, as well as the treatment

Figure 8-3
Goals and Training Guidelines for Point-of-Entry Staff (Non–Substance-Abuse Treatment Providers)

Goals	Guidelines
Attitudes	• To be nonjudgmental, supportive, and respectful • To be culturally responsive and appropriate
Skills	• To actively listen and express concern • To treat all women with respect and dignity • To engage women in nonthreatening discussions • To routinely screen for alcohol and substance use and abuse (e.g., complete a behavioral checklist, identify behavioral signs) • To recognize signs of intoxication and symptoms of mental disorders • To facilitate appropriate referrals for women who abuse substances
Knowledge	• To understand women's lives in sociocultural, psychological, economic, and political contexts • To learn about the etiology, symptoms, consequences, and course of substance use disorders among women • To know the available treatment and support resources for women who abuse substances and how to make a referral • To continue to learn drug language and culture • To understand the diverse experiences of women from different cultural groups, sexual orientations, and gender identities

experience. Some clients need to feel empowered to assume new roles, make decisions and a new life, and remain substance free. Treatment staff can help clients find acceptance, understand their conflicts, and reach comfortable roles. Figure 8-4 defines the attitudes, skills, and knowledge that training should instill in an audience of substance abuse treatment counselors.

Supervision

The consensus panel recommends that staff supervision be built into an agency's procedures on two levels: administrative supervision (timesheets, policies, etc.) and clinical supervision. Clinical supervision provides a method to address countertransference issues or other problems when a staff member's values, attitudes, and/or expectations might interfere with the therapeutic process. Clinical supervisors can help counselors foster therapeutic alliances and help providers learn to use the therapeutic relationship to model and foster mutuality, respect, and connection for women (Finkelstein 1996; Finkelstein et al. 1997). Literature from cross-cultural psychology and social work shows that therapeutic relationships with those who have substance use problems are stronger and more effective if the counselor understands the client's historical, cultural, and economic background (Pedersen et al. 1989; Sue and Sue 2003). Research in psychology shows that counselors' gender and ethnicity can affect the diagnoses they assign (Loring and Powell 1988). This speaks to the need for ongoing clinical

Figure 8-4
Goals and Training Guidelines for Substance Abuse Treatment Counselors

Goals	Guidelines
Attitudes	<ul><li>To main tain a nonjudgmental, supportive, and respectful manner</li><li>To understand the diverse experience of women from different cultural groups, abilities, sexual orientations, and gender identities (e.g., be aware of attitudes toward race, sex, and disability)</li><li>To be committed to women's issues</li><li>To uphold a sense of hope</li><li>To demonstrate unconditional acceptance of and positive regard for the client</li></ul>
Skills	<ul><li>To engage women with empathy, warmth, and sincerity</li><li>To develop a treatment alliance with female clients that is mutual and collaborative, individualized, and continually negotiated</li><li>To have clear professional boundaries (neither distant nor abandoning) and maintain confidentiality</li><li>To remain consistent in caring and availability and possess the ability to set limits in a calm and supportive manner</li><li>To conduct assessments that are thorough and trauma informed</li><li>To develop individually focused and outcome-oriented treatment plans</li><li>To work with multidisciplinary teams</li><li>To perform crisis intervention</li><li>To apply trauma coping skills</li><li>To tolerate one's own distress in hearing trauma information</li><li>To deliver client-led treatment (e.g., help the client learn how to manage her distress without shutting down or becoming overwhelmed—a central focus of treatment)</li><li>To maintain and ensure self-care</li><li>To support clients' cultural and racial identities and sexual orientations</li><li>To ask for and participate in supervision, in part to explore personal biases in ongoing processes, and to be invested in ongoing training</li><li>To be a visible advocate for women who use/abuse substances for stigma reduction and for treatment (within treatment teams, the community, and the system)</li><li>To be an appropriate role model for women, including on the topic of parenting</li><li>To develop professional, respectful, mutually supportive, and collaborative relationships with coworkers</li></ul>

Knowledge	<ul><li>To be culturally informed and knowledgeable</li><li>To be trauma informed, including awareness of the prevalence and impact of trauma on women's lives</li><li>To understand the psychological growth and development of women</li><li>To recognize the centrality of relationships for women, particularly parenting and social roles and the socialization process</li><li>To be knowledgeable about the physiology of women as it relates to substance use and abuse</li><li>To understand the etiology of substance abuse in women</li><li>To be familiar with the co-occurring disorders that commonly occur in women</li><li>To understand the context of abuse and patterns of use for women</li><li>To identify the consequences of substance abuse (e.g., legal, general health, infectious diseases, family and relationships, psychological)</li><li>To understand the treatment and recovery experience of women</li><li>To identify family dynamics (e.g., family of origin, parenting, child development)</li><li>To be familiar with a woman's process of recovery</li><li>To be knowledgeable about relapse prevention for women; relapse triggers such as family reunification; recovery resources; maintaining a safe place for the client; and loss, grief, and mourning</li><li>To understand issues related to sexuality, sexual orientation, and gender identity for women and their relationship to substance abuse</li><li>To know confidentiality rules and guidelines</li></ul>

supervision of counselors and to the need for training individuals to be effective supervisors (Cramer 2002). Supervisors also can support staff members who are in recovery and working as volunteers or mentors.

Clinical supervision for trauma

The management of the powerful effect associated with trauma presents challenges for counselors. As a result of their intense daily contact with trauma survivors, counselors are vulnerable to many symptoms and conditions including:

Vicarious traumatization. The experiences of trauma frequently are overwhelming for clients. As counselors listen to the life experiences of their clients, they too are at risk of becoming overwhelmed. Counselors can develop symptoms of depression, such as sleep disturbance, loss of appetite, or loss of pleasure in usually enjoyable activities. Programs can take various steps to lessen the effect of vicarious traumatization:

- *Training.* Staff training on trauma issues (including vicarious traumatization) and on the connections between trauma, substance abuse, and mental illness, help staff address trauma experiences.
- *Supervision.* Regular clinical supervision helps counselors unburden themselves. The sooner a counselor's distress is addressed, the easier it is to manage. Understanding the counselor's emotional vulnerabilities when she works with women who were traumatized is essential to providing effective treatment and allowing staff to work well, safely, and consistently.
- *Debriefing.* Managers and supervisors need to ensure that counselors debrief after hearing painful and intense histories from their clients and to watch for signs of counselors becoming overwhelmed.

- *Self-care.* Agency support should include awareness and education about signs of burnout, breaks from work, vacations, and varied schedules (i.e., with periods of less exposure to trauma histories).
- *Employee services.* Through peer support groups, an agency can acknowledge that vicarious traumatization is taking place and that its employees' ability to do their jobs well is important.
- *Staff appreciation.* Program managers and supervisors should be aware that staff members perform an important function as role models; they need to let staff members know they are valued. Counselors need to be examples of assertive, appropriate, high-functioning adults.

Supervision for counselors can be understood in a rock-climbing metaphor. The client has survived a terrible experience; it is as if she were on a high and windy ledge, still alive, but unable to find her way back to safety. To help her, the counselor must go out on the ledge; calling to her from safe ground will not do. To manage the task, the counselor must be tied to a supervisor, much as a rock climber is tied to another climber, to keep from falling (Cramer 2002).

Strategies for Organizational Change

A program seeking to become woman-centered cannot limit the transformation process to simply adopting superficial elements of the treatment culture (Markoff et al. 2005), such as creating a female-only program without changing program structure, integrating services, or building collaborative relationships across community agencies. Rather, it must use numerous strategies and endorse a change model to ensure organizational change is deep, pervasive, and across systems. The consensus panel recommends the following:

- *Training and education.* Staff members need help in identifying their biases and assumptions. Such training does not have to be intensive or expensive to be effective. For example, agencies can trade speakers.

- *Policies and procedures.* It is critical that programs have clear policies and procedures, and that women are informed of these policies and procedures at the beginning of their treatment. Programs must be consistent in how they implement policies and procedures. This is important from both a program management perspective and a clinical treatment perspective. Having clear, reasonable standards that are implemented uniformly creates a safe and predictable environment for clients.

  Drug and alcohol testing and searches for contraband must be done respectfully, letting the client know it is part of treatment and seeking her cooperation. It is necessary to spend time building a relationship with the client and to give her an opportunity to admit to a relapse or to remove items that are not permitted in a residential community.

  Staff must reinforce policies and rules uniformly and without preferential treatment. Fairness and justice are critical for women in treatment, and they must be modeled by the staff.

  Rules and punitive restrictions must be germane to treatment. For example, some programs do not allow women to talk to their children for the first 30 days of treatment. Such a blanket rule is inappropriate for children and shows disrespect for the importance of the mother–child relationship. Arbitrary rules are disempowering for women and not part of a collaborative relationship. The treatment milieu is a model for parent–child relationships, in which the use of arbitrary rules is discouraged. Following rules and procedures should not result in acts that retraumatize women. For example, it could be frightening for some women to have counselors check rooms at night while the women are sleeping.
- *Top-down support for change.* Advocacy for the program's philosophy of treatment is essential. It must be top down and explicit.
- *Hiring, retention, and promotion.* Programs must reflect women's needs, possibly

including onsite daycare for staff, sick-child care, support (both financial and technical) for staff to become certified as addiction counselors, onsite training, and a good health benefits package. The programs should consider ways in which male staff members can contribute to woman-centered programming. Staff members are more likely to support staffing policies and procedures when they are involved in their development.

- *Consumer input.* The development of consumer advisory boards allows clients to share their input and lets them know their opinions are valued and respected.

- *Relationships.* Positive relationships are of immeasurable value to women. How staff members relate to one another is part of the treatment milieu. Administrators need to model respectful relationships with clients and staff and incorporate support services for staff issues, such as mediation for staff conflicts and peer support groups for handling job stress.

- *The environment is a message.* Women recover best in a homelike atmosphere that is warm and welcoming for them and their children. The program environment needs to reflect the diverse cultures of the staff and clients; all groups can participate in designing, arranging, and furnishing the facility.

- *Adopt a change model.* Administrators and supervisors need to develop a change plan to maintain a steadfast course in adopting new policies and procedures and in integrating services. Anticipation of roadblocks, methods for creating buy-in with staff, and strategies for building interagency relationships are a few issues that need consideration. Relevant resources to help support and guide change include the Relational Systems Change Model (Markoff et al. 2005a) and *The Change Book: A Blueprint of Technology Transfer* (Addiction Technology Transfer Center [ATTC] 2004).

- *Collaborative relationships.* Establishing a collaborative relationship with the client provides the woman with an experience of mutuality and shared power in a relationship, which in itself is part of healing.

At all times, staff members should work respectfully and in partnership with the client, and should:

Set a positive tone for the treatment relationship. Counselors get a good start by showing respect for the clients' personal needs and comfort. For example, one treatment agency keeps a book that highlights the stories of women who have successfully completed treatment. Another offers clients food and drink. During a long client-assessment session, a counselor can offer a client a break instead of waiting for the client to ask for one. If possible, during the break the counselor should interact with the client so that she does not feel alone. However, if she requests it, the client should have private time.

Treat substance abuse as a health issue, not a moral one. A client who feels judged is more likely to leave treatment. Let clients know how they can be involved in their treatment, explain the process to them, explain the roles of the treatment staff members, and explain when clients will make decisions with staff about their treatment (i.e., during treatment planning, reassessments, discharge).

Allow time to hear the client's stories. Too often, a client's low self-esteem is made even lower by cues that there is not enough time to listen to her.

Do what is necessary to ensure that the client understands the assessment and treatment processes. For a client with cognitive impairment, this can involve breaking down the process into short sessions, repeating or explaining questions, proceeding more slowly, using less abstract language, or presenting information in an alternative format.

Seek feedback from the client on how her treatment plan is working. Inquire where she is in relation to her goals for treatment, her life, and her feelings about her progress. Implement formal strategies to obtain client feedback on a regular basis instead of gathering this data at the termination of treatment.

When addressing noncompliance with clients, involve them in identifying the problem and its solution. Use policies that are educational rather than punitive. For example, encourage clients to examine the behaviors they need to change, how staff can help them in this process, an agreeable timeframe for doing so, and so on.

State substance abuse treatment standards for women

To provide general guidance in establishing and providing services for women, administrators and clinical staff benefit from reviewing available State standards or protocols for women, pregnant women, and women and children programs for substance abuse treatment (for review, see CSAT 2007). Figure 8-5 provides examples of State standards of gender-specific treatment across the continuum of care.

	Figure 8-5
	State Standard Examples of Gender-Specific Treatment
Gender-Specific Women Services	**State Standard Examples**
Treatment Approach	• A relational or cultural approach that focuses on the relevance and centrality of relationships for women must be a vital ingredient in treatment • Selected treatment approaches shall be grounded in evidence-based or best practices for women
Screening/ Assessment	• Screening and assessments shall involve the use of tools, including the Addiction Severity Index and Stages of Change/Readiness Assessment • Assessments shall evaluate barriers to treatment and related services • Assessment and documentation of a client's need for prenatal care shall be included in the assessment process • History and assessment of interpersonal violence shall be evaluated • Sensitivity to retraumatization must be taken into consideration in the assessment process • Assessment shall be a collaborative process across agencies
Treatment Planning	• Planning shall include participation of significant others and other agencies; i.e., child welfare, correction, and other social service agencies
Treatment Programs	• Emotional and physical safety of women shall take precedence over all other considerations in the delivery of services • Women-only therapeutic environments shall be made available • Treatment shall include psychoeducation on the impact of gender on development and functioning in society • Treatment must be strength-based

Figure 8-5

State Standard Examples of Gender-Specific Treatment (continued)

Treatment Services	• Services must provide prenatal and childcare services • Treatment shall include smoking cessation strategies and programs • Services shall include child safety, parenting, and nutrition services • Wrap-around and integrated interagency and intra-agency services must be an integral part of treatment delivery services
Trauma-Informed and Integrated Trauma Services	• Treatment considerations shall incorporate an understanding of the way symptoms of trauma affect treatment, progress in treatment, and the relationship among counselor, program, and client
Co-Occurring Disorders	• Treatment must include symptom management strategies • Services for mental health and substance abuse treatment shall be integrated and coordinated
Staffing	• The program must provide gender-specific staff • Treatment services shall involve a majority of women as staff members
Support Systems	• The program shall make use of peer supports • Referrals shall be made to female-dominated support groups where available
Staff Training	• Formal staff training in women's treatment needs must include family counseling, trauma-informed services, prenatal education, etc.
Program Evaluation	• Program must measure short- and long-term impact of interventions, including educational attainment, employment, housing, parenting and reunification with children, and physical and mental health

Source: Adapted from Connecticut Treatment Guidelines 2007; Colorado Alcohol and Drug Abuse Division Substance Use Disorder Treatment Rules 2006; Oklahoma Department of Mental Health and Substance Abuse Services Standards and Criteria for Alcohol and Drug Treatment Programs 2008; and Oregon Department of Human Services Standards for Outpatient and Residential Alcohol and Drug Treatment Programs 2008.

Guidance to States: Treatment Standards for Women with Substance Use Disorders

This document serves as a comprehensive guide to assist States in creating their own treatment standards for women with substance use disorders. It provides a summary of existing State standards and incorporates other relevant resources pertinent to women's treatment needs across multiple service systems. Specific concerns for special populations are addressed, such as pregnant women, women with children, and women involved in the criminal justice system (The National Association of State Alcohol and Drug Abuse Directors 2008; see http://www.nasadad.org/resource.php?base_id=1482).

Appendix A: Bibliography

Abs, R., Verhelst, J., Maeyaert, J., Van Buyten, J.P., Opsomer, F., Adriaensen, H., Verlooy, J., Van Havenbergh, T., Smet, M., and Van Acker, K. Endocrine consequences of long-term intrathecal administration of opioids. *Journal of Clinical Endocrinology and Metabolism* 85(6):2215–2222, 2000.

Ackard, D.M., and Neumark-Sztainer, D. Multiple sexual victimizations among adolescent boys and girls: Prevalence and associations with eating behaviors and psychological health. *Journal of Child Sexual Abuse* 12(1):17–37, 2003.

Acker, C. Neuropsychological deficits in alcoholics: the relative contributions of gender and drinking history. *British Journal of Addiction* 81(3):395–403, 1986.

Adams, H., and Phillips, L. Experiences of two-spirit lesbian and gay Native Americans: An argument for standpoint theory in identity research. *Identity* 6(3):273-291, 2006.

Addiction Technology Transfer Center. *The Change Book: A Blueprint for Technology Transfer*. 2nd ed. Kansas City, MO: Addiction Technology Transfer Center, 2004.

Adler, N.E., and Coriell, M. Socioeconomic status and women's health. In: Gallant, S.J., Keita, G.P., and Royak-Schaler, R., eds. *Health Care for Women: Psychological, Social, and Behavioral Influences*. Washington, DC: American Psychological Association Press, 1997. pp. 11–23.

Agrawal, A., Gardner, C.O., Prescott, C.A., and Kendler, K.S. The differential impact of risk factors on illicit drug involvement in females. *Social Psychiatry and Psychiatric Epidemiology* 40(6):454–466, 2005.

Aguirre-Molina, M., Molina, C.W., and Zambrana, R.E. *Health Issues in the Latino Community*. San Francisco: Jossey-Bass, 2001.

Alati, R., Al, M.A., Williams, G.M., O'Callaghan, M., Najman, J.M., and Bor, W. In utero alcohol exposure and prediction of alcohol disorders in early adulthood: a birth cohort study. *Archives of General Psychiatry* 63(9):1009–1016, 2006.

Alegria, M., Canino, G., Rios, R., Vera, M., Calderon, J., Rusch, D., and Ortega, A.N. Mental health care for Latinos: Inequalities in use of specialty mental health services among Latinos, African Americans, and Non-Latino Whites. *Psychiatric Services* 53(12):1547–1555, 2002.

Alexander, M.J. Women with co-occurring addictive and mental disorders: An emerging profile of vulnerability. *American Journal of Orthopsychiatry* 66(1):61–70, 1996.

Allen, D.N., Frantom, L.V., Forrest, T.J., and Strauss, G.P. Neuropsychology of substance use disorders. In: Snyder, P.J., Nussbaum, P.D., and Robins, D.L., eds. *Clinical Neuropsychology: A Pocket Handbook for Assessment, 2nd ed.* 1-59147-283-0 (paperback). American Psychological Association: Washington, 2006. pp. 649–673.

Allen, J.P. The interrelationship of alcoholism assessment and treatment. *Alcohol Health and Research World* 15:178–185, 1991.

Allen, K. Barriers to treatment for addicted African-American women. *Journal of the National Medical Association* 87(10):751–756, 1995.

Altarriba, J., and Bauer, L.M. Counseling the Hispanic client: Cuban Americans, Mexican Americans, and Puerto Ricans. *Journal of Counseling & Development* 76(4):389-396, 1998.

Alvarez, L.R., and Ruiz, P. Substance abuse in the Mexican American population. In: Straussner, S.L.A., ed. *Ethnocultural Factors in Substance Abuse Treatment.* New York: Guilford Press, 2001. pp. 111–136.

Amaro, H., and Aguiar, M. Programa Mama / Mom's Project: A community-based outreach model for addicted women. In: Szapocznik, J., Orlandi, M.A., and Epstein, L.G., eds. *A Hispanic/Latino Family Approach to Substance Abuse Prevention.* CSAP Cultural Competence Series 2. HHS Publication No. (SMA) 95-3034. Rockville, MD: Center for Substance Abuse Prevention, 1995. pp. 125–153.

Amaro, H., and de la Torre, A. Public health needs and scientific opportunities in research on Latinas. *American Journal of Public Health* 92(4):525–529, 2002.

Amaro, H., and Hardy-Fanta, C. Gender relations in addiction and recovery. *Journal of Psychoactive Drugs* 27(4):325–337, 1995.

Amaro, H., Chernoff, M., Brown, V., Arevalo, S., and Gatz, M. Does integrated trauma-informed substance abuse treatment increase treatment retention? *Journal of Community Psychology* 35(7):845–862, 2008.

Amaro, H., Larson, M.J., Gampel, J., Richardson, E., Savage, A., and Wagler, D. Racial/ethnic differences in social vulnerability among women with co-occurring mental health and substance abuse disorders: Implications for treatment services. *Journal of Community Psychology* 33(4):495–511, 2005.

Amaro, H., Larson, M.J., Zhang, A., Acevedo, A., Dai, J., and Matsumoto, A. Effects of trauma intervention on HIV sexual risk behaviors among women with co-occurring disorders in substance abuse treatment. *Journal of Community Psychology* 35(7):895–908, 2007.

Amaro, H., Nieves, R., Johannes, S.W., and Labault Cabeza, N.M. Substance abuse treatment: Critical issues and challenges in the treatment of Latina women. *Hispanic Journal of Behavioral Sciences* 21(3):266–282, 1999.

Amaro, H., Whitaker, R., Coffman, G., and Heeren, T. Acculturation and marijuana and cocaine use: Findings from HHANES 1982–84. *American Journal of Public Health* 80(Supplement):54–60, 1990.

American Association of Community Psychiatrists. LOCUS - Level of Care Utilization System, Psychiatric and Addiction Services. Adult Version, 2000.

American Psychiatric Association. *Diagnostic and Statistical Manual of Mental Disorders.* 4th ed. Washington, DC: American Psychiatric Association, 1994.

American Psychiatric Association. *Diagnostic and Statistical Manual of Mental Disorders.* 4th Text Revision ed. Washington, DC: American Psychiatric Association, 2000*a*.

American Psychiatric Association. *Position Statement on Therapies Focused on Memories of Childhood Physical and Sexual Abuse.* Washington, DC: American Psychiatric Association, 2000*b*.

American Psychological Association - Presidential Task Force on Violence and the Family. *Violence and the Family: Report of the American Psychological Association Presidential Task Force on Violence and the Family.* Washington, DC: American Psychological Association, 1996.

American Society of Addiction Medicine. *Patient Placement Criteria for the Treatment of Substance-Related Disorders: ASAM PPC-2.* 2d ed. Chevy Chase, MD: American Society of Addiction Medicine, 1996.

American Society of Addiction Medicine. *Patient Placement Criteria for the Treatment of Substance-Related Disorders: ASAM PPC-2R.* 2d - Revised ed. Chevy Chase, MD: American Society of Addiction Medicine, 2001.

Ames, G., and Mora, J. Alcohol problem prevention in Mexican American populations. In: Gilbert, M.J., ed. *Alcohol Consumption Among Mexicans and Mexican Americans: A Binational Perspective.* Los Angeles: University of California, 1988. pp. 253–281.

Ammendola, A., Gemini, D., Iannaccone, S., Argenzio, F., Ciccone, G., Ammendola, E., Serio, L., Ugolini, G., and Bravaccio, F. Gender and peripheral neuropathy in chronic alcoholism: Clinical-electroneurographic study. *Alcohol and Alcoholism* 35(4):368–371, 2000.

Amodeo, M., and Jones, L.K. Viewing alcohol and other drug use cross culturally: A cultural framework for clinical practice. *Families in Society* 78(3):240–254, 1997.

Anda, R.F., Whitfield, C.L., Felitti, V.J., Chapman, D., Edwards, V.J., Dube, S.R., and Williamson, D.F. Adverse childhood experiences, alcoholic parents, and later risk of alcoholism and depression. *Psychiatric Services* 53(8):1001–1009, 2002.

Andersen, A., Due, P., Holstein, B.E., and Iversen, L. Tracking drinking behaviour from age 15-19 years. *Addiction* 98(11):1505-1511, 2003.

Andersen, M. Health needs of drug dependent clients: Focus on women. *Women and Health* 5(1):23–33, 1980.

Anderson, F., Paluzzi, P., Lee, J., Huggins, G., and Huggins, G. Illicit use of clonidine in opiate-abusing pregnant women. *Obstetrics and Gynecology* 90(5):790–794, 1997.

Anderson, S.C. Substance abuse and dependency in gay men and lesbians. In: Peterson, K.J., ed. *Health Care for Lesbians and Gay Men: Confronting Homophobia and Heterosexism.* Binghamton, NY: Haworth Press, 1996. pp. 59–77.

Andrykowski, M.A., Cordova, M.J., Studts, J.L., and Miller, T.W. Posttraumatic stress disorder after treatment for breast cancer: Prevalence of diagnosis and use of the PTSD Checklist--Civilian Version (PCL--C) as a screening instrument. *Journal of Consulting and Clinical Psychology* 66(3):586–590, 1998.

Antai-Otong, D. Women and alcoholism: Gender-related medical complications: Treatment considerations. *Journal of Addictions Nursing* 17(1):33–45, 2006.

Appel, P.W., Ellison, A.A., Jansky, H.K., and Oldak, R. Barriers to enrollment in drug abuse treatment and suggestions for reducing them: opinions of drug injecting street outreach clients and other system stakeholders. *American Journal of Drug and Alcohol Abuse* 30(1):129–153, 2004.

Aquilino, W.S. Interview mode effects in surveys of drug and alcohol use: A field experiment. *Public Opinion Quarterly* 58(2):210–240, 1994.

Arborelius, E., and Damstrom, T.K. Why is it so difficult for general practitioners to discuss alcohol with patients? *Family Practice* 12(4):419–422, 1995.

Archie, C. Methadone in the management of narcotic addiction in pregnancy. *Current Opinion in Obstetrics and Gynecology* 10(6):435–440, 1998.

Arfken, C.L., Klein, C., di Menza, S., and Schuster, C.R. Gender differences in problem severity at assessment and treatment retention. *Journal of Substance Abuse Treatment* 20(1):53–57, 2001.

Arnett, J.J. The developmental context of substance use in emerging adulthood. *Journal of Drug Issues* 35(2):235–254, 2005.

Ashley, O.S., Sverdlov, L., and Brady, T.M. Length of stay among female clients in substance abuse treatment. *Health Services Utilization by Individuals With Substance Abuse and Mental Disorders* Council, C. L. (HHS Publication No. SMA 04-3949, Analytic Series A-25) Rockville, MD: Substance Abuse and Mental Health Services Administration, 2004.

Augustyn, M., Parker, S., Groves, B., and Zuckerman, B. Silent victims: Children who witness violence. *Contemporary Pediatrics* 12(8):35–37, 1995.

Ayala, J., and Coleman, H. Predictors of depression among lesbian women. *Journal of Lesbian Studies* 4(3):71–86, 2000.

Babor, T.F., and Grant M. From clinical research to secondary prevention: International collaboration in the development of the Alcohol Use Disorders Identification Test (AUDIT). *Alcoholism and Health Research World* 13:371–374, 1989.

Babor, T.F., McRee, B.G., Kassebaum, P.A., Grimaldi, P.L., Ahmed, K., and Bray, J. Screening, Brief Intervention, and Referral to Treatment (SBIRT): Toward a public health approach to the management of substance abuse. *Substance Abuse* 28(3):7–30, 2007.

Baca, C.T., Alverson, D.C., Manuel, J.K., and Blackwell, G.L. Telecounseling in rural areas for alcohol problems. *Alcoholism Treatment Quarterly* 25(4):31–45, 2007.

Bachu, A., and O'Connell, M. Fertility of American Women: June 2000. *Current Population Reports.P20-543RV* Washington, DC: U.S. Census Bureau, 2001.

Bagnardi, V., Blangiardo, M., La Vecchia, C., and Corrao, G. Alcohol consumption and the risk of cancer: A meta-analysis. *Alcohol Research and Health* 25(4):263–270, 2001.

Balcazar, H., and Qian, Z. Immigrant families and sources of stress. In: McKenry, P.C., and Price, S.J., eds. *Families and Change: Coping with Stressful Events and Transitions*. 2d ed. Thousand Oaks, CA: Sage Publications, 2000. pp. 359–377.

Balsam, K.F., Huang, B., Fieland, K.C., Simoni, J.M., and Walters, K.L. Culture, trauma, and wellness: a comparison of heterosexual and lesbian, gay, bisexual, and two-spirit Native Americans. *Cultural Diversity & Ethnic Minority Psychology* 10(3):287-301, 2004.

Barnes, J.S., and Bennett, C.E. *The Asian Population: 2000. Census 2000 Brief* Washington, DC: U.S. Census Bureau, 2002.

Barnes-Josiah, D.L. Undoing racism in public health: A blueprint for action in urban MCH. CityMatCH at the University of Nebraska Medical Center. Omaha, NE, 2004.

Baron, M. Addiction treatment for Mexican American families. In: Krestan, J.A., ed. *Bridges to Recovery: Addiction, Family Therapy, and Multicultural Treatment*. New York: The Free Press, 2000. pp. 219–252.

Barsky, A.J., Peekna, H.M., and Borus, J.F. Somatic symptom reporting in women and men. *Journal of General Internal Medicine* 16(4):266–275, 2001.

Bassuk, E.L., Melnick, S., and Browne, A. Responding to the needs of low-income and homeless women who are survivors of family violence. *Journal of the American Medical Women's Association* 53(2):57–64, 1998.

Bateman, D.A., and Chiriboga, C.A. Dose-response effect of cocaine on newborn head circumference. *Pediatrics* 106(3):E33, 2000.

Battle, C.L., Zlotnick, C., Najavits, L.M., Gutierrez, M., and Winsor, C. Posttraumatic stress disorder and substance use disorder among incarcerated women. In: Ouimette, P., and Brown, P.J., eds. *Trauma and Substance Abuse: Causes, Consequences, and Treatment of Comorbid Disorders*. Washington, DC: American Psychological Association, 2003. pp. 209–225.

Bauer, C.R., Langer, J.C., Shankaran, S., Bada, H.S., Lester, B., Wright, L.L., Krause-Steinrauf, H., Smeriglio, V.L., Finnegan, L.P., Maza, P.L., and Verter, J. Acute neonatal effects of cocaine exposure during pregnancy. *Archives of Pediatrics & Adolescent Medicine* 159(9):824–834, 2005.

Beatty, L.A. Substance abuse, disabilities, and black women: An issue worth exploring. *Women & Therapy* 26(3-4):223–236, 2003.

Beauvais, F., Wayman, J.C., Jumper Thurman, P., Plested, B., and Helm, H. Inhalant abuse among American Indian, Mexican American, and non-Latino white adolescents. *American Journal of Drug and Alcohol Abuse* 28(1):171–187, 2002.

Beck, A.J. *Prisoners in 1999*. NCJ 183476 Washington, DC: Bureau of Justice Statistics, 2000.

Beck, A.J., and Harrison, P.M. Prisoners in 2000. *Bureau of Justice Statistics Bulletin* Washington, DC: Bureau of Justice Statistics, 2001.

Beck, A.J., Karberg, J.C., and Harrison, P.M. *Prison and Jail Inmates at Midyear 2001*. NCJ 191702 Washington, DC: Bureau of Justice Statistics, 2002.

Beck, A.T. *Beck Anxiety Inventory*. San Antonio, TX: The Psychological Corporation, 1993.

Beck, A.T., Steer, R.A., and Brown, G.K. *Beck Depression Inventory - II Manual*. San Antonio, TX: The Psychological Corporation, 1996*a*.

Beck, R.W., Jijon, C.R., and Edwards, J.B. The relationships among gender, perceived financial barriers to care, and health status in a rural population. *Journal of Rural Health* 12(3):188–189, 1996*b*.

Becker, U., Deis, A., Sorensen, T.I., Gronbaek, M., Borch-Johnsen, K., Muller, C.F., Schnohr, P., and Jensen, G. Prediction of risk of liver disease by alcohol intake, sex, and age: A prospective population study. *Hepatology* 23(5):1025–1029, 1996.

Becker, M.A., and Gatz, M. Introduction to the impact of co-occurring disorders and violence on women: Findings from the SAMHSA Women, Co-occurring Disorders and Violence Study. *Journal of Behavior Health Services & Research* 32(2):111–112, 2005.

Beckman, L.J. Treatment needs of women with alcohol problems. *Alcohol Health and Research World* 18(3):206–211, 1994.

Beckman, L.J., and Amaro, H. Personal and social difficulties faced by women and men entering alcoholism treatment. *Journal of Studies on Alcohol* 47(2):135–145, 1986.

Bell, B.P., Mast, E.E., Terrault, N., and Hutin, Y.J. Prevention of hepatitis C in women. *Emerging Infectious Diseases* 10(11):2035–2036, 2004.

Bell, E.C., Baker, G.B., Poag, C., Bellavance, F., Khudabux, J., and Le Melledo, J.M. Response to flumazenil in the late luteal phase and follicular phase of the menstrual cycle in healthy control females. *Psychopharmacology (Berl)* 172(3):248–254, 2004.

Bell, G.L., and Lau, K. Perinatal and neonatal issues of substance abuse. *Pediatric Clinics of North America* 42(2):261–281, 1995.

Bell, P. *Chemical Dependency and the African-American: Counseling Strategies and Community Issues*. 2nd ed. Center City, MN: Hazelden, 2002.

Benshoff, J.J., Harrawood, L.K., and Koch, D.S. Substance abuse and the elderly: Unique issues and concerns. *Journal of Rehabilitation* 69(2): 2003.

Bergmark, K.H. Drinking in the Swedish gay and lesbian community. *Drug and Alcohol Dependence* 56(2):133–143, 1999.

Berkowitz, G., Peterson, S., Smith, E.M., Taylor, T., and Brindis, C. Community and treatment program challenges for chemically dependent American Indian and Alaska Native women. *Contemporary Drug Problems* 25(2):347–371, 1998.

Bernstein, D.P. Childhood trauma and drug addiction: Assessment, diagnosis, and treatment. *Alcoholism Treatment Quarterly* 18(3):19–30, 2000.

Besharov, D.J., and Hanson, K.W. *When Drug Addicts Have Children: Reorienting Child Welfare's Response*. Washington, DC: Child Welfare League of America, 1994.

Beutler, L.E., Machado, P.P., and Neufeldt, S.A. Therapist variables. In: Bergin, A.E., and Garfield, S.L., eds. *Handbook of Psychotherapy and Behavior Change*. 4th ed. Oxford: John Wiley and Sons, 1994. pp. 229–269.

Bickelhaupt, E.E. Alcoholism and drug abuse in gay and lesbian persons: A review of incidence studies. *Journal of Gay and Lesbian Social Services* 2(1):5–14, 1995.

Black, S.A., and Markides, K.S. Acculturation and alcohol consumption in Puerto Rican, Cuban-American, and Mexican-American women in the United States. *American Journal of Public Health* 83(6):890–893, 1993.

Blanchard, E.B., Jones-Alexander, J., Buckley, T.C., and Forneris, C.A. Psychometric properties of the PTSD Checklist (PCL). *Behaviour Research & Therapy* 34(8):669–673, 1996.

Block, R.I., Farinpour, R., and Schlechte, J.A. Effects of chronic marijuana use on testosterone, luteinizing hormone, follicle stimulating hormone, prolactin and cortisol in men and women. *Drug and Alcohol Dependence* 28(2):121–128, 1991.

Bloom, B., Owen, B., and Covington, S. *Gender-Responsive Strategies: Research, Practice, and Guiding Principles for Women Offenders*. Washington, DC: National Institute of Corrections, 2003.

Blow, F.C., and Barry, K.L. Use and misuse of alcohol among older women. *Alcohol Research and Health* 26(4):308–315, 2002.

Blum, L.N., Nielsen, N.H., and Riggs, J.A. Alcoholism and alcohol abuse among women: Report of the Council on Scientific Affairs. American Medical Association. *Journal of Women's Health* 7(7):861–871, 1998.

Blume, S. Sexuality and stigma. *Alcohol Health and Research World* 15(2):139–146, 1991.

Blume, S.B. Women and alcohol: Issues in social policy. In: Wilsnack, R.W., and Wilsnack, S.C., eds. *Gender And Alcohol: Individual And Social Perspectives*. New Brunswick, NJ: Rutgers Center of Alcohol Studies, 1997. pp. 462–489.

Blumenthal, S.J. Women and substance abuse: A new national focus. In: Wetherington, C.L., and Roman, A.B., eds. *Drug Addiction Research and the Health of Women*. NIH Publication No. 98-4290. Rockville, MD: National Institute on Drug Abuse, 1998. pp. 13–32.

Bobo, J.K., Schilling, R.F., Gilchrist, L.D., and Schinke, S.P. The double triumph: Sustained sobriety and successful cigarette smoking cessation. *Journal of Substance Abuse Treatment* 3(1):21–25, 1986.

Bolnick, J.M., and Rayburn, W.F. Substance use disorders in women: special considerations during pregnancy. *Obstetrics and Gynecology Clinics of North America* 30(3):545–58, vii, 2003.

Borrelli, B., Papandonatos, G., Spring, B., Hitsman, B., and Niaura, R. Experimenter-defined quit dates for smoking cessation: adherence improves outcomes for women but not for men. *Addiction* 99(3):378–385, 2004.

Bottorff, J.L., Johnson, J.L., Irwin, L.G., and Ratner, P.A. Narratives of smoking relapse: The stories of postpartum women. *Research in Nursing and Health* 23(2):126–134, 2000.

Boyd, M.B., Mackey, M.C., Phillips, K.D., and Tavakoli, A. Alcohol and other drug disorders, comorbidity and violence in rural African American women. *Issues in Mental Health Nursing* 27(10):1017–1036, 2006.

Boyd, M.R. Substance abuse in rural women. *Nursing Connections* 11(2):33–45, 1998.

Boyd, M.R. Vulnerability to alcohol and other drug disorders in rural women. *Archives of Psychiatric Nursing* 17(1):33–41, 2003.

Boyd, M.R., and Mackey, M.C. Alienation from self and others: The psychosocial problem of rural alcoholic women. *Archives of Psychiatric Nursing* 14(3):134–141, 2000*a*.

Boyd, M.R., and Mackey, M.C. Running away to nowhere: Rural women's experiences of becoming alcohol dependent. *Archives of Psychiatric Nursing* 14(3):142–149, 2000*b*.

Boyd-Franklin, N. *Black Families In Therapy: A Multisystems Approach*. New York: Guilford Press, 1989.

Boyd-Franklin, N., and Lockwood, T.W. Spirituality and religion: Implications for psychotherapy with African American families. In: Walsh, F., ed. Spiritual Resources In Family Therapy (2nd ed.). 978-1-60623-022-0 (hardcover). Guilford Press: New York, 2009. pp. 141-155.

Bradley, K.A., Badrinath, S., Bush, K., Boyd-Wickizer, J., and Anawalt, B. Medical risks for women who drink alcohol. *Journal of General Internal Medicine* 13(9):627–639, 1998*a*.

Bradley, K.A., Boyd-Wickizer, J., Powell, S.H., and Burman, M.L. Alcohol screening questionnaires in women: A critical review. *JAMA* 280(2):166–171, 1998*b*.

Bradley, K.A., Bush, K.R., McDonell, M.B., Malone, T., and Fihn, S.D. Screening for problem drinking: Comparison of CAGE and AUDIT. Ambulatory Care Quality Improvement Project (ACQUIP). Alcohol Use Disorders Identification Test. *Journal of General Internal Medicine* 13(6):379–388, 1998*c*.

Brady, K. *Anxiety and Substance Abuse.* 154th Annual Meeting of the American Psychiatric Association May 5 – 10, 2001, New Orleans, Louisiana, 2001*a*.

Brady, K.T. Comorbid posttraumatic stress disorder and substance use disorders. *Psychiatric Annals* 31(5):313–319, 2001*b*.

Brady, K.T., and Randall, C.L. Gender differences in substance use disorders. *Psychiatric Clinics of North America* 22(2):241–252, 1999.

Brady, K.T., Dansky, B.S., Back, S.E., Foa, E.B., and Carroll, K.M. Exposure therapy in the treatment of PTSD among cocaine-dependent individuals: Preliminary findings. *Journal of Substance Abuse Treatment* 21(1):47–54, 2001.

Brady, K.T., Killeen, T.K., Brewerton, T., and Lucerini, S. Comorbidity of psychiatric disorders and posttraumatic stress disorder. *Journal of Clinical Psychiatry* 61(Suppl 7):22–32, 2000.

Brady, T.M., and Ashley, O.S. Women In Substance Abuse Treatment: Results from the Alcohol and Drug Services Study (ADSS). (HHS Publication No. SMA 04-3968, Analytic Series A-26). Rockville, MD: Substance Abuse and Mental Health Services Administration, Office of Applied Studies, 2005.

Brecht, M.L., O'Brien, A., Mayrhauser, C.V., and Anglin, M.D. Methamphetamine use behaviors and gender differences. *Addictive Behaviors* 29(1):89–106, 2004.

Brems, C. Substance use, mental health, and health in Alaska: Emphasis on Alaska Native peoples. *Arctic Medical Research* 55(3):135–147, 1996.

Brennan, P.L., Moos, R.H., and Kim, J.Y. Gender differences in the individual characteristics and life contexts of late-middle-aged and older problem drinkers. *Addiction* 88(6):781–790, 1993.

Breslau, N., Davis, G.C., Andreski, P., and Peterson, E. Traumatic events and posttraumatic stress disorder in an urban population of young adults. *Archives of General Psychiatry* 48(3):216–222, 1991.

Breslau, N., Davis, G.C., Andreski, P., Peterson, E.L., and Schultz, L.R. Sex differences in posttraumatic stress disorder. *Archives of General Psychiatry* 54(11):1044–1048, 1997.

Bride, B.E. Single-gender treatment of substance abuse: Effect on treatment retention and completion. *Social Work Research* 25(4):223–232, 2001.

Brindis, C.D., and Theidon, K.S. The role of case management in substance abuse treatment services for women and their children. *Journal of Psychoactive Drugs* 29(1):79–88, 1997.

Brome, D.R., Ownes, M.D., Allen, K., and Vevaina, T. An examination of spirituality among African American women in recovery from substance abuse. *Journal of Black Psychology* 26(4):470–486, 2000.

Bronfenbrenner, U. Ecological systems theory. *Annals of Child Development* 6:187–249, 1989.

Brook, D.W., Brook, J.S., Richter, L., Masci, J.R., and Roberto, J. Needle sharing: a longitudinal study of female injection drug users. *American Journal of Drug and Alcohol Abuse* 26(2):263-281, 2000.

Brook, J., Whiteman, M., Balka, E., Win, P., and Gursen, M. Similar and different precursors to drug use and delinquency among African Americans and Puerto Ricans. *Journal of Genetic Psychology* 159(1):13–29, 1998.

Brown, E., Frank, D., and Friedman, A. *Supplementary Administration Manual for the Expanded Female Version of the Addiction Severity Index (ASI) Instrument The ASI-F.* HHS Publication Number 96-8056. U.S. Department of Health and Human Services, Substance Abuse and Mental Health Services Administration, Center for Substance Abuse Treatment, 1997.

Brown, E.R., Ponce, N., and Rice, T. *The State of Health Insurance in California: Recent Trends, Future Prospects.* Los Angeles: UCLA Center for Health Policy Research, 2001.

Brown, P.J., Recupero, P.R., and Stout, R. PTSD substance abuse comorbidity and treatment utilization. *Addictive Behaviors* 20(2):251–254, 1995.

Brown, P.J., Stout, R.L., and Mueller, T. Posttraumatic stress disorder and substance abuse relapse among women: A pilot study. *Psychology of Addictive Behaviors* 10(2):124–128, 1996.

Brown, S.P., Lipford-Sanders, J., and Shaw, M. Kujichagulia: Uncovering the secrets of the heart: Group work with African American women on predominantly white campuses. *Journal for Specialists in Group Work* 20(3):151–158, 1995a.

Brown, T.G., Kokin, M., Seraganian, P., and Shields, N. The role of spouses of substance abusers in treatment: Gender differences. *Journal of Psychoactive Drugs* 27(3):223–229, 1995b.

Brown, V.B. *Changing And Improving Services For Women And Children: Strategies Used And Lessons Learned.* Los Angeles, CA: Prototypes Systems Change Center, 2000.

Brown, V.B., Najavits, L.M., Cadiz, S., Finkelstein, N., Heckman, J.P., and Rechberger, E. Implementing an evidence-based practice: Seeking Safety Group. *Journal of Psychoactive Drugs* 39(3):231–240, 2007.

Brownridge, D.A. Partner violence against women with disabilities: Prevalence, risk, and explanations. *Violence Against Women* 12(9):805–822, 2006.

Brudenell, I. Parenting an infant during alcohol recovery. *Journal of Pediatric Nursing* 15(2):82–88, 2000.

Bryant, J., and Treloar, C. The gendered context of initiation to injecting drug use: evidence for women as active initiates. *Drug And Alcohol Review* 26(3):287–293, 2007.

Buchsbaum, D.G., Buchanan, R.G., Lawton, M.J., Elswick, R.K., Jr., and Schnoll, S.H. A program of screening and prompting improves short-term physician counseling of dependent and nondependent harmful drinkers. *Archives of Internal Medicine* 153(13):1573–1577, 1993.

Bulik, C., and Sullivan, P. Comorbidity of eating disorders and substance-related disorders. In: Kranzler, H.R., and Rounsaville, B., eds. *Dual Diagnosis and Treatment: Substance Abuse and Cormorbid Medical and Psychiatric Disorders.* New York: Marcel Dekker, 1998. pp. 365–392.

Bulik, C.M., Klump, K.L., Thornton, L., Kaplan, A.S., Devlin, B., Fichter, M.M., Halmi, K.A., Strober, M., Woodside, D.B., Crow, S., Mitchell, J.E., Rotondo, A., Mauri, M., Cassano, G.B., Keel, P.K., Berrettini, W.H., and Kaye, W.H. Alcohol use disorder comorbidity in eating disorders: A multicenter study. *Journal of Clinical Psychiatry* 65(7):1000–1006, 2004.

Bureau of Justice Statistics. *Compendium of Federal Justice Statistics, 2004.* Washington, DC: U.S. Department of Justice, 2006.

Bureau of the Census (Current Population Survey, March 2002, Ethnic and Hispanic Statistics Branch, Population Division). Table 15.1 Poverty status of families in 2001 by family type and by Hispanic origin and race of householder: March 2002 http://www.census.gov/population/socdemo/hispanic/ppl-165/tab15-1.pdf [Accessed September 17, 2008].

Burkett, G., Gomez-Marin, O., Yasin, S.Y., and Martinez, M. Prenatal care in cocaine-exposed pregnancies. *Obstetrics and Gynecology* 92(2):193–200, 1998.

Burkett, G., Yasin, S.Y., Palow, D., LaVoie, L., and Martinez, M. Patterns of cocaine binging: Effect on pregnancy. *American Journal of Obstetrics and Gynecology* 171(2):372–379, 1994.

Burling, T.A., Burling, A.S., and Latini, D. A controlled smoking cessation trial for substance-dependent inpatients. *Journal of Consulting & Clinical Psychology* 69(2):295–304, 2001.

Burns, L., Mattick, R.P., Lim, K., and Wallace, C. Methadone in pregnancy: treatment retention and neonatal outcomes. *Addiction* 102(2):264–270, 2007.

Burt, V.K., and Stein, K. Epidemiology of depression throughout the female life cycle. *Journal of Clinical Psychiatry* 63(Suppl7):9–15, 2002.

Bushy, A. Mental health and substance abuse: Challenges in providing services to rural clients. In: Center for Substance Abuse Treatment, ed. *Bringing Excellence To Substance Abuse Services In Rural And Frontier America*. Technical Assistance Publication Series 20. Rockville, MD: Center for Substance Abuse Treatment, 1997. pp. 45–53.

Butler, A.C., Chapman, J.E., Forman, E.M., and Beck, A.T. The empirical status of cognitive-behavioral therapy: a review of meta-analyses. *Clinical Psychology Review* 26(1):17–31, 2006.

Caetano, R. Alcohol use among Hispanic groups in the United States. *American Journal of Drug and Alcohol Abuse* 14(3):293–308, 1988.

Caetano, R. Drinking patterns and alcohol problems in a national sample of U.S. Hispanics. In: Spiegler, D., Tate, D., Aitken, S., and Christian, C., eds. *Alcohol Use Among U.S. Ethnic Minorities: Proceedings Of A Conference On The Epidemiology Of Alcohol Use And Abuse Among Ethnic Minority Groups, September 1985*. NIAAA Research Monograph No. 18. HHS Publication No. (ADM) 89-1435. Rockville, MD: National Institute on Alcohol Abuse and Alcoholism, 1989. pp. 147–162.

Caetano, R. Drinking and alcohol-related problems among minority women. *Alcohol Health and Research World* 18(3):233–241, 1994.

Caetano, R., Ramisetty-Mikler, S., Vaeth, P.A.C., and Harris, T.R. Acculturation stress, drinking, and intimate partner violence among Hispanic couples in the U.S. *Journal of Interpersonal Violence* 22(11):1431–1447, 2007.

Caetano, R., Ramisetty-Mikler, S., Wallisch, L.S., McGrath, C., and Spence, R.T. Acculturation, drinking, and alcohol abuse and dependence among Hispanics in the Texas-Mexico border. *Alcoholism: Clinical & Experimental Research* 32(2):314-321, 2008.

Caldwell, T.M., Rodgers, B., Jorm, A.F., Christensen, H., Jacomb, P.A., Korten, A.E., and Lynskey, M.T. Patterns of association between alcohol consumption and symptoms of depression and anxiety in young adults. *Addiction* 97(5):583–594, 2002.

Camp, J.M., and Finkelstein, N. Parenting training for women in residential substance abuse treatment: Results of a demonstration project. *Journal of Substance Abuse Treatment* 14(5):411–422, 1997.

Canino, G. Alcohol use and misuse among Hispanic women: Selected factors, processes, and studies. *International Journal of the Addictions* 29(9):1083–1100, 1994.

Canino, G., Vega, W.A., Sribney, W.M., Warner, L.A., and Alegria, M. Social Relationships, social assimilation, and substance use disorders among adult Latinos in the U.S. *Journal of Drug Issues* 38(1):69–101, 2008.

Carlson, B.E., Matto, H., Smith, C.A., and Eversman, M. A pilot study of reunification following drug abuse treatment: Recovering the mother role. *Journal of Drug Issues* 36(4):877–902, 2006.

Carmen, E.H. Inner city community mental health: The interplay of abuse and race in chronic mentally ill women. In: Willie, C.V., Rieker, P.P., Kramer, B.M., and Brown, B.S., eds. *Mental Health: Racism and Sexism*. Pittsburgh, PA: University of Pittsburgh Press, 1995. pp. 217–236.

Carmichael, S.L., and Ahluwalia, I.B. Correlates of postpartum smoking relapse: Results from the pregnancy risk assessment monitoring system (PRAMS). *American Journal of Preventive Medicine* 19(3):193–196, 2000.

Carney, C.P., and Jones, L.E. The influence of type and severity of mental illness on receipt of screening mammography. *Journal of General Internal Medicine* 21(10):1097–1104, 2006.

Carr, A., and McNulty, M. Eating disorders. In: Carr, A., and McNulty, M., eds. *The Handbook Of Adult Clinical Psychology: An Evidence-Based Practice Approach*. 978-1-58391-854-8 (paperback); 978-1-58391-853-1 (hardcover). Routledge/Taylor & Francis Group: New York, 2006. pp. 724–765.

Carroll, J.F.X., and McGinley, J.J. A screening form for identifying mental health problems in alcohol/other drug dependent persons. *Alcoholism Treatment Quarterly* 19(4):33–47, 2001.

Carter, R.E., Haynes, L.F., Back, S.E., Herrin, A.E., Brady, K.T., Leimberger, J.D., Sonne, S.C., Hubbard, R.L., and Liepman, M.R. Improving the transition from residential to outpatient addiction treatment: Gender differences in response to supportive telephone calls. *American Journal of Drug and Alcohol Abuse* 34(1):47–59, 2008.

Case, P., Austin, S.B., Hunter, D.J., Manson, J.E., Malspeis, S., Willett, W.C., and Spiegelman, D. Sexual orientation, health risk factors, and physical functioning in the Nurses' Health Study II. *Journal of Women's Health (Larchmt.)* 13(9):1033–1047, 2004.

Catalano, S. Intimate partner violence in the United States. *Bureau of Justice Statistics* Washington, DC: U.S. Department of Justice, 2007.

Center for Substance Abuse Prevention. *Maternal Substance Use Assessment Methods Reference Manual: A Review Of Screening And Clinical Assessment Instruments For Examining Maternal Use Of Alcohol, Tobacco, And Other Drugs*. CSAP Special Report 13. HHS Publication No. (SMA)93–2059. Rockville, MD: Substance Abuse and Mental Health Services Administration, 1993.

Center for Substance Abuse Prevention. *Substance Abuse Resource Guide: Lesbian, Gay, Bisexual, And Transgender Populations*. Revised 2000 ed. Rockville, MD: Center for Substance Abuse Prevention, 2000.

Center for Substance Abuse Treatment. *Improving Treatment for Drug-Exposed Infants*. Treatment Improvement Protocol (TIP) Series 5. HHS Publication No. (SMA) 95-3057. Rockville, MD: Substance Abuse and Mental Health Services Administration, 1993a.

Center for Substance Abuse Treatment. *Pregnant, Substance-Using Women*. Treatment Improvement Protocol (TIP) Series 2. HHS Publication No. (SMA) 93-1998. Rockville, MD: Substance Abuse and Mental Health Services Administration, 1993b.

Center for Substance Abuse Treatment. *Screening for Infectious Diseases Among Substance Abusers*. Treatment Improvement Protocol (TIP) Series 6. HHS Publication No. (SMA) 95-3060. Rockville, MD: Substance Abuse and Mental Health Services Administration, 1993*c*.

Center for Substance Abuse Treatment. *Practical Approaches in the Treatment of Women Who Abuse Alcohol and Other Drugs*. HHS Publication No. (SMA) 94-3006. Washington, DC: U.S. Government Printing Office, 1994*a*.

Center for Substance Abuse Treatment. *Simple Screening Instruments for Outreach for Alcohol and Other Drug Abuse and Infectious Diseases*. Treatment Improvement Protocol (TIP) Series 11. HHS Publication No. (SMA) 94-2094. Rockville, MD: Substance Abuse and Mental Health Services Administration, 1994*b*.

Center for Substance Abuse Treatment. *Alcohol and Other Drug Screening of Hospitalized Trauma Patients*. Treatment Improvement Protocol (TIP) Series 16. HHS Publication No. (SMA) 95-3041. Rockville, MD: Substance Abuse and Mental Health Services Administration, 1995*a*.

Center for Substance Abuse Treatment. *Combining Alcohol and Other Drug Treatment with Diversion for Juveniles in the Justice System*. Treatment Improvement Protocol (TIP) Series 21. HHS Publication No. (SMA) 95-3051. Rockville, MD: Substance Abuse and Mental Health Services Administration, 1995*b*.

Center for Substance Abuse Treatment. *Developing State Outcomes Monitoring Systems for Alcohol and Other Drug Abuse Treatment*. Treatment Improvement Protocol (TIP) Series 14. HHS Publication No. (SMA) 95-3031. Rockville, MD: Substance Abuse and Mental Health Services Administration, 1995*c*.

Center for Substance Abuse Treatment. *The Role and Current Status of Patient Placement Criteria in the Treatment of Substance Use Disorders*. Treatment Improvement Protocol (TIP) Series 13. HHS Publication No. (SMA) 95-3021. Rockville, MD: Substance Abuse and Mental Health Services Administration, 1995*d*.

Center for Substance Abuse Treatment. *The Tuberculosis Epidemic: Legal and Ethical Issues for Alcohol and Other Drug Abuse Treatment Providers*. Treatment Improvement Protocol (TIP) Series 18. HHS Publication No. (SMA) 95-3047. Rockville, MD: Substance Abuse and Mental Health Services Administration, 1995*e*.

Center for Substance Abuse Treatment. *Treatment Drug Courts: Integrating Substance Abuse Treatment With Legal Case Processing*. Treatment Improvement Protocol (TIP) Series 23. HHS Publication No. (SMA) 96-3113. Rockville, MD: Substance Abuse and Mental Health Services Administration, 1996.

Center for Substance Abuse Treatment. *A Guide to Substance Abuse Services for Primary Care Clinicians*. Treatment Improvement Protocol (TIP) Series 24. HHS Publication No. (SMA) 97-3139. Rockville, MD: Substance Abuse and Mental Health Services Administration, 1997*a*.

Center for Substance Abuse Treatment. *Substance Abuse Treatment and Domestic Violence*. Treatment Improvement Protocol (TIP) Series 25. HHS Publication No. (SMA) 97-3163. Rockville, MD: Substance Abuse and Mental Health Services Administration, 1997*b*.

Center for Substance Abuse Treatment. *Supplementary Administration Manual For The Expanded Female Version Of The Addiction Severity Index (ASI) Instrument*. HHS Publication No. (SMA) 96-8056. Rockville, MD: Substance Abuse and Mental Health Services Administration, 1997*c*.

Center for Substance Abuse Treatment. *Comprehensive Case Management for Substance Abuse Treatment*. Treatment Improvement Protocol (TIP) Series 27. HHS Publication No. (SMA) 98-3222. Rockville, MD: Substance Abuse and Mental Health Services Administration, 1998*a*.

Center for Substance Abuse Treatment. *Continuity of Offender Treatment for Substance Use Disorders From Institution to Community*. Treatment Improvement Protocol (TIP) Series 30. HHS Publication No. (SMA) 98-3245. Rockville, MD: Substance Abuse and Mental Health Services Administration, 1998*b*.

Center for Substance Abuse Treatment. *Naltrexone and Alcoholism Treatment*. Treatment Improvement Protocol (TIP) Series 28. HHS Publication No. (SMA) 98-3206. Rockville, MD: Substance Abuse and Mental Health Services Administration, 1998*c*.

Center for Substance Abuse Treatment. *Substance Abuse Among Older Adults*. Treatment Improvement Protocol (TIP) Series 26. HHS Publication No. (SMA) 98-3179. Rockville, MD: Substance Abuse and Mental Health Services Administration, 1998*d*.

Center for Substance Abuse Treatment. *Substance Use Disorder Treatment for People With Physical and Cognitive Disabilities*. Treatment Improvement Protocol (TIP) Series 29. HHS Publication No. (SMA) 98-3249. Rockville, MD: Substance Abuse and Mental Health Services Administration, 1998*e*.

Center for Substance Abuse Treatment. *Brief Interventions and Brief Therapies for Substance Abuse*. Treatment Improvement Protocol (TIP) Series 34. HHS Publication No. (SMA) 99-3353. Rockville, MD: Substance Abuse and Mental Health Services Administration, 1999*a*.

Center for Substance Abuse Treatment. *Enhancing Motivation for Change in Substance Abuse Treatment*. Treatment Improvement Protocol (TIP) Series 35. HHS Publication No. (SMA) 99-3354. Rockville, MD: Substance Abuse and Mental Health Services Administration, 1999*b*.

Center for Substance Abuse Treatment. *Screening and Assessing Adolescents for Substance Use Disorders*. Treatment Improvement Protocol (TIP) Series 31. HHS Publication No. (SMA) 99-3282. Rockville, MD: Substance Abuse and Mental Health Services Administration, 1999*c*.

Center for Substance Abuse Treatment. *Treatment of Adolescents With Substance Use Disorders*. Treatment Improvement Protocol (TIP) Series 32. HHS Publication No. (SMA) 99-3283. Rockville, MD: Substance Abuse and Mental Health Services Administration, 1999*d*.

Center for Substance Abuse Treatment. *Treatment for Stimulant Use Disorders*. Treatment Improvement Protocol (TIP) Series 33. HHS Publication No. (SMA) 99-3296. Rockville, MD: Substance Abuse and Mental Health Services Administration, 1999*e*.

Center for Substance Abuse Treatment. *Integrating Substance Abuse Treatment and Vocational Services*. Treatment Improvement Protocol (TIP) Series 38. HHS Publication No. (SMA) 00-3470. Rockville, MD: Substance Abuse and Mental Health Services Administration, 2000*a*.

Center for Substance Abuse Treatment. *Substance Abuse Treatment for Persons With Child Abuse and Neglect Issues*. Treatment Improvement Protocol (TIP) Series 36. HHS Publication No. (SMA) 00-3357. Rockville, MD: Substance Abuse and Mental Health Services Administration, 2000*b*.

Center for Substance Abuse Treatment. *Substance Abuse Treatment for Persons With HIV/AIDS*. Treatment Improvement Protocol (TIP) Series 37. HHS Publication No. (SMA) 00-3459. Rockville, MD: Substance Abuse and Mental Health Services Administration, 2000*c*.

Center for Substance Abuse Treatment. Benefits of Residential Substance Abuse Treatment for Pregnant and Parenting Women: Highlights from a Study of 50 Demonstration Programs of the Center for Substance Abuse Treatment. Rockville, MD: Center for Substance Abuse Treatment 2001a.

Center for Substance Abuse Treatment. *A Provider's Introduction To Substance Abuse Treatment For Lesbian, Gay, Bisexual, And Transgender Individuals.* HHS Publication No. (SMA) 01-3498. Rockville, MD: Substance Abuse and Mental Health Services Administration, 2001b.

Center for Substance Abuse Treatment. *Telling Their Stories: Reflections Of The 11 Original Grantees That Piloted Residential Treatment For Women And Children For CSAT.* HHS Publication No. (SMA) 01-3529. Rockville, MD: Substance Abuse and Mental Health Services Administration, 2001c.

Center for Substance Abuse Treatment. *Helping Yourself Heal: A Recovering Woman's Guide To Coping With Childhood Abuse Issues.* HHS Publication No. (SMA) 03-3789. Rockville, MD: Substance Abuse and Mental Health Services Administration, 2003a.

Center for Substance Abuse Treatment. *Lessons Learned: Residential Substance Abuse Treatment For Women And Their Children.* HHS Publication No. (SMA) 03-3787. Rockville, MD: U.S. Department of Health and Human Services, Substance Abuse and Mental Health Services Administration, Center for Substance Abuse Treatment, 2003b.

Center for Substance Abuse Treatment. *Clinical Guidelines for the Use of Buprenorphine in the Treatment of Opioid Addiction.* Treatment Improvement Protocol (TIP) Series 40. HHS Publication No. (SMA) 04-3939. Rockville, MD: Substance Abuse and Mental Health Services Administration, 2004a.

Center for Substance Abuse Treatment. *Substance Abuse Treatment and Family Therapy.* Treatment Improvement Protocol (TIP) Series 39. HHS Publication No. (SMA) 04-3957. Rockville, MD: Substance Abuse and Mental Health Services Administration, 2004b.

Center for Substance Abuse Treatment. *Medication-Assisted Treatment For Opioid Addiction In Opioid Treatment Programs.* Rockville, MD: Substance Abuse and Mental Health Services Administration, 2005a.

Center for Substance Abuse Treatment. *Medication-Assisted Treatment for Opioid Addiction.* Treatment Improvement Protocol (TIP) Series 43. HHS Publication No. SMA 05-4048. Rockville, MD: Substance Abuse and Mental Health Services Administration, 2005b.

Center for Substance Abuse Treatment. *Substance Abuse Treatment for Adults in the Criminal Justice System.* Treatment Improvement Protocol (TIP) Series 44. HHS Publication No. (SMA) 05-4056. Rockville, MD: Substance Abuse and Mental Health Services Administration, 2005c.

Center for Substance Abuse Treatment. *Substance Abuse Treatment: Group Therapy.* Treatment Improvement Protocol (TIP) Series 41. HHS Publication No. SMA 05-4056. Rockville, MD: Substance Abuse and Mental Health Services Administration, 2005d.

Center for Substance Abuse Treatment. *Substance Abuse Treatment for Persons with Co-Occurring Disorders.* Treatment Improvement Protocol (TIP) Series 42. HHS Publication No. SMA 05-3992. Rockville, MD: Substance Abuse and Mental Health Services Administration, 2005e.

Center for Substance Abuse Treatment. *Detoxification and Substance Abuse Treatment.* Treatment Improvement Protocol (TIP) Series 45. HHS Publication No. SMA 06-4131. Rockville, MD: Substance Abuse and Mental Health Services Administration, 2006a.

Center for Substance Abuse Treatment. *Substance Abuse: Administrative Issues in Intensive Outpatient Treatment.* Treatment Improvement Protocol (TIP) Series 46. HHS Publication No. SMA 06-4151. Rockville, MD: Substance Abuse and Mental Health Services Administration, 2006*b*.

Center for Substance Abuse Treatment. *Substance Abuse: Clinical Issues in Intensive Outpatient Treatment.* Treatment Improvement Protocol (TIP) Series 47. HHS Publication No. 06-4182. Rockville, MD: Substance Abuse and Mental Health Services Administration, 2006*c*.

Center for Substance Abuse Treatment. State substance abuse treatment standards for women: A review of the current landscape. Prepared for Discussion at the NASADAD-WTC 2007 Annual Meeting June 6, 2007, Burlington, Vermont. 2007.

Center for Substance Abuse Treatment. *Managing Depressive Symptoms in Substance Abuse Clients During Early Recovery.* Treatment Improvement Protocol (TIP) Series 48. HHS Publication No. SMA 08-4353 Rockville, MD: Substance Abuse and Mental Health Services Administration, 2008.

Center for Substance Abuse Treatment. *Addressing Suicidal Thoughts and Behaviors With Clients in Substance Abuse Treatment.* Treatment Improvement Protocol (TIP) Series 50. HHS Publication No. SMA 09-4381. Rockville, MD: Substance Abuse and Mental Health Services Administration, 2009*a*.

Center for Substance Abuse Treatment. *Incorporating Alcohol Pharmacotherapies Into Medical Practice.* Treatment Improvement Protocol (TIP) Series 49. HHS Publication No. SMA 09-4380. Rockville, MD: Substance Abuse and Mental Health Services Administration, 2009*b*.

Center for Substance Abuse Treatment. *Improving Cultural Competence in Substance Abuse Treatment.* Treatment Improvement Protocol (TIP) Series. Rockville, MD: Substance Abuse and Mental Health Services Administration, in development *a*.

Center for Substance Abuse Treatment. *Management of Chronic Pain in People With Substance Use Disorders.* Treatment Improvement Protocol (TIP) Series. Rockville, MD: Substance Abuse and Mental Health Services Administration, in development *b*.

Center for Substance Abuse Treatment. *Relapse Prevention and Recovery in Substance Abuse Treatment Settings.* Treatment Improvement Protocol (TIP) Series. Rockville, MD: Substance Abuse and Mental Health Services Administration, in development *c*

Center for Substance Abuse Treatment. *Substance Abuse Treatment: Addressing the Specific Needs of Women.* Treatment Improvement Protocol (TIP) Series. Rockville, MD: Substance Abuse and Mental Health Services Administration, in development *d*.

Center for Substance Abuse Treatment. *Substance Abuse Treatment with American Indians and Alaska Natives.* Treatment Improvement Protocol (TIP) Series. Rockville, MD: Substance Abuse and Mental Health Services Administration. In development *e*.

Center for Substance Abuse Treatment. *Substance Abuse Treatment and Men's Issues.* Treatment Improvement Protocol (TIP) Series. Rockville, MD: Substance Abuse and Mental Health Services Administration, in development *f*.

Center for Substance Abuse Treatment. *Substance Abuse Treatment With People Who Are Homeless.* Treatment Improvement Protocol (TIP) Series. Rockville, MD: Substance Abuse and Mental Health Services Administration, in development *g*.

Center for Substance Abuse Treatment. *Substance Abuse Treatment and Trauma*. Treatment Improvement Protocol (TIP) Series. Rockville, MD: Substance Abuse and Mental Health Services Administration, in development *h*.

Center for Substance Abuse Treatment. *Supervision and the Professional Development of the Substance Abuse Counselor*. Treatment Improvement Protocol (TIP) Series. Rockville, MD: Substance Abuse and Mental Health Services Administration, in development *i*.

Center for Substance Abuse Treatment. *Viral Hepatitis and Substance Abuse*. Treatment Improvement Protocol (TIP) Series. Rockville, MD: Substance Abuse and Mental Health Services Administration, in development *j*.

Center on Alcoholism, *Substance Abuse and Addictions. Religious Practice and Beliefs Instrument*. Albuquerque, NM: University of New Mexico, 2004.

Centers for Disease Control and Prevention. Public Health Service task force recommendations for the use of antiretroviral drugs in pregnant women infected with HIV-1 for maternal health and for reducing perinatal HIV-1 transmission in the United States. *Morbidity and Mortality Weekly Report* 47(RR-2):1–30, 1998.

Centers for Disease Control & Prevention. Women and Smoking: A Report of the Surgeon General, 2001. *Pattern of Tobacco Use Among Women and Girls - Fact Sheet* Atlanta, GA: Center for Disease Control & Prevention, Office of Smoking and Health 2001.

Centers for Disease Control and Prevention. Drug-Associated HIV Transmission Continues in the United States. Atlanta, GA: 2002.

Centers for Disease Control and Prevention. Cigarette smoking among adults - United States, 2002. *MMWR* 53(20):427–446. Washington, D.C.: Centers for Disease Control and Prevention, 2004.

Centers for Disease Control and Prevention. HIV/AIDS among African Americans. *Fact Sheet - HIV/AIDS Among African Americans*. Atlanta, GA: Centers for Disease Control and Prevention (CDC) 2005.

Centers for Disease Control and Prevention. HIV/AIDS among Women. Atlanta, GA: Centers for Disease Control and Prevention, 2007*a*.

Centers for Disease Control and Prevention. HIV/AIDS Surveillance Report, 2005: Cases of HIV infection and AIDS in the United States and Dependent Areas, 2005. Volume 17 Atlanta, GA: U.S. Department of Health and Human Services, Centers for Disease Control and Prevention, 2007*b*.

Centers for Disease Control and Prevention. Hepatitis C fact sheet. 2008. http://cdc.gov/hepatitis/hcv/pdfs/hepcgeneralfactsheet.pdf [Accessed October 2, 2008].

Chabrol, H., Teissedre, F., Saint-Jean, M., Teisseyre, N., Roge, B., and Mullet, E. Prevention and treatment of post-partum depression: A controlled randomized study on women at risk. *Psychological Medicine* 32(6):1039–1047, 2002.

Chamberlin, J., and Schene, A.H. A working definition of empowerment. *Psychiatric Rehabilitation Journal* 20(4):43–46, 1997.

Chan, A.W., Pristach, E.A., Welte, J.W., and Russell, M. Use of the TWEAK test in screening for alcoholism/heavy drinking in three populations. *Alcoholism: Clinical & Experimental Research* 17(6):1188–1192, 1993.

Chan, C.S. Issues of identity development among Asian-American lesbians and gay men. *Journal of Counseling and Development* 68(1):16–20, 1989.

Chan, C.S. Don't ask, don't tell, don't know: The formation of a homosexual identity and sexual expression among Asian American lesbians. In: Greene, B., ed. *Ethnic And Cultural Diversity Among Lesbians And Gay Men.* Thousand Oaks, CA: Sage Publications, 1997. pp. 240–248.

Chang, G. Brief interventions for problem drinking and women. *Journal of Substance Abuse Treatment* 23(1):1–7, 2002.

Chang, G., Goetz, M.A., Wilkins-Haug, L., and Berman, S. A brief intervention for prenatal alcohol use: An in-depth look. *Journal of Substance Abuse Treatment* 18(4):365–369, 2000.

Chang, G., McNamara, T.K., Haimovici, F., and Hornstein, M.D. Problem drinking in women evaluated for infertility. *American Journal of Addiction* 15(2):174–179, 2006.

Chang, G., Wilkins-Haug, L., Berman, S., and Goetz, M.A. The TWEAK: Application in a prenatal setting. *Journal of Studies on Alcohol* 60(3):306–309, 1999.

Chang, G., Wilkins-Haug, L., Berman, S., Goetz, M.A., Behr, H., and Hiley, A. Alcohol use and pregnancy: Improving identification. *Obstetrics and Gynecology* 91(6):892–898, 1998.

Chang, P. Treating Asian/Pacific American addicts and their families. In: Krestan, J.-A., ed. *Bridges To Recovery: Addiction, Family Therapy, And Multicultural Treatment.* New York: Free Press, 2000. pp. 192–218.

Chang, Y.-Y.J. Comorbidity of depression and substance use disorders: The role of depression as a risk factor for post-treatment relapse, 1997.

Chasnoff, I.J., McGourty, R.F., Bailey, G.W., Hutchins, E., Lightfoot, S.O., Pawson, L.L., Fahey, C., May, B., Brodie, P., McCulley, L., and Campbell, J. The 4P's Plus screen for substance use in pregnancy: clinical application and outcomes. *Journal of Perinatology* 25(6):368–374, 2005.

Chasnoff, I.J., Neuman, K., Thornton, C., and Callaghan, M.A. Screening for substance use in pregnancy: A practical approach for the primary care physician. *American Journal of Obstetrics and Gynecology* 184(4):752–758, 2001.

Chatham, L.R., Hiller, M.L., Rowan-Szal, G.A., Joe, G.W., and Simpson, D.D. Gender differences at admission and follow-up in a sample of methadone maintenance clients. *Substance Use & Misuse* 34(8):1137–1165, 1999.

Chavkin, W., and Breitbart, V. Substance abuse and maternity: The United States as a case study. *Addiction* 92(9):1201–1205, 1997.

Chen, H., Guarnaccia, P.J., and Chung, H. Self-attention as a mediator of cultural influences on depression. *International Journal of Social Psychiatry* 49(3):192-203, 2003.

Chen, X., Burgdorf, K., Dowell, K., Roberts, T., Porowski, A., and Herrell, J.M. Factors associated with retention of drug abusing women in long-term residential treatment. *Evaluation and Program Planning* 27(2):205–212, 2004.

Chen, C.M., Yoon, Y.H., Yi, H.y., and Lucas, D.L. Alcohol and hepatitis C mortality among males and females in the United States: A life table analysis. *Alcoholism: Clinical and Experimental Research* 31(2):285–292, 2007.

Cherry, D.K., and Woodwell, D.A. National Ambulatory Medical Care Survey: 2000 Summary. *Advance Data From Vital and Health Statistics, No.328* Hyattsville, MD: National Center for Health Statistics 2002.

Chilcoat, H.D., and Breslau, N. Alcohol disorders in young adulthood: Effects of transitions into adult roles. *Journal of Health and Social Behavior* 37(4):339–349, 1996.

Child Welfare League of America. *Crack And Other Addictions: Old Realities And New Challenge For Child Welfare.* Washington, DC: Child Welfare League of America, 1990.

Child Welfare League of America. *Children at the Front: A Different View of the War on Alcohol and Drugs.* Washington, DC: Child Welfare League of America, 1992.

Chisholm, D., Rehm, J., Van, O.M., and Monteiro, M. Reducing the global burden of hazardous alcohol use: a comparative cost-effectiveness analysis. *Journal of Studies on Alcohol* 65(6):782–793, 2004.

Choi, S., and Ryan, J.P. Co-occurring problems for substance abusing mothers in child welfare: Matching services to improve family reunification. *Children and Youth Services Review* 29(11):1395–1410, 2007.

Chou, S.P., Grant, B.F., and Dawson, D.A. Medical consequences of alcohol consumption--United States, 1992. *Alcoholism: Clinical and Experimental Research* 20(8):1423–1429, 1996.

Chung, R.H., Kim, B.S., and Abreu, J.M. Asian American multidimensional acculturation scale: development, factor analysis, reliability, and validity. *Cultural Diversity and Ethnic Minority Psychology* 10(1):66–80, 2004.

Clark, J.J., Leukefeld, C., Godlaski, T., Brown, C., Garrity, J., and Hays, L. Developing, implementing, and evaluating a treatment protocol for rural substance abusers. *Journal of Rural Health* 18(3):396–406, 2002.

Claus, R.E., Orwin, R.G., Kissin, W., Krupski, A., Campbell, K., and Stark, K. Does gender-specific substance abuse treatment for women promote continuity of care? *Journal of Substance Abuse Treatment* 32(1):27–39, 2007.

Cochran, S.D., Ackerman, D., Mays, V.M., and Ross, M.W. Prevalence of non-medical drug use and dependence among homosexually active men and women in the US population. *Addiction* 99(8):989–998, 2004.

Cochran, S.D., and Mays, V.M. Relation between psychiatric syndromes and behaviorally defined sexual orientation in a sample of the US population. *American Journal of Epidemiology* 151(5):516–523, 2000.

Cochran, S.D., Keenan, C., Schober, C., and Mays, V.M. Estimates of alcohol use and clinical treatment needs among homosexually active men and women in the U.S. population. *Journal of Consulting and Clinical Psychology* 68(6):1062–1071, 2000.

Cochran, S.D., Mays, V.M., Alegria, M., Ortega, A.N., and Takeuchi, D. Mental health and substance use disorders among Latino and Asian American lesbian, gay, and bisexual adults. *Journal of Consulting and Clinical Psychology* 75(5):785-794, 2007.

Cochran, S.D., Mays, V.M., Bowen, D., Gage, S., Bybee, D., Roberts, S.J., Goldstein, R.S., Robison, A., Rankow, E.J., and White, J. Cancer-related risk indicators and preventive screening behaviors among lesbians and bisexual women. *American Journal of Public Health* 91(4):591–597, 2001.

Cocozza, J.J., Jackson, E.W., Hennigan, K., Morrissey, J.P., Reed, B.G., Fallot, R., and Banks, S. Outcomes for women with co-occurring disorders and trauma: program-level effects. *Journal of Substance Abuse Treatment* 28(2):109–119, 2005.

Cohen, J.B., Dickow, A., Horner, K., Zweben, J.E., Balabis, J., Vandersloot, D., and Reiber, C. Abuse and violence history of men and women in treatment for methamphetamine dependence. *American Journal of Addiction* 12(5):377–385, 2003.

Cohen, L.R., and Hien, D.A. Treatment outcomes for women with substance abuse and PTSD who have experienced complex trauma. *Psychiatric Services* 57(1):100–106, 2006.

Cohen, L.S., Viguera, A.C., Bouffard, S.M., Nonacs, R.M., Morabito, C., Collins, M.H., and Ablon, J.S. Venlafaxine in the treatment of postpartum depression. *Journal of Clinical Psychology* 62(8):592–596, 2001.

Cohen, M. *Counseling Addicted Women.* Thousand Oaks, CA: Sage Publications, 2000.

Cohen, R.A., Hao, C., and Coriaty-Nelson, Z. Health insurance coverage: Estimates from the National Health Interview Survey, January - June 2004. Atlanta, GA: Centers for Disease Control and Prevention, 2004.

Cohen-Smith, D., and Severson, H.H. A comparison of male and female smokeless tobacco use. *Nicotine & Tobacco Research* 1(3):211–218, 1999.

Cohn, J.A. HIV-1 infection in injection drug users. *Infectious Disease Clinics of North America* 16(3):745–770, 2002.

Coleman, V.E. Lesbian battering: The relationship between personality and the perpetration of violence. *Violence and Victims* 9(2):139–152, 1994.

Collins, R.L., and McNair, L.D. Minority women and alcohol use. *Alcohol Research & Health* 26(4):251–256, 2002.

Colorado Department of Human Services, and Alcohol and Drug Abuse Division (ADAD). Substance use disorder treatment rules. Denver, CO: Colorado Department of Human Services, Alcohol and Drug Abuse Division (ADAD), 2006.

Comfort, M., and Kaltenbach, K. The psychosocial history: An interview for pregnant and parenting women in substance abuse treatment and research. In: Rahdert, E.R., ed. *Treatment For Drug-Exposed Women And Their Children: Advances In Research Methodology.* NIDA Research Monograph 166. NIH Publication No. 96-3632. Rockville, MD: National Institute on Drug Abuse, 1996. pp. 133–142.

Comfort, M., and Kaltenbach, K.A. Predictors of treatment outcomes for substance-abusing women: A retrospective study. *Substance Abuse* 21(1):33–45, 2000.

Comfort, M., Hagan, T., and Kaltenbach, K. *Psychosocial History.* Philadelphia, PA: Thomas Jefferson University, Jefferson Medical Center, Family Center, 1996.

Comfort, M., Loverro, J., and Kaltenbach, K. A search for strategies to engage women in substance abuse treatment. *Social Work in Health Care* 31(4):59–70, 2000.

Comfort, M., Zanis, D.A., Whiteley, M.J., Kelly-Tyler, A., and Kaltenbach, K.A. Assessing the needs of substance abusing women: Psychometric data on the psychosocial history. *Journal of Substance Abuse Treatment* 17(1–2):79–83, 1999.

Connecticut Department of Mental Health and Addiction Services, Women's Services Practice Improvement Collaborative, compiled by David J. Berkowitz. *Treatment Guidelines: Gender Responsive Treatment Of Women With Substance Use Disorders.* January 23, 2007 Revision Hartford, CT: Connecticut Department of Mental Health and Addiction Services, 2007.

Conners, N.A., Bradley, R.H., Mansell, L.W., Liu, J.Y., Roberts, T.J., Burgdorf, K., and Herrell, J.M. Children of mothers with serious substance abuse problems: An accumulation of risks. *American Journal of Drug and Alcohol Abuse* 30(1):85–100, 2004.

Conners, N.A., Grant, A., Crone, C.C., and Whiteside-Mansell, L. Substance abuse treatment for mothers: Treatment outcomes and the impact of length of stay. *Journal of Substance Abuse Treatment* 31(4):447–456, 2006.

Conway, K.P., and Montoya, I.D. Symposium: What is the directionality of the onset of co-morbid substance use and other psychiatric disorders? Bethesda, MD: National Institute on Drug Abuse, 2007.

Cooley, M.E., Blood, E., Hoskinson, R., and Garvey, A. Gender differences in smoking relapse. *Oncology Nursing Forum* 33(2):401-402, 2006.

Corcos, M., Nezelof, S., Speranza, M., Topa, S., Girardon, N., Guilbaud, O., TaÇeb, O., Bizouard, P., Halfon, O., Venisse, J.L., Perez-Diaz, F., Flament, M., and Jeammet, P. Psychoactive substance consumption in eating disorders. *Eating Behaviors* 2(1):27–38, 2001.

Corliss, H.L., Grella, C.E., Mays, V.M., and Cochran, S.D. Drug use, drug severity, and help-seeking behaviors of lesbian and bisexual women. *Journal of Women's Health (Larchmt.)* 15(5):556–568, 2006.

Corse, S.J., McHugh, M.K., and Gordon, S.M. Enhancing provider effectiveness in treating pregnant women with addictions. *Journal of Substance Abuse Treatment* 12(1):3–12, 1995.

Cottrell, B.H. Vaginal douching. *Journal of Obstetric, Gynecologic, and Neonatal Nursing* 32(1):12–18, 2003.

Coughey, K., Feighan, K., Cheney, R., and Klein, G. Retention in an aftercare program for recovering women. *Substance Use and Misuse* 33(4):917–933, 1998.

Cournoyer, L.G., Brochu, S., Landry, M., and Bergeron, J. Therapeutic alliance, patient behaviour and dropout in a drug rehabilitation programme: the moderating effect of clinical subpopulations. *Addiction* 102(12):1960–1970, 2007.

Covington, S. A case for gender-responsive drug treatment. *Clinical Psychiatry News* 35(8):15, 2007.

Covington, S.S. *A Woman's Way through the Twelve Steps.* Center City, MN: Hazelden, 1994.

Covington, S.S. Women, addiction, and sexuality. In: Straussner, S.L.A., and Zelvin, E., eds. *Gender and Addictions: Men and Women in Treatment.* Northvale, NJ: Jason Aronson, 1997. pp. 71–95.

Covington, S.S. Women in prison: Approaches in the treatment of our most invisible population. *Women & Therapy* 21(1):141–155, 1998.

Covington, S.S. *Helping Women Recover: A Program for Treating Addiction.* San Francisco: Jossey-Bass, 1999*a*.

Covington, S.S. *Helping Women Recover: A Program for Treating Addiction. Special Edition for Use in Correctional Settings.* San Francisco: Jossey-Bass, 1999*b*.

Covington, S.S. *Awakening Your Sexuality: A Guide for Recovering Women.* Center City, MN: Hazelden, 2000.

Covington, S.S. *A Woman's Journey Home: Challenges for Female Offenders and Their Children.* Washington, DC: Urban Institute 2002*a*.

Covington, S.S. Helping women recover: Creating gender-responsive treatment. In: Straussner, S.L.A., and Brown, S., eds. *Handbook of Women's Addiction Treatment: Theory and Practice*. San Francisco: Jossey-Bass, 2002*b*. pp. 52–72.

Covington, S.S. *Beyond Trauma: A Healing Journey for Women: Facilitator's Guide*. Center City, Minnesota: Hazelden, 2003*a*.

Covington, S.S. *Beyond Trauma: A Healing Journey for Women: Participant's Workbook*. Center City, Minnesota: Hazelden, 2003*b*.

Covington, S. S. *Women and Addiction: A Gender-Responsive Approach*. Clinical Innovators Series. Center City, MN: Hazelden, 2007.

Covington, S.S. *Helping Women Recover: A Program for Treating Addiction*. (Rev. ed.) San Francisco: Jossey-Bass, 2008*a*.

Covington, S.S. *Helping Women Recover: A Program for Treating Addiction. Special Edition for Use in Correctional Settings*. (Rev. ed.) San Francisco: Jossey-Bass, 2008*b*.

Covington, S.S., and Bloom, B.E. Gendered justice: Women in the criminal justice system. In: Bloom, B.E., ed. *Gendered Justice: Addressing the Female Offender*. Durham, NC: Carolina Academic Press, 2003. pp. 3–24.

Covington, S.S., and Surrey, J.L. The relational model of women's psychological development: Implications for substance abuse. In: Wilsnack, R.W., and Wilsnack, S.C., eds. *Gender and Alcohol: Individual and Social Perspectives*. New Brunswick, NJ: Rutgers Center of Alcohol Studies, 1997. pp. 335–351.

Cowan, G., and Ullman, J.B. Ingroup rejection among women: The role of personal inadequacy. *Psychology of Women Quarterly* 30(4):399–409, 2006.

Coyhis, D. Culturally specific addiction recovery for Native Americans. In: Krestan, J., ed. *Bridges To Recovery: Addiction, Family Therapy, And Multicultural Treatment*. New York: The Free Press, 2000. pp. 77–114.

Coyne, C.M., Jarrett, M.E., Burr, R.L., and Murphy, S.A. Women's physical and psychological symptoms during early phase recovery from alcoholism: A longitudinal study. *Journal of Addictions Nursing* 17(2):83–93, 2006.

Cramer, M. *Issues in the treatment of dual diagnosis: PTSD and substance abuse in women*. Presentation to DATA of Rhode Island, Providence, RI, October, 2000.

Cramer, M. Under the influence of unconscious process: Countertransference in the treatment of PTSD and substance abuse in women. *American Journal of Psychotherapy* 56(2):194–210, 2002.

Crits-Christoph, P., Baranackie, K., Kurcias, J.S., and Beck, A.T. Meta-analysis of therapist effects in psychotherapy outcome studies. *Psychotherapy Research* 1(2):81–91, 1991.

Cuellar, I., Harris, L.C., and Jasso, R. An acculturation scale for Mexican American normal and clinical populations. *Hispanic Journal of Behavioral Sciences*. 2(3):199–217, 1980.

Cuijpers, P., van Straten A., and Warmerdam, L. Behavioral activation treatments of depression: A meta-analysis. *Clinical Psychology Review* 27(3):318–326, 2007.

Cunningham, J.A., Sobell, L.C., Gavin, D.R., Sobell, M.B., and Breslin, F.C. Assessing motivation for change: Preliminary development and evaluation of a scale measuring the costs and benefits of changing alcohol or drug use. *Psychology of Addictive Behaviors* 11(2):107–114, 1997.

Curtis, C.E., Jason, L.A., Olson, B.D., and Ferrari, J.R. Disordered eating, trauma, and sense of community: Examining women in substance abuse recovery homes. *Women & Health* 41(4):87–100, 2005.

Cutrona, C.E., Cadoret, R.J., Suhr, J.A., Richards, C.C., Troughton, E., Schutte, K., and Woodworth, G. Interpersonal variables in the prediction of alcoholism among adoptees: evidence for gene-environment interactions. *Comprehensive Psychiatry* 35(3):171–179, 1994.

Daley, M., Argeriou, M., and McCarty, D. Substance abuse treatment for pregnant women: A window of opportunity? *Addictive Behaviors* 23(2):239–249, 1998.

Dallam, S.J. The identification and management of self-mutilating patients in primary care. *Nurse Practitioner* 22(5):151–165, 1997.

Dansky, B.S., Brewerton, T.D., and Kilpatrick, D.G. Comorbidity of bulimia nervosa and alcohol use disorders: Results from the National Women's Study. *International Journal of Eating Disorders* 27(2):180–190, 2000.

Dashe, J.S., Jackson, G.L., Olscher, D.A., Zane, E.H., and Wendel, G.D., Jr. Opioid detoxification in pregnancy. *Obstetrics and Gynecology* 92(5):854–858, 1998.

D'Avanzo, C., Dunn, P., Murdock, J., and Naegle, M. Developing culturally informed strategies for substance-related interventions. In: Naegle, M.A., and D'Avanzo, C.E., eds. *Addictions And Substance Abuse: Strategies For Advanced Practice Nursing.* Upper Saddle River, NJ: Prentice Hall Health, 2001. pp. 59–74.

D'Avanzo, C.E., Frye, B., and Froman, R. Culture, stress and substance use in Cambodian refugee women. *Journal of Studies on Alcohol* 55(4):420–426, 1994.

Davidson, P.R., and Parker, K.C. Eye movement desensitization and reprocessing (EMDR): A meta-analysis. *Journal of Consulting and Clinical Psychology* 69(2):305–316, 2001.

Davis, T.M., Bush, K.R., Kivlahan, D.R., Dobie, D.J., and Bradley, K. Screening for substance abuse and psychiatric disorders among women patients in a VA Health Care System. *Psychiatric Services* 54:214–218, 2003.

Dawson, D.A., Grant, B.F., Chou, S.P., and Stinson, F.S. The impact of partner alcohol problems on women's physical and mental health. *Journal of Studies on Alcohol and Drugs* 68(1):66–75, 2007.

Day, N., Cornelius, M., Goldschmidt, L., Richardson, G., Robles, N., and Taylor, P. The effects of prenatal tobacco and marijuana use on offspring growth from birth through 3 years of age. *Neurotoxicology and Teratology* 14(6):407–414, 1992.

Dayton, T. *Trauma and Addiction: Ending the Cycle of Pain Through Emotional Literacy.* Deerfield Beach, FL: Health Communications, 2000.

de Mello, M.F., de Jesus Mari, J., Bacaltchuk, J., Verdeli, H., and Neugebauer, R. A systematic review of research findings on the efficacy of interpersonal therapy for depressive disorders. *European Archives of Psychiatry and Clinical Neuroscience* 255(2):75–82, 2005.

Dean, L., Meyer, I.H., Robinson, K., Sell, R.L., Sember, R., Silenzio, V.M.B., Bowen, D.J., Bradford, J., Rothblum, E., Scout, White, J., Dunn, P., Lawrence, A., Wolfe, D., and Xavier, J. Lesbian, gay, bisexual, and transgender health: Findings and concerns. *Journal of the Gay and Lesbian Medical Association* 4(3):101–151, 2000.

Dempsey, P., Bird, D.C., and Hartley, D. Rural mental health and substance abuse. In: Ricketts, T.C., ed. *Rural Health in the United States.* New York: Oxford University Press, 1999. pp. 159–178.

DeNavas-Walt, C., Proctor, B.D., and Mills, R.J. Income, Poverty, and Health Insurance Coverage in the United States: 2003. *U.S. Census Bureau, Current Population Reports, P60-226*, Washington, D.C.: U.S. Government Printing Office, 2004.

Dennerstein, L. *Factors associated with the experience of menopause and related therapy.* Presented at First World Congress on Women's Mental Health, Berlin, Germany, March 27–31, 2001a.

Dennerstein, L. *How does women's mental health differ from that of men?* Plenary speech presented at First World Congress on Women's Mental Health, Berlin, Germany, March 27–31, 2001b.

Derauf, C., LaGasse, L.L., Smith, L.M., Grant, P., Shah, R., Arria, A., Huestis, M., Haning, W., Strauss, A., Grotta, S.D., Liu, J., and Lester, B.M. Demographic and psychosocial characteristics of mothers using methamphetamine during pregnancy: Preliminary results of the infant development, environment, and lifestyle study (IDEAL). *American Journal of Drug and Alcohol Abuse* 33(2):281–289, 2007.

Derogatis, L.R., and Melisaratos, N. The Brief Symptom Inventory: An introductory report. *Psychological Medicine* 13(3):595–605, 1983.

Devaud, L.L., Risinger, F.O., and Selvage, D. Impact of the Hormonal Milieu on the Neurobiology of Alcohol Dependence and Withdrawal. *Journal of General Psychology* 133(4):337–356, 2006.

DeVoe, D. Feminist and nonsexist counseling: Implications for the male counselor. *Journal of Counseling & Development* 69(1):33–36, 1990.

Diamant, A.L., Wold, C., Spritzer, K., and Gelberg, L. Health behaviors, health status, and access to and use of health care: A population-based study of lesbian, bisexual, and heterosexual women. *Archives of Family Medicine* 9(10):1043–1051, 2000.

Dick, D.M., Pagan, J.L., Holliday, C., Viken, R., Pulkkinen, L., Kaprio, J., and Rose, R.J. Gender differences in friends' influences on adolescent drinking: a genetic epidemiological study. *Alcoholism: Clinical & Experimental Research* 31(12):2012–2019, 2007.

DiNitto, D.M., and Crisp, C. Addictions and women with major psychiatric disorders. In: Straussner, S.L.A., and Brown, S., eds. *The Handbook of Addiction Treatment for Women: Theory and Practice.* San Francisco: Jossey-Bass, 2002. pp. 423–450.

Dixit, A.R., and Crum, R.M. Prospective study of depression and the risk of heavy alcohol use in women. *American Journal of Psychiatry* 157(5):751–758, 2000.

Dobie, D.J., Kivlahan, D.R., Maynard, C., Bush, K.R., Davis, T.M., and Bradley, K.A. Posttraumatic stress disorder in female veterans: association with self-reported health problems and functional impairment. *Archives of Internal Medicine* 164(4):394–400, 2004.

Dole, V.P., and Nyswander, M.E. Rehabilitation of heroin addicts after blockade with methadone. *New York State Journal of Medicine* 66(15):2011–2017, 1966a.

Dole, V.P., Nyswander, M.E., and Kreek, M.J. Narcotic blockade. *Archives of Internal Medicine* 118(4):304–309, 1966b.

Donaldson, P.L. Perinatal drug and alcohol addiction: The role of the primary care provider. *Lippincotts Primary Care Practice* 4(3):349–358, 2000.

Dorgan, J.F., Baer, D.J., Albert, P.S., Judd, J.T., Brown, E.D., Corle, D.K., Campbell, W.S., Hartman, J.J., Tejpar, A.A., Clevidence Beverly a., Giffen, C.A., Chandler, D.W., Stanczyk, F.Z., and Taylor, P.R. Serum hormones and the alcohol-breast cancer association in postmenopausal women. *Journal of the National Cancer Institute* 93(9):710–715, 2001.

Drabble, L. Elements of effective services for women in recovery: Implications for clinicians and program supervisors. In: Underhill, B.L., and Finnegan, D.G., eds. *Chemical Dependency: Women At Risk*. New York: Harrington Park Press/Haworth Press, 1996. pp. 1–21.

Drabble, L., and Underhill, B. Elements of effective intervention and treatment for lesbians. In: Straussner, S.L.A., and Brown, S., eds. *The Handbook of Addiction Treatment for Women: Theory and Practice*. San Francisco: Jossey-Bass, 2002. pp. 399–422.

Drake, R.E., Mercer-McFadden, C., Mueser, K.T., McHugo, G.J., and Bond, G.R. Review of integrated mental health and substance abuse treatment for patients with dual disorders. *Schizophrenia Bulletin* 24(4):589–608, 1998.

Dube, S.R., Miller, J.W., Brown, D.W., Giles, W.H., Felitti, V.J., Dong, M., and Anda, R.F. Adverse childhood experiences and the association with ever using alcohol and initiating alcohol use during adolescence. *Journal of Adolescent Health* 38(4):444–10, 2006.

Duszynski, K.R., Nieto, F.J., and Valente, C.M. Reported practices, attitudes, and confidence levels of primary care physicians regarding patients who abuse alcohol and other drugs. *Maryland Medical Journal* 44(6):439–446, 1995.

Eaton, D.K., Kann, L., Kinchen, S., Shanklin, S., Ross, J., Hawkins, J., Harris, W.A., Lowry, R., McManus, T., Chyen, D., Lim, C., Brener, N.D., and Wechsler, H. *Youth Risk Behavior Surveillance--United States, 2007*. 57: No. SS-4:1–133. Atlanta, GA: Centers for Disease Control and Prevention, 2008.

Eggert, J., Theobald, H., and Engfeldt, P. Effects of alcohol consumption on female fertility during an 18-year period. *Fertility and Sterility* 81(2):379–383, 2004.

Ehrmin, J.T. Unresolved feelings of guilt and shame in the maternal role with substance-dependent African American women. *Journal of Nursing Scholarship* 33(1):47–52, 2001.

El-Bassel, N., Gilbert, L., Frye, V., Wu, E., Go, H., Hill, J., and Richman, B.L. Physical and Sexual Intimate Partner Violence Among Women in Methadone Maintenance Treatment. Source. *Psychology of Addictive Behaviors*. 18(2):180–183, 2004.

El-Bassel, N., Gilbert, L., Wu, E., Go, H., and Hill, J. Relationship Between Drug Abuse and Intimate Partner Violence: A Longitudinal Study Among Women Receiving Methadone. *American Journal of Public Health* 95(3):465–470, 2005.

Eliason, M.J., and Skinstad, A.H. Drug and alcohol intervention for older women: A pilot study. *Journal of Gerontological Nursing* 27(12):18–24, 2001.

Ellickson, P.L., Hays, R.D., and Bell, R.M. Stepping through the drug use sequence: Longitudinal scalogram analysis of initiation and regular use. *Journal of Abnormal Psychology* 101(3):441–451, 1992.

Elliott, D.E., Bjelajac, P., Fallot, R.D., Markoff, L.S., and Reed, B.G. Trauma-informed or trauma-denied: Principles and implementation of trauma-informed services for women. *Journal of Community Psychology* 33(4):461–477, 2005.

El-Mohandes, A., Herman, A.A., Nabil El-Khorazaty, M., Katta, P.S., White, D., and Grylack, L. Prenatal care reduces the impact of illicit drug use on perinatal outcomes. *Journal of Perinatology* 23(5):354–360, 2003.

Epstein, E.E., Fischer-Elber, K., and Al-Otaiba, Z. Women, aging, and alcohol use disorders. *Journal of Women and Aging* 19(1–2):31–48, 2007.

Evans, J., Hahn, J., Page-Shafer, K., Lum, P., Stein, E., Davidson, P., and Moss, A. Gender differences in sexual and injection risk behavior among active young injection drug users in San Francisco (the UFO study). *Journal of Urban Health* 80(1):137–146, 2003.

Evans, K., and Sullivan, J.M. *Treating Addicted Survivors of Trauma*. New York: Guilford Press, 1995.

Evans, S.M. The role of estradiol and progesterone in modulating the subjective effects of stimulants in humans. *Experimental and Clinical Psychopharmacology* 15(5):418–426, 2007.

Evans, S.M., and Foltin, R.W. Exogenous progesterone attenuates the subjective effects of smoked cocaine in women, but not in men. *Neuropsychopharmacology* 31(3):659–674, 2006.

Evans, S.M., Haney, M., and Foltin, R.W. The effects of smoked cocaine during the follicular and luteal phases of the menstrual cycle in women. *Psychopharmacology* 159(4):397–406, 2002.

Evans-Campbell, T. Historical trauma in American Indian/Native Alaska communities: A multilevel framework for exploring impacts on individuals, families, and communities. *Journal of Interpersonal Violence* 23(3):316–338, 2008.

Evans-Campbell, T., Fredriksen-Goldsen, K.I., Walters, K.L., and Stately, A. Caregiving experiences among American Indian two-spirit men and women: Contemporary and historical roles. *Journal of Gay & Lesbian Social Services: Issues in Practice, Policy & Research* 18(3-4):75-92, 2005.

Ewing, H. *A Practical Guide to Intervention in Health and Social Services with Pregnant and Postpartum Addicts and Alcoholics: Theoretical Framework, Brief Screening Tool, Key Interview Questions, and Strategies for Referral to Recovery Resources*. State of California Grant for Training and Cross-Training in Health, Social Services, and Alcohol/Drug Services, 1990.

Ewing, J.A. Detecting alcoholism. The CAGE questionnaire. *JAMA: The Journal of the American Medical Association* 252(14):1905–1907, 1984.

Eyler, F.D., and Behnke, M. Early development of infants exposed to drugs prenatally. *Clinics in Perinatology* 26(1):107–150, vii, 1999.

Eyler, F.D., Behnke, M., Garvan, C.W., Woods, N.S., Wobie, K., and Conlon, M. Newborn evaluations of toxicity and withdrawal related to prenatal cocaine exposure. *Neurotoxicology and Teratology* 23(5):399–411, 2001.

Fals-Stewart, W., Birchler, G.R., and O'Farrell, T.J. Drug-abusing patients and their intimate partners: Dyadic adjustment, relationship stability, and substance use. *Journal of Abnormal Psychology* 108(1):11–23, 1999.

Fals-Stewart, W., O'Farrell, T.J., Birchler, G.R., Cordova, J., and Kelley, M.L. Behavioral couples therapy for alcoholism and drug abuse: Where we've been, where we are, and where we're going. *Journal of Cognitive Psychotherapy* 19(3):229-246, 2005.

Federal Interagency Forum on Aging-Related Statistics. *Older Americans 2004: Key Indicators of Well-being*. November. Federal Interagency Forum on Aging-Related Statistics. Washington, D.C.: U.S. Government Printing Office, 2004.

Feinberg, F. Substance-abusing mothers and their children: Treatment for the family. In: Combrinck-Graham, L., ed. *Children in Families at Risk: Maintaining the Connections*. New York: Guilford Press, 1995. pp. 228–247.

Felitti, V.J., Anda, R.F., Nordenberg, D., Williamson, D.F., Spitz, A.M., Edwards, V., Koss, M.P., and Marks, J.S. Relationship of childhood abuse and household dysfunction to many of the leading causes of death in adults. The Adverse Childhood Experiences (ACE) Study. *American Journal of Preventive Medicine* 14(4):245-258, 1998.

Fernandez-Sola, J., and Nicolas-Arfelis, J.M. Gender differences in alcoholic cardiomyopathy. *The Journal of Gender-Specific Medicine: JGSM : The Official Journal of the Partnership for Women's Health at Columbia.* 5(1):41–47, 2002.

Ferreyra, N. Substance abuse and women with disabilities. Barker, L. T., Magill, K., MacKinnon, J. Dougal., Ridley, B., and Freeman, A. Cupolo. *Practitioner's Guide To Primary Care For Women With Physical Disabilities.* Oakland, CA: Berkeley Policy Associates and Alta Bates Summit Medical Center, 2005.

Fetzer Institute/National Institute on Aging Workgroup. *Multidimensional Measurement Of Religiousness/Spirituality For Use In Health Research: A Report Of The Fetzer Institute/National Institute On Aging Workgroup.* Kalamazoo, MI: Fetzer Institute, 1999.

Fetzer Institute/National Institute on Aging Workgroup. *Multidimensional Measurement Of Religiousness/Spirituality For Use In Health Research: A Report of the Fetzer Institute/National Institute on Aging Workgroup.* Kalamazoo, MI: Fetzer Institute, 2003.

Fields, J., and Casper, L.M. America's Families and Living Arrangements. *Current Population Reports* March 2000. P20-537 Washington, DC: U.S. Census Bureau, 2000.

Fillmore, K.M., Leino, E.V., Motoyoshi, M., Shoemaker, C., Terry, H., Ager, C.R., and Ferrer, H.P. Patterns and trends in women's and men's drinking. In: Wilsnack, R.W., and Wilsnack, S.C., eds. *Gender and Alcohol: Individual and Social Perspectives.* New Brunswick, NJ: Rutgers Center of Alcohol Studies, 1997. pp. 21–48.

Finch, B.K., Kolody, B., and Vega, W.A. Perceived discrimination and depression among Mexican-origin adults in California. *Journal of Health and Social Behavior* 41(3):295–313, 2000.

Finkelhor, D., Hotaling, G., Lewis, I.A., and Smith, C. Sexual abuse in a national survey of adult men and women: Prevalence, characteristics, and risk factors. *Child Abuse and Neglect* 14(1):19–28, 1990.

Finkelstein, N. The relational model. In: *Pregnancy and Exposure to Alcohol and Other Drug Use.* CSAP Technical Report 7. Rockville, MD: Center for Substance Abuse Prevention, 1993*a*. pp. 47–59.

Finkelstein, N. Treatment programming for alcohol and drug-dependent pregnant women. *International Journal of the Addictions* 28(13):1275–1309, 1993*b*.

Finkelstein, N. Treatment issues for alcohol- and drug-dependent pregnant and parenting women. *Health & Social Work* 19(1):7–15, 1994.

Finkelstein, N. Using the relational model as a context for treating pregnant and parenting chemically dependent women. In: Underhill, B.L., and Finnegan, D.G., eds. *Chemical Dependency: Women at Risk.* New York: Harrington Park Press/Haworth Press, 1996. pp. 23–44.

Finkelstein, N., Brown, K.N., and Laham, C.Q. Alcoholic mothers and guilt: Issues for caregivers. *Alcohol Health and Research World* 6(1):45–49, 1981.

Finkelstein, N., Kennedy, C., Thomas, K., and Kearns, M. *Gender-Specific Substance Abuse Treatment.* Rockville, MD: Center for Substance Abuse Prevention, 1997.

Finkelstein, N., VandeMark, N., Fallot, R., Brown, V., Cadiz, S., and Heckman, S. Enhancing substance abuse recovery through integrated trauma treatment. Sarasota, FL: National Trauma Consortium, 2004.

Fiorentine, R., and Anglin, M.D. Does increasing the opportunity for counseling increase the effectiveness of outpatient drug treatment? *American Journal of Drug and Alcohol Abuse* 23(3):369–382, 1997.

Fiorentine, R., Anglin, M.D., Gil-Rivas, V., and Taylor, E. Drug treatment: Explaining the gender paradox. *Substance Use and Misuse* 32(6):653–678, 1997.

Fischer, G., Ortner, R., Rohrmeister, K., Jagsch, R., Baewert, A., Langer, M., and Aschauer, H. Methadone versus buprenorphine in pregnant addicts: A double-blind, double-dummy comparison study. *Addiction* 101(2):275–281, 2006.

Fitzgerald, L.F., and Harmon, L.W. Women's career development: A postmodern update. In: Leong, F.T.L., and Barak, A., eds. *Contemporary Models In Vocational Psychology: A Volume In Honor Of Samuel H. Osipow.* 0-8058-2666-1 (hardcover); 0-8058-2667-X (paperback). Lawrence Erlbaum Associates Publishers: Mahwah, 2001. pp. 207–230.

Fitzgerald, L.F., Fassinger, R.E., and Betz, N.E. Theoretical advances in the study of women's career development. In: Walsh, W.B., and Osipow, S.H., eds. *Handbook Of Vocational Psychology: Theory, Research, And Practice (2nd ed.).* Contemporary topics in vocational psychology. 0-8058-1374-8 (hardcover). Lawrence Erlbaum Associates, 1995. pp. 67–109.

Fitzsimons, H.E., Tuten, M., Vaidya, V., and Jones, H.E. Mood disorders affect drug treatment success of drug-dependent pregnant women. *Journal of Substance Abuse Treatment* 32(1):19–25, 2007.

Flannery, B., Fishbein, D., Krupitsky, E., Langevin, D., Verbitskaya, E., Bland, C., Bolla, K., Egorova, V., Bushara, N., Tsoy, M., and Zvartau, E. Gender differences in neurocognitive functioning among alcohol-dependent Russian patients. *Alcoholism: Clinical & Experimental Research* 31(5):745–754, 2007.

Flensborg-Madsen, T., Knop, J., Mortensen, E.L., Becker, U., and Gronbaek, M. Amount of alcohol consumption and risk of developing alcoholism in men and women. *Alcohol and Alcoholism* 42(5):442–447, 2007.

Flores, E., Tschann, J.M., Dimas, J.M., Bachen, E.A., Pasch, L.A., and de Groat, C.L. Perceived discrimination, perceived stress, and mental and physical health among Mexican-origin adults. *Hispanic Journal of Behavioral Sciences* 30(4):401–424, 2008.

Foa, E.B., and Rothbaum, B.O. *Treating the Trauma of Rape: Cognitive-Behavioral Therapy for PTSD.* New York: Guilford Press, 1998.

Foa, E.B., Hembree, E.A., and Rothbaum, B.O. *Prolonged Exposure Therapy For PTSD: Emotional Processing Of Traumatic Experiences: Therapist Guide.* Treatments that work. Oxford University Press: New York, 2007.

Ford, J., Kasimer, N., MacDonald, M., and Savill, G. *Trauma Adaptive Recovery Group Education and Therapy (TARGET): Participant Guidebook and Leader Manual.* Farmington, CT: University of Connecticut Health Center, 2000.

Fortenberry, J.D., McFarlane, M., Bleakley, A., Bull, S., Fishbein, M., Grimley, D.M., Malotte, C.K., and Stoner, B.P. Relationships of stigma and shame to gonorrhea and HIV screening. *American Journal of Public Health* 92(3):378–381, 2002.

Frajzyngier, V., Neaigus, A., Gyarmathy, V.A., Miller, M., and Friedman, S.R. Gender differences in injection risk behaviors at the first injection episode. *Drug and Alcohol Dependence* 89(2–3):145–152, 2007.

Frank, D.A., Augustyn, M., Knight, W.G., Pell, T., and Zuckerman, B. Growth, development, and behavior in early childhood following prenatal cocaine exposure. *Journal of the American Medical Association* 285(12):1613–1625, 2001.

Frank, J.B., Weihs, K., Minerva, E., and Lieberman, D.Z. Women's mental health in primary care: Depression, anxiety, somatization, eating disorders, and substance abuse. *Medical Clinics of North America* 82(2):359–389, 1998.

Franklin, T.R., Ehrman, R., Lynch, K.G., Harper, D., Sciortino, N., O'Brien, C.P., and Childress, A.R. Menstrual cycle phase at quit date predicts smoking status in an NRT treatment trial: A retrospective analysis. *Journal of Women's Health (15409996)* 17(2):287–292, 2008.

Franko, D.L., Dorer, D.J., Keel, P.K., Jackson, S., Manzo, M.P., and Herzog, D.B. How do eating disorders and alcohol use disorder influence each other? *International Journal of Eating Disorders* 38(3):200–207, 2005.

French, G.M., Groner, J.A., Wewers, M.E., and Ahijevych, K. Staying smoke free: An intervention to prevent postpartum relapse. *Nicotine & Tobacco Research* 9(6):663–670, 2007.

Frezza, M., di Padova, C., Pozzato, G., Terpin, M., Baraona, E., and Lieber, C.S. High blood alcohol levels in women: The role of decreased gastric alcohol dehydrogenase activity and first-pass metabolism. *New England Journal of Medicine* 322(2):95–99, 1990.

Fried, P.A., and Smith, A.M. A literature review of the consequences of prenatal marihuana exposure: An emerging theme of a deficiency in aspects of executive function. *Neurotoxicology and Teratology* 23(1):1–11, 2001.

Fullilove, M.T., Fullilove, R.E., Smith, M., and Winkler, K. Violence, trauma, and posttraumatic stress disorder among women drug users. *Journal of Traumatic Stress* 6(4):533–543, 1993.

Funkhouser, E., Pulley, L., Lueschen, G., Costello, C., Hook, E., III, and Vermund, S.H. Douching beliefs and practices among black and white women. *Journal of Women's Health and Gender-Based Medicine* 11(1):29–37, 2002.

Galbraith, S. *And So I Began to Listen to Their Stories: Working with Women in the Criminal Justice System.* Delmar, NY: National Gains Center, 1998.

Gale, T.C., White, J.A., and Welty, T.K. Differences in detection of alcohol use in a prenatal population (on a Northern Plains Indian Reservation) using various methods of ascertainment. *South Dakota Journal of Medicine* 51(7):235–240, 1998.

Galea, S., and Vlahov, D. Social determinants and the health of drug users: Socioeconomic status, homelessness, and incarceration. *Public Health Reports* 117 Suppl 1:S135–S145, 2002.

Galen, L.W., Brower, K.J., Gillespie, B.W., and Zucker, R.A. Sociopathy, gender, and treatment outcome among outpatient substance abusers. *Drug and Alcohol Dependence* 61(1):23–33, 2000.

Garner, D.M., Olmstead, M.P., Bohr, Y., and Garfinkel, P.E. The Eating Attitudes Test: Psychometric features and clinical correlates. *Psychological Medicine* 12:871–878, 1982.

Garner, D.M., Rosen, L.W., and Barry, D. Eating disorders among athletes: Research and recommendations. *Child and Adolescent Psychiatric Clinics of North America* 7(4):839–857, 1998.

Gary, L.E., and Littlefield, M.B. The protective factor model: Strengths-oriented prevention for African-American families. In: Brisbane, F.L., Epstein, L.G., Pacheco, G., and Quinlan, J.W., eds. *Cultural Competence for Health Care Professionals Working with African-American Communities: Theory and Practice.* CSAP Cultural Competence Series 7. HHS Publication No. (SMA) 98-3238. Rockville, MD: Center for Substance Abuse Prevention, 1998. pp. 81–105.

Gavaler, J.S., and Arria, A.M. Increased susceptibility of women to alcoholic liver disease: Artifactual or real? In: Hall, P.M., ed. *Alcoholic Liver Disease: Pathology and Pathogenesis.* 2nd ed. London, UK: Edward Arnold, 1995. pp. 123–133.

Gear, R.W., Gordon, N.C., Heller, P.H., Paul, S., Miaskowski, C., and Levine, J.D. Gender difference in analgesic response to the kappa-opioid pentazocine. *Neuroscience Letters* 205(3):207–209, 1996.

Gee, G.C. A Multilevel Analysis of the Relationship Between Institutional and Individual Racial Discrimination and Health Status. *American Journal of Public Health* 92(4):615–623, 2002.

Gehart, D.R., and Lyle, R.R. Client experience of gender in therapeutic relationships: an interpretive ethnography. *Family Process* 40(4):443–458, 2001.

George, W.H., Gournic, S.J., and McAfee, M.P. Perceptions of postdrinking female sexuality: Effects of gender, beverage choice, and drink payment. *Journal of Applied Social Psychology* 18(15, Pt 1):1295–1317, 1988.

Giglia, R., and Binns, C. Alcohol and lactation: A systematic review. *Nutrition & Dietetics* 63:103–116, 2006.

Gilbert, M.J. Acculturation and changes in drinking patterns among Mexican-American women: Implications for prevention. *Alcohol Health and Research World* 15(3):234–238, 1991.

Gilbert, M.J., and Collins, R.L. Ethnic variation in women's and men's drinking. In: Wilsnack, R.W., and Wilsnack, S.C., eds. *Gender and Alcohol: Individual and Social Perspectives.* New Brunswick, NJ: Rutgers Center of Alcohol Studies, 1997. pp. 357–378.

Gilligan, C. *In a Different Voice: Psychological Theory and Women's Development.* Cambridge, MA: Harvard University Press, 1982.

Gilligan, C., Lyons, N., Hanmer, T.J., and Emma Willard School. *Making Connections: The Relational Worlds of Adolescent Girls at Emma Willard School.* Cambridge, Mass: Harvard University Press, 1990.

Gilman, S.E., Cochran, S.D., Mays, V.M., Hughes, M., Ostrow, D., and Kessler, R.C. Risk of psychiatric disorders among individuals reporting same-sex sexual partners in the National Comorbidity Survey. *American Journal of Public Health* 91(6):933–939, 2001.

Gil-Rivas, V., Fiorentine, R., and Anglin, M.D. Sexual abuse, physical abuse, and posttraumatic stress disorder among women participating in outpatient drug abuse treatment. *Journal of Psychoactive Drugs* 28(1):95–102, 1996.

Gil-Rivas, V., Fiorentine, R., Anglin, M.D., and Taylor, E. Sexual and physical abuse: Do they compromise drug treatment outcomes? *Journal of Substance Abuse Treatment* 14(4):351–358, 1997.

Gim Chung, R.H., Kim, B.S.K., and Abreu, J.M. Asian American Multidimensional Acculturation Scale: Development, Factor Analysis, Reliability, and Validity. *Cultural Diversity and Ethnic Minority Psychology* 10(1):66–80, 2004.

Gloria, A.M., and Peregoy, J.J. Counseling Latino alcohol and other substance users/abusers: Cultural considerations for counselors. *Journal of Substance Abuse Treatment* 13(2):119–126, 1996.

Goldberg, B. *A Framework for Systems Change: Evaluation of the Milwaukee Family Services Coordination Initiative.* Madison, WI: Wisconsin Department of Health and Family Services, Division of Supportive Living, Bureau of Substance Abuse Services, 2000.

Goldschmidt, L., Day, N.L., and Richardson, G.A. Effects of prenatal marijuana exposure on child behavior problems at age 10. *Neurotoxicology and Teratology* 22(3):325–336, 2000.

Goode, T.D., Dunne, C., and Bronheim, S.M. *The Evidence Base for Cultural and Linguistic Competency in Health Care.* October New York, NY: The Commonwealth Fund 2006.

Gopaul-McNicol, S.A., and Brice-Baker, J. *Cross-Cultural Practice: Assessment, Treatment, and Training.* New York: John Wiley & Sons, 1998.

Gordon, M.T., and Riger, S. *The Female Fear.* New York: The Free Press, 1989.

Gottheil, E., Sterling, R.C., and Weinstein, S.P. Outreach engagement efforts: Are they worth the effort? *American Journal of Drug and Alcohol Abuse* 23(1):61–66, 1997.

Graham, K., Massak, A., Demers, A., and Rehm, J. Does the association between alcohol consumption and depression depend on how they are measured? *Alcoholism: Clinical & Experimental Research* 31(1):78–88, 2007.

Grant, B.F., Dawson, D.A., Stinson, F.S., Chou, S.C., Dufour, M.C., and Pickering, R.P. The 12-Month prevalence and trends in DSM-TR-IV alcohol abuse and dependence. *Alcohol Research & Health* 29(2):79–91, 2006.

Grant, B.F., Stinson, F.S., Hasin, D.S., Dawson, D.A., Chou, S.P., and Anderson, K. Immigration and lifetime prevalence of DSM-IV Psychiatric disorders among Mexican Americans and Non-Hispanic Whites in the United States: Results from the National Epidemiologic Survey on Alcohol and Related Conditions. *Archives of General Psychiatry* 61(12):1226–1233, 2004.

Gray, M., and Littlefield, M.B. Black women and addiction. In: Straussner, S.L.A., and Brown, S., eds. *The Handbook of Addiction Treatment for Women: Theory and Practice.* San Francisco: Jossey-Bass, 2002. pp. 301–322.

Grayson, C.E., and Nolen-Hoeksema, S. Motives to drink as mediators between childhood sexual assault and alcohol problems in adult women. *Journal of Traumatic Stress* 18(2):137–145, 2005.

Green, C.A., Polen, M.R., Dickinson, D.M., Lynch, F.L., and Bennett, M.D. Gender differences in predictors of initiation, retention, and completion in an HMO-based substance abuse treatment program. *Journal of Substance Abuse Treatment* 23(4):285–295, 2002.

Green, C.A., Polen, M.R., Lynch, F.L., Dickinson, D.M., and Bennett, M.D. Gender differences in outcomes in an HMO-based substance abuse treatment program. *Journal of Addictive Diseases.* 23(2):47–70, 2004.

Green, J.H. Fetal Alcohol Spectrum Disorders: understanding the effects of prenatal alcohol exposure and supporting students. *J Sch Health* 77(3):103–108, 2007.

Greene, B. Ethnic minority lesbians and gay men: Mental health and treatment issues. In: Greene, B., ed. *Ethnic and Cultural Diversity Among Lesbians and Gay Men.* Thousand Oaks, CA: Sage Publications, 1997. pp. 216–239.

Greenfeld, L.A., and Snell, T.L. *Women Offenders*. Bureau of Justice Statistics Special Report. NCJ 175688. Washington, DC: Bureau of Justice Statistics, 1999.

Greenfield, L., Burgdorf, K., Chen, X., Porowski, A., Roberts, T., and Herrell, J. Effectiveness of long-term residential substance abuse treatment for women: findings from three national studies. *American Journal of Drug and Alcohol Abuse* 30(3):537–550, 2004.

Greenfield, S.F. Women and substance use disorders. In: Jensvold, M.F., and Halbreich, U., eds. *Psychopharmacology and Women: Sex, Gender, and Hormones*. Washington, DC: American Psychiatric Press, 1996. pp. 299–321.

Greenfield, S.F., and O'Leary, G. Sex differences in substance use disorders. In: Lewis-Hall, F., and Williams, T.S., eds. *Psychiatric Illness in Women: Emerging Treatments and Research*. Washington, DC: American Psychiatric Publishing, Inc, 2002. pp. 467–533.

Greenfield, S.F., Brooks, A.J., Gordon, S.M., Green, C.A., Kropp, F., McHugh, R.K., Lincoln, M., Hien, D., and Miele, G.M. Substance abuse treatment entry, retention, and outcome in women: A review of the literature. *Drug and Alcohol Dependence* 86(1):1–21, 2007*a*.

Greenfield, S.F., Trucco, E.M., McHugh, R.K., Lincoln, M., and Gallop, R.J. The Women's Recovery Group Study: a Stage I trial of women-focused group therapy for substance use disorders versus mixed-gender group drug counseling. *Drug and Alcohol Dependence* 90(1):39–47, 2007*b*.

Grella, C.E. Background and overview of mental health and substance abuse treatment systems: Meeting the needs of women who are pregnant or parenting. *Journal of Psychoactive Drugs* 28(4):319–343, 1996.

Grella, C.E. Services for perinatal women with substance abuse and mental health disorders: The unmet need. *Journal of Psychoactive Drugs* 29(1):67–78, 1997.

Grella, C.E. Women in residential drug treatment: Differences by program type and pregnancy. *Journal of Health Care for the Poor and Underserved* 10(2):216–229, 1999.

Grella, C.E., and Joshi, V. Gender differences in drug treatment careers among clients in the national Drug Abuse Treatment Outcome Study. *American Journal of Drug and Alcohol Abuse* 25(3):385–406, 1999.

Grella, C.E., Annon, J.J., and Anglin, M.D. Ethnic differences in HIV risk behaviors, self-perceptions, and treatment outcomes among women in methadone maintenance treatment. *Journal of Psychoactive Drugs* 27(4):421–433, 1995.

Grella, C.E., Joshi, V., and Hser, Y.I. Program variation in treatment outcomes among women in residential drug treatment. *Evaluation Review* 24(4):364–383, 2000.

Grella, C.E., Scott, C.K., and Foss, M.A. Gender differences in long-term drug treatment outcomes in Chicago PETS. *Journal of Substance Abuse Treatment* 28(Suppl1):S3–S12, 2005.

Grice, D.E., Brady, K.T., Dustan, L.R., Malcolm, R., and Kilpatrick, D.G. Sexual and physical assault history and posttraumatic stress disorder in substance-dependent individuals. *American Journal on Addictions* 4(4):297–305, 1995.

Grieco, E.M. The Native Hawaiian and Other Pacific Islander Population: 2000. *Census 2000 Brief* Washington, DC: U.S. Census Bureau 2001.

Griffin, M.L., Mendelson, J.H., Mello, N.K., and Lex, B.W. Marihuana use across the menstrual cycle. *Drug and Alcohol Dependence* 18(2):213–224, 1986.

Griffiths, E.J., Lorenz, R.P., Baxter, S., and Talon, N.S. Acute neurohumoral response to electroconvulsive therapy during pregnancy: A case report. *Journal of Reproductive Medicine* 34(11):907–911, 1989.

Grosenick, J.K., and Hatmaker, C.M. Perceptions of the importance of physical setting in substance abuse treatment. *Journal of Substance Abuse Treatment* 18(1):29–39, 2000.

Gross, M., and Brown, V. Outreach to injection drug-using women. In: Brown, B.S., and Beschner, G.M., eds. *Handbook on Risk of AIDS: Injection Drug Users and Sexual Partners.* Westport, CT: Greenwood Press, 1993. pp. 445–463.

Gruber, K., Fleetwood, T., and Herring, M. In-home continuing care services for substance affected families: The Bridges Program. *Social Work* 46(3):267–277, 2001.

Grucza, R.A., Bucholz, K.K., Rice, J.P., and Bierut, L.J. Secular trends in the lifetime prevalence of alcohol dependence in the United States: a re-evaluation. *Alcoholism: Clinical & Experimental Research* 32(5):763–770, 2008.

Gutierres, S.E., and Todd, M. The impact of childhood abuse on treatment outcomes of substance users. *Professional Psychology: Research and Practice* 28(4):348–354, 1997.

Hagedorn, H., Dieperink, E., Dingmann, D., Durfee, J., Ho, S.B., Isenhart, C., Rettmann, N., and Willenbring, M. Integrating hepatitis prevention services into a substance use disorder clinic. *Journal of Substance Abuse Treatment* 32(4):391–398, 2007.

Hall, J.M. Lesbians in alcohol recovery surviving childhood sexual abuse and parental substance misuse. *International Journal of Psychiatric Nursing Research* 5(1):507–515, 1999.

Hall, J.M. Core issues for female child abuse survivors in recovery from substance misuse. *Qualitative Health Research* 10(5):612–631, 2000.

Hall, P.M. Pathological spectrum of alcoholic liver disease. In: Hall, P.M., ed. *Alcoholic Liver Disease: Pathology and Pathogenesis.* 2nd ed. London, UK: Edward Arnold, 1995. pp. 41–68.

Haller, D.L., and Miles, D.R. Psychopathology is associated with completion of residential treatment in drug dependent women. *Journal of Addictive Diseases* 23(1):17–28, 2004.

Haller, D.L., Miles, D.R., and Dawson, K.S. Psychopathology influences treatment retention among drug-dependent women. *Journal of Substance Abuse Treatment* 23(4):431–436, 2002.

Hamajima, N., Hirose, K., Tajima, K., Rohan, T., Calle, E.E., Heath, C.W., et al. Alcohol, tobacco and breast cancer: Collaborative reanalysis of individual data from 53 epidemiological studies, including 58,515 women with breast cancer and 95,067 women without the disease. *British Journal of Cancer* 87(11):1234–1245, 2002.

Handmaker, N.S., and Wilbourne, P. Motivational interventions in prenatal clinics. *Alcohol Research and Health* 25(3):219–229, 2001.

Hankin, J., McCaul, M.E., and Heussner, J. Pregnant, alcohol-abusing women. *Alcoholism: Clinical and Experimental Research* 24(8):1276–1286, 2000.

Hanlon, J.T., Fillenbaum, G.G., Ruby, C.M., Gray, S., and Bohannon, A. Epidemiology of over-the-counter drug use in community dwelling elderly: United States perspective. *Drugs and Aging* 18(2):123–131, 2001.

Hanna, E., Dufour, M.C., Elliott, S., and Stinson, F. Dying to be equal: Women, alcohol, and cardiovascular disease. *British Journal of Addiction* 87(11):1593–1597, 1992.

Harned, M.S., Najavits, L.M., and Weiss, R.D. Self-harm and suicidal behavior in women with comorbid PTSD and substance dependence. *American Journal of Addiction* 15(5):392–395, 2006.

Harris, B., Lovett, L., Newcombe, R.G., Read, G.F., Walker, R., and Riad-Fahmy, D. Maternity blues and major endocrine changes: Cardiff puerperal mood and hormone study II. *British Medical Journal* 308(6934):949–953, 1994.

Harris, M. Modifications in service delivery and clinical treatment for women diagnosed with severe mental illness who are also the survivors of sexual abuse trauma. *Journal of Mental Health Administration* 21(4):397–406, 1994.

Harris, M., and Community Connections Trauma Work Group. *Trauma Recovery and Empowerment: A Clinician's Guide for Working with Women in Groups.* New York: Simon & Schuster, 1998.

Harris, M., and Fallot, R.D. Designing trauma-informed addictions services. In: Harris, M., and Fallot, R.D., eds. *Using Trauma Theory to Design Service Systems.* New Directions for Mental Health Services, No. 89. San Francisco: Jossey-Bass, 2001*a*. pp. 57–73.

Harris, M., and Fallot, R.D. Envisioning a trauma-informed service system: A vital paradigm shift. In: Harris, M., and Fallot, R.D., eds. *Using Trauma Theory to Design Service Systems.* New Directions for Mental Health Services, No. 89. San Francisco: Jossey-Bass, 2001*b*. pp. 3–22.

Harrison, P.M., and Beck, A.J. Prisoners in 2001. *Bureau of Justice Statistics Bulletin* Washington, DC: Bureau of Justice Statistics, 2002.

Harrison, P.M., and Karberg, J.C. *Prison and Jail Inmates at Midyear 2002.* Washington, DC: Bureau of Justice Statistics, 2003.

Haskett, M.E., Miller, J.W., Whitworth, J.M., and Huffman, J.M. Intervention with cocaine-abusing mothers. *Families in Society* 73(8):451–461, 1992.

Haswell, D.E., and Graham, M. Self-inflicted injuries: Challenging knowledge, skill, and compassion. *Canadian Family Physician* 42:1756–1758, 1761–1764, 1996.

Havens, J.R., Cornelius, L.J., Ricketts, E.P., Latkin, C.A., Bishai, D., Lloyd, J.J., Huettner, S., and Strathdee, S.A. The effect of a case management intervention on drug treatment entry among treatment-seeking injection drug users with and without comorbid antisocial personality disorder. *Journal of Urban Health* 84(2):267–271, 2007.

Hawke, J.M., Jainchill, N., and De Leon, G. The prevalence of sexual abuse and its impact on the onset of drug use among adolescents in therapeutic community drug treatment. *Journal of Child & Adolescent Substance Abuse* 9(3):35–49, 2000.

Heath, A.C., Slutske, W.S., and Madden, P.A.F. Gender differences in the genetic contribution to alcoholism risk and to alcohol consumption patterns. In: Wilsnack, R.W., and Wilsnack, S.C., eds. *Gender and Alcohol: Individual and Social Perspectives.* New Brunswick, NJ: Rutgers Center of Alcohol Studies, 1997. pp. 114–149.

Heffernan, K. The nature and predictors of substance use among lesbians. *Addictive Behaviors* 23(4):517–528, 1998.

Heflin, C.M. *Dynamics of Material Hardship in the Women's Employment Survey.* Paper presented at the annual meeting of the American Sociological Association, Montreal Convention Center, Montreal, Quebec, Canada, 2006.

Heintges, T., and Wands, J.R. Hepatitis C virus: epidemiology and transmission. *Hepatology* 26(3):521–526, 1997.

Henderson, D.J. Drug abuse and incarcerated women: A research review. *Journal of Substance Abuse Treatment* 15(6):579–587, 1998.

Henderson, D.J., Boyd, C., and Mieczkowski, T. Gender, relationships, and crack cocaine: A content analysis. *Research in Nursing and Health* 17(4):265–272, 1994.

Herman, J.L. *Trauma and Recovery*. Rev. ed. New York: Basic Books, 1997.

Hernandez-Avila, C.A., Rounsaville, B.J., and Kranzler, H.R. Opioid-, cannabis- and alcohol-dependent women show more rapid progression to substance abuse treatment. *Drug and Alcohol Dependence* 74(3):265–272, 2004.

Herzog, D.B., Franko, D.L., Dorer, D.J., Keel, P.K., Jackson, S., and Manzo, M.P. Drug abuse in women with eating disorders. *International Journal of Eating Disorders* 39(5):364–368, 2006.

Hewitt, P.L., and Norton, G.R. The Beck Anxiety Inventory: A psychometric analysis. *Psychological Assessment* 5(4):408–412, 1993.

Hiebert-Murphy, D., and Woytkiw, L. A model for working with women dealing with child sexual abuse and addictions: The Laurel Centre, Winnipeg, Manitoba, Canada. *Journal of Substance Abuse Treatment* 18(4):387–394, 2000.

Hien, D.A., Cohen, L.R., Miele, G.M., Litt, L.C., and Capstick, C. Promising treatments for women with comorbid PTSD and substance use disorders. *American Journal of Psychiatry* 161(8):1426–1432, 2004.

Highleyman, L. Women and HCV. *HCV Advocate* San Francisco, CA: Hepatitis C Support Project 2005.

Hill, R.B. *The Strengths of Black Families*. New York: Emerson Hall Publishers, 1972.

Hillhouse, M.P., and Fiorentine, R. 12–Step program participation and effectiveness: Do gender and ethnic differences exist? *Journal of Drug Issues* 31(3):767–780, 2001.

Hoek, H. The distribution of eating disorders. In: Brownell, K.D., and Fairburn, C.G., eds. *Eating Disorders and Obesity: A Comprehensive Handbook*. New York: Guilford Press, 1995. pp. 207–211.

Hoek, H.W., and van Hoeken, D. Review of the prevalence and incidence of eating disorders. *International Journal of Eating Disorders* 34(4):383–396, 2003.

Hoffman, E.H., Blackburn, C., and Cullari, S. Brief residential treatment for nicotine addiction: a five-year follow-up study. *Psychological Reports* 89(1):99–105, 2001.

Hofmann, S.G., and Smits, J.A. Cognitive–behavioral therapy for adult anxiety disorders: a meta-analysis of randomized placebo-controlled trials. *Journal of Clinical Psychiatry* 69(4):621–632, 2008.

Holcomb-McCoy, C. Group mentoring with urban African American female adolescents. *E-Journal of Teaching and Learning in Diverse Settings* 2(1):161–176. Baton Rouge, LA: Southern University and A&M College 2004.

Holdcraft, L.C., and Comtois, K.A. Description of and preliminary data from a women's dual diagnosis community mental health program. *Canadian Journal of Community Mental Health* 21(2):91–109, 2002.

Holderness, C.C., Brooks-Gunn, J., and Warren, M.P. Co-morbidity of eating disorders and substance abuse: Review of the literature. *International Journal of Eating Disorders* 16(1):1–34, 1994.

Holman, C.D.J., English, D.R., Milne, E., and Winter, M.G. Meta-analysis of alcohol and all-cause mortality: A validation of NHMRC recommendations. *Medical Journal of Australia* 164(3):141–145, 1996.

Hommer, D., Momenan, R., Rawlings, R., Ragan, P., Williams, W., Rio, D., and Eckardt, M. Decreased corpus callosum size among alcoholic women. *Archives of Neurology* 53(4):359–363, 1996.

Hommer, D.W., Momenan, R., Kaiser, E., and Rawlings, R.R. Evidence for a gender-related effect of alcoholism on brain volumes. *American Journal of Psychiatry* 158(2):198–204, 2001.

Hope, S., Rodgers, B., and Power, C. Marital status transitions and psychological distress: Longitudinal evidence from a national population sample. *Psychological Medicine* 29(2):381–389, 1999.

Horrell, S.C.V. Effectiveness of cognitive–behavioral therapy with adult ethnic minority clients: A review. *Professional Psychology: Research and Practice* 39(2):160–168, 2008.

Horwitz, A.V., White, H.R., and Howell-White, S. The use of multiple outcomes in stress research: A case study of gender differences in responses to marital dissolution. *Journal of Health and Social Behavior* 37(3):278–291, 1996.

Howell, E.M., and Chasnoff, I.J. Perinatal substance abuse treatment: Findings from focus groups with clients and providers. *Journal of Substance Abuse Treatment* 17(1–2):139–148, 1999.

Howland, R.H. The treatment of persons with dual diagnoses in a rural community. *Psychiatric Quarterly* 66(1):33–49, 1995.

Hser, Y.I., Anglin, M.D., and Booth, M.W. Sex differences in addict careers: 3. Addiction. *American Journal of Drug and Alcohol Abuse* 13(3):231–251, 1987.

Hser, Y.I., Evans, E., Huang, D., and Anglin, D.M. Relationship between drug treatment services, retention, and outcomes. *Psychiatric Services* 55(7):767–774, 2004.

Hser, Y.I., Polinsky, M.L., Maglione, M., and Anglin, M.D. Matching clients' needs with drug treatment services. *Journal of Substance Abuse Treatment* 16(4):299–305, 1999.

Hudson, J.I., Hiripi, E., Pope, H.G., Jr., and Kessler, R.C. The prevalence and correlates of eating disorders in the National Comorbidity Survey Replication. *Biological Psychiatry* 61(3):348–358, 2007.

Hudson, J.I., Weiss, R.D., Pope, H.G., Jr., McElroy, S.K., and Mirin, S.M. Eating disorders in hospitalized substance abusers. *American Journal of Drug and Alcohol Abuse* 18(1):75–85, 1992.

Hughes, P.H., Coletti, S.D., Neri, R.L., Urmann, C.F., Stahl, S., Sicilian, D.M., and Anthony, J.C. Retaining cocaine-abusing women in a therapeutic community: The effect of a child live-in program. *American Journal of Public Health* 85(8 Pt 1):1149–1152, 1995.

Hughes, T.L., and Eliason, M. Substance use and abuse in lesbian, gay, bisexual and transgender populations. *Journal of Primary Prevention* 22(3):263–298, 2002.

Hughes, T.L., and Jacobson, K.M. Sexual orientation and women's smoking. *Current Women's Health Report* 3(3):254–261, 2003.

Hughes, T.L., and Norris, J. Sexuality, sexual orientation, and violence: Pieces in the puzzle of women's use and abuse of alcohol. In: McElmurry, F.J., and Parker, R.S., eds. *Annual Review of Women's Health: Vol. II.* New York: National League for Nursing Press, 1995. pp. 285–317.

Hughes, T.L., and Wilsnack, S.C. Use of alcohol among lesbians: Research and clinical implications. *American Journal of Orthopsychiatry* 67(1):20–36, 1997.

Hughes, T.L., Haas, A.P., Razzano, L., Cassidy, R., and Matthews, A. Comparing lesbians' and heterosexual women's mental health: Findings from a multi-site study. *Journal of Gay and Lesbian Social Services* 11(1):57–76, 2000.

Hughes, T.L., Johnson, T.P., Wilsnack, S.C., and Szalacha, L.A. Childhood risk factors for alcohol abuse and psychological distress among adult lesbians. *Child Abuse and Neglect* 31(7):769–789, 2007.

Hurd, Y.L., Wang, X., Anderson, V., Beck, O., Minkoff, H., and Dow-Edwards, D. Marijuana impairs growth in mid-gestation fetuses. *Neurotoxicology and Teratology* 27(2):221–229, 2005.

Hurt, H., Brodsky, N.L., Betancourt, L., Braitman, L.E., Malmud, E., and Giannetta, J. Cocaine-exposed children: Follow-up through 30 months. *Journal of Developmental and Behavioral Pediatrics* 16(1):29–35, 1995.

Hurt, H., Malmud, E., Betancourt, L.M., Brodsky, N.L., and Giannetta, J.M. A prospective comparison of developmental outcome of children with in utero cocaine exposure and controls using the Battelle Developmental Inventory. *Journal of Developmental and Behavioral Pediatrics* 22(1):27–34, 2001.

Hussong, R.G., Bird, K., and Murphy, C.V. Substance abuse among American Indian women of childbearing age. *IHS Primary Care Provider* 19(12):196–199, 1994.

Hyman, S.M., Paliwal, P., and Sinha, R. Childhood maltreatment, perceived stress, and stress-related coping in recently abstinent cocaine dependent adults. *Psychology of Addictive Behaviors* 21(2):233–238, 2007.

Hyman, S.M., Paliwal, P., Chaplin, T.M., Mazure, C.M., Rounsaville, B.J., and Sinha, R. Severity of childhood trauma is predictive of cocaine relapse outcomes in women but not men. *Drug and Alcohol Dependence* 92(1–3):208–216, 2008.

Hymbaugh, K., Miller, L.A., Druschel, C.M., Podvin, D.W., Meaney, F.J., and Boyle, C.A. A multiple source methodology for the surveillance of fetal alcohol syndrome--The Fetal Alcohol Syndrome Surveillance Network (FASSNet). *Teratology* 66 Suppl 1:S41–S49, 2002.

Indian Health Service. Demographic statistics section of regional differences in Indian health 2000–2001: Tables only. Rockville, MD: Indian Health Service, 2002.

International Longevity Center-USA. Caregiving in America. New York, NY: 2006.

Jacobson, J.O., Robinson, P.L., and Bluthenthal, R.N. Racial disparities in completion rates from publicly funded alcohol treatment: economic resources explain more than demographics and addiction severity. *Health Services Research* 42(2):773–794, 2007.

Janes, J. Their own worst enemy? Management and prevention of self-harm. *Professional Nurse* 9(12):838–841, 1994.

Janoff-Bulman, R. *Shattered Assumptions: Towards a New Psychology of Trauma*. New York: Free Press, 1992.

Jansson, L.M., Svikis, D.S., Breon, D., and Cieslak, R. Intensity of Case Management Services: Does More Equal Better for Drug-Dependent Women and Their Children? *Social Work in Mental Health* 3(4):63–78, 2005.

Jarvis, M.A., and Schnoll, S.H. Methadone use during pregnancy. In: Chiang, C.N., and Finnegan, L.P., eds. *Medications Development for the Treatment of Pregnant Addicts and Their Infants*. NIDA Research Monograph 149. NIH Publication No. 95–3891. Rockville, MD: National Institute on Drug Abuse, 1995. pp. 58–77.

Jarvis, T.J., Copeland, J., and Walton, L. Exploring the nature of the relationship between child sexual abuse and substance use among women. *Addiction* 93(6):865–875, 1998.

Jennison, K.M., and Johnson, K.A. Alcohol dependence in adult children of alcoholics: Longitudinal evidence of early risk. *Journal of Drug Education* 28(1):19–37, 1998.

Jennison, K.M., and Johnson, K.A. Parental alcoholism as a risk factor for DSM-IV defined alcohol abuse and dependence in American women: The protective benefits of dyadic cohesion in marital communication. *American Journal of Drug and Alcohol Abuse* 27(2):349–374, 2001.

Jessup, M. Addiction in women: Prevalence, profiles, and meaning. *Journal of Obstetric, Gynecologic, and Neonatal Nursing* 26(4):449–458, 1997.

Jessup, M., Humphreys, J., Brindis, C., and Lee, K. Extrinsic barriers to substance abuse treatment among pregnant drug dependent women. *Journal of Drug Issues* 23(2):285–304, 2003.

Joe, G.W., Rowan-Szal, G.A., Greener, J.M., and Simpson, D.D. The TCU Brief Intake and Client Problem Index (CPI). Poster presented at the American Methadone Treatment Association conference, San Francisco, April 2000.

Joe, G.W., Simpson, D.D., and Broome, K.M. Retention and patient engagement models for different treatment modalities in DATOS. *Drug and Alcohol Dependence* 57(2):113–125, 1999.

Joe, G.W., Simpson, D.D., Dansereau, D.F., and Rowan-Szal, G.A. Relationships between counseling rapport and drug abuse treatment outcomes. *Psychiatric Services* 52(9):1223–1229, 2001.

Joe, K.A. "Ice is strong enough for a man but made for a woman:" A social cultural analysis of crystal methamphetamine use among Asian Pacific Americans. *Crime, Law, and Social Change* 22:269–289, 1995.

Joe, K.A. Lives and times of Asian-Pacific American women drug users: An ethnographic study of their methamphetamine use. *Journal of Drug Issues* 26(1):199–218, 1996.

Joe, S., Baser, R.E., Breeden, G., Neighbors, H.W., and Jackson, J.S. Prevalence of and risk factors for lifetime suicide attempts among blacks in the United States. *JAMA* 296(17):2112–2123, 2006.

John, U., Meyer, C., Rumpf, H.J., and Hapke, U. Psychiatric comorbidity including nicotine dependence among individuals with eating disorder criteria in an adult general population sample. *Psychiatry Research* 141(1):71–79, 2006.

Johnson, H.L., Glassman, M.B., Fiks, K.B., and Rosen, T.S. Path analysis of variables affecting 36-month outcome in a population of multi-risk children. *Infant Behavior and Development* 10(4):451–465, 1987.

Johnson, J.L., and Leff, M. Children of substance abusers: Overview of research findings. *Pediatrics* 103(5 Pt 2):1085–1099, 1999.

Johnson, P.B., Richter, L., Kleber, H.D., McLellan, A.T., and Carise, D. Telescoping of drinking-related behaviors: Gender, racial/ethnic, and age comparisons. *Substance Use & Misuse* 40(8):1139–1151, 2005.

Johnson, T.P., and Hughes, T.L. Reliability and concurrent validity of the cage screening questions: A Comparison of lesbians and heterosexual women. *Substance Use & Misuse* 40(5):657–669, 2005.

Jones, H.E., and Johnson, R.E. Pregnancy and substance abuse. *Current Opinion in Psychiatry* 14:187–193, 2001.

Jones, H.E., Haug, N., Silverman, K., Stitzer, M., and Svikis, D. The effectiveness of incentives in enhancing treatment attendance and drug abstinence in methadone-maintained pregnant women. *Drug and Alcohol Dependence* 61(3):297–306, 2001.

Jones, H. E., Johnson, R. E., Jasinski, D. R., O'Grady, K. E., Chisholm, C. A., Choo, R. E. et al. Buprenorphine versus methadone in the treatment of pregnant opioid-dependent patients: Effects on the neonatal abstinence syndrome. *Drug and Alcohol Dependence*, 79, 2005. pp. 1-10.

Jones, K.L., and Smith, D.W. Recognition of the fetal alcohol syndrome in early infancy. *Lancet* 2(7836):999–1001, 1973.

Jones-Webb, R.J., Hsiao, C.Y., and Hannan, P. Relationships between socioeconomic status and drinking problems among black and white men. *Alcoholism: Clinical and Experimental Research* 19(3):623–627, 1995.

Jonker, J., De Jong, C.A., de Weert-van Oene, G.H., and Gijs, L. Gender-role stereotypes and interpersonal behavior: How addicted inpatients view their ideal male and female therapist. *Journal of Substance Abuse Treatment* 19(3):307–312, 2000.

Jordan, J.V., and Hartling, L.M. New developments in relational-cultural theory. In: Ballou, M., and Brown, L.S., eds. *Rethinking Mental Health and Disorders: Feminists Perspectives*. New York: Guilford Publications, 2002. pp. 48-70.

Jordan, K.M., and Deluty, R.H. Coming out for lesbian women: Its relation to anxiety, positive affectivity, self-esteem and social support. *Journal of Homosexuality* 35(2):41–63, 1998.

Jumper Thurman, P., and Plested, B. Health needs of American Indian women. *Drug Addiction Research and the Health of Women*. (eds.) Wetherington, Cora Lee and Roman, Adele B. 553–562. Bethesda, MD: National Institute on Drug Abuse, 1998.

Kail, B.L., and Elberth, M. Moving the Latina substance abuser toward treatment: The role of gender and culture. *Journal of Ethnicity in Substance Abuse* 1(3):3–16, 2002.

Kalarchian, M.A., Marcus, M.D., Levine, M.D., Courcoulas, A.P., Pilkonis, P.A., Ringham, R.M., Soulakova, J.N., Weissfeld, L.A., and Rofey, D.L. Psychiatric disorders among bariatric surgery candidates: Relationship to obesity and functional health status. *American Journal of Psychiatry* 164(2):328–334, 2007.

Kaltenbach, K. The effects of maternal cocaine abuse on mothers and newborns. *Current Psychiatry Reports* 2(6):514–518, 2000.

Kaltenbach, K., Berghella, V., and Finnegan, L. Opioid dependence during pregnancy: Effects and management. *Obstetrics and Gynecology* 25(1):139–151, 1998.

Kaltenbach, K.A. Effects of in-utero opiate exposure: New paradigms for old questions. *Drug and Alcohol Dependence* 36(2):83–87, 1994.

Kaltenbach, K.A. Exposure to opiates: Behavioral outcomes in preschool and school-age children. In: Wetherington, C.L., Smeriglio, V.L., and Finnegan, L.P., eds. *Behavioral Studies of Drug-Exposed Offspring: Methodological Issues in Human and Animal Research*. NIDA Research Monograph 164. NIH Publication No. 96-4105. Rockville, MD: National Institute on Drug Abuse, 1996. pp. 230–241.

Kamimori, G.H., Sirisuth, N., Greenblatt, D.J., and Eddington, N.D. The influence of the menstrual cycle on triazolam and indocyanine green pharmacokinetics. *Journal of Clinical Pharmacology* 40(7):739–744, 2000.

Karberg, J.C., and James, D.J. Substance Dependence, Abuse, and Treatment of Jail Inmates, 2002. *Bureau of Justice Statistics: Special Report* JulyNCJ209588 Washington, DC: U. S. Department of Justice, 2005.

Karenga, M. *Kwanzaa; A Celebration of Family, Community, and Culture*. Los Angeles: University of Sankore Press, 1998.

Kaskutas, L.A., Zhang, L., French, M.T., and Witbrodt, J. Women's programs versus mixed-gender day treatment: Results from a randomized study. *Addiction* 100(1):60–69, 2005.

Kasl, C.D. *Many Roads, One Journey: Moving Beyond the Twelve Steps.* New York: Harper Perennial, 1992.

Katz, E.C., Chutuape, M.A., Jones, H., Jasinski, D., Fingerhood, M., and Stitzer, M. Abstinence incentive effects in a short-term outpatient detoxification program. *Experimental and Clinical Psychopharmacology* 12(4):262-268, 2004.

Kauffman, E., Dore, M.M., and Nelson-Zlupko, L. The role of women's therapy groups in the treatment of chemical dependence. *American Journal of Orthopsychiatry* 65(3):355–363, 1995.

Kayemba-Kay's, S., and Laclyde, J.P. Buprenorphine withdrawal syndrome in newborns: a report of 13 cases. *Addiction* 98(11):1599–1604, 2003.

Kaysen, D., Dillworth, T.M., Simpson, T., Waldrop, A., Larimer, M.E., and Resick, P.A. Domestic violence and alcohol use: Trauma-related symptoms and motives for drinking. *Addictive Behaviors* 32(6):1272-1283, 2007.

Keefe, S.E., and Padilla, A.M. *Chicano Ethnicity.* Albuquerque, NM: University of New Mexico Press, 1987.

Kelly, B.C., and Parsons, J.T. Prescription drug misuse among club drug-using young adults. *American Journal of Drug and Alcohol Abuse* 33(6):875–884, 2007.

Kelly, P.J., Blacksin, B., and Mason, E. Factors affecting substance abuse treatment completion for women. *Issues in Mental Health Nursing* 22(3):287–304, 2001a.

Kelly, R., Zatzick, D., and Anders, T. The detection and treatment of psychiatric disorders and substance use among pregnant women cared for in obstetrics. *American Journal of Psychiatry* 158(2):213–219, 2001b.

Kelly, S. Cognitive–behavioral therapy with African Americans. In: Hays, P.A., and Iwamasa, G.Y., eds. *Culturally Responsive Cognitive–Behavioral Therapy: Assessment, Practice, and Supervision.* Washington, DC: American Psychological Association, 2006. pp. 97–116.

Kendler, K.S., and Prescott, C.A. Cannabis use, abuse, and dependence in a population-based sample of female twins. *American Journal of Psychiatry* 155(8):1016–1022, 1998.

Kendler, K.S., Bulik, C.M., Silberg, J., Hettema, J.M., Myers, J., and Prescott, C.A. Childhood sexual abuse and adult psychiatric and substance use disorders in women: An epidemiological and co twin control analysis. *Archives of General Psychiatry* 57(10):953–959, 2000.

Kendler, K.S., Gardner, C.O., and Prescott, C.A. Religion, psychopathology, and substance use and abuse; A multimeasure, genetic-epidemiologic study. *American Journal of Psychiatry* 154(3):322–329, 1997.

Kendler, K.S., Heath, A.C., Neale, M.C., Kessler, R.C., and Eaves, L.J. A population-based twin study of alcoholism in women. *JAMA* 268(14):1877–1882, 1992.

Kendler, K.S., Liu, X.Q., Gardner, C.O., McCullough, M.E., Larson, D., and Prescott, C.A. Dimensions of religiosity and their relationship to lifetime psychiatric and substance use disorders. *American Journal of Psychiatry* 160(3):496-503, 2003.

Kendler, K.S., Thornton, L.M., and Prescott, C.A. Gender differences in the rates of exposure to stressful life events and sensitivity to their depressogenic effects. *American Journal of Psychiatry* 158(4):587–593, 2001.

Kennedy, C., Finkelstein, N., Hutchins, E., and Mahoney, J. Improving screening for alcohol use during pregnancy: the Massachusetts ASAP program. *Maternal & Child Health Journal* 8(3):137–147, 2004.

Kesmodel, U., Wisborg, K., Olsen, S.F., Henriksen, T.B., and Secher, N.J. Moderate alcohol intake during pregnancy and the risk of stillbirth and death in the first year of life. *American Journal of Epidemiology* 155(4):305–312, 2002.

Kessler, R.C., Borges, G., and Walters, E.E. Prevalence of and risk factors for lifetime suicide attempts in the National Comorbidity Survey. *Archives of General Psychiatry* 56(7):617–626, 1999.

Kessler, R.C., Crum, R.M., Warner, L.A., Nelson, C.B., Schulenberg, J., and Anthony, J.C. Lifetime co-occurrence of DSM-III-R alcohol abuse and dependence with other psychiatric disorders in the National Comorbidity Survey. *Archives of General Psychiatry* 54(4):313–321, 1997a.

Kessler, R.C., McGonagle, K.A., Zhao, S., Nelson, C.B., Hughes, M., Eshleman, S., Wittchen, H.U., and Kendler, K.S. Lifetime and 12-month prevalence of DSM-III-R psychiatric disorders in the United States. *Archives of General Psychiatry* 51(1):8–19, 1994.

Kessler, R.C., Sonnega, A., Bromet, E., Hughes, M., and Nelson, C.B. Posttraumatic stress disorder in the National Comorbidity Survey. *Archives of General Psychiatry* 52(12):1048–1060, 1995.

Kessler, R.C., Zhao, S., Blazer, D.G., and Swartz, M. Prevalence, correlates, and course of minor depression and major depression in the national comorbidity survey. *Journal of Affective Disorders* 45(1-2):19–30, 1997b.

Key, J., Hodgson, S., Omar, R.Z., Jensen, T.K., Thompson, S.G., Boobis, A.R., Davies, D.S., and Elliott, P. Meta-analysis of studies of alcohol and breast cancer with consideration of the methodological issues. *Cancer Causes and Control* 17(6):759–770, 2006.

Killeen, T., Hien, D., Campbell, A., Brown, C., Hansen, C., Jiang, H., Kristman-Valente, A., Neuenfeldt, C., Rocz-de la, L.N., Sampson, R., Suarez-Morales, L., Wells, E., Brigham, G., and Nunes, E. Adverse events in an integrated trauma-focused intervention for women in community substance abuse treatment. *Journal of Substance Abuse Treatment*, 2008.

Kilpatrick, D.G., Acierno, R., Resnick, H.S., Saunders, B.E., and Best, C.L. A 2-year longitudinal analysis of the relationships between violent assault and substance use in women. *Journal of Consulting and Clinical Psychology* 65(5):834–847, 1997.

Kitano, K.J., and Louie, L.J. Asian and Pacific Islander women and addiction. In: Straussner, S.L.A., and Brown, S., eds. *The Handbook Of Addiction Treatment For Women: Theory And Practice*. San Francisco: Jossey-Bass, 2002. pp. 348–373.

Klein, H., Elifson, K.W., and Sterk, C.E. Perceived temptation to use drugs and actual drug use among women. *Journal of Drug Issues* 33(1):161–192, 2003.

Kleiner, K.D., Gold, M.S., Frost-Pineda, K., Lenz-Brunsman, B., Perri, M.G., and Jacobs, W.S. Body Mass Index and Alcohol Use. *Journal of Addictive Diseases* 23(3):105–118, 2004.

Klitzner, M., Fisher, D., Stewart, K., and Gilbert, S. *Substance Abuse: Early Intervention for Adolescents*. Princeton, NJ: The Robert Wood Johnson Foundation, 1992.

Knight, D.K., and Simpson, D.D. Influences of family and friends on client progress during drug abuse treatment. *Journal of Substance Abuse* 8(4):417–429, 1996.

Knight, D.K., Logan, S., and Simpson, D.D. Predictors of program completion for women in residential substance abuse treatment. *American Journal of Drug and Alcohol Abuse* 27(1):1–18, 2001a.

Knight, D.K., Wallace, G.L., Joe, G.W., and Logan, S.M. Change in psychosocial functioning and social relations among women in residential substance abuse treatment. *Journal of Substance Abuse* 13(4):533–547, 2001*b*.

Knight, K. TCU Drug Screen II. Fort Worth, TX: Texas Christian University, Institute of Behavioral Research, 2002.

Knight, K., Simpson, D.D., and Hiller, M.L. Screening and referral for substance abuse treatment in the criminal justice system. In: Leukefeld, C.G., Tims, F.M., and Farabee, D., eds. *Treatment of Drug Offenders: Policies and Issues*. New York: Springer Publishing Company, 2002. pp. 259–272.

Koegel, P., Sullivan, G., Burnam, A., Morton, S.C., and Wenzel, S. Utilization of mental health and substance abuse services among homeless adults in Los Angeles. *Medical Care* 37(3):306–317, 1999.

Koh, A.S. Use of preventive health behaviors by lesbian, bisexual, and heterosexual women: Questionnaire survey. *Western Journal of Medicine* 172(6):379–384, 2000.

Kohn, L.P., Oden, T., Munoz, R.F., Robinson, A., and Leavitt, D. Adapted cognitive behavioral group therapy for depressed low-income African American women. *Community Mental Health Journal* 38(6):497–504, 2002.

Kornstein, S.G., Schatzberg, A.F., Thase, M.E., Yonkers, K.A., McCullough, J.P., Keitner, G.I., Gelenberg, A.J., Ryan, C.E., Hess, A.L., Harrison, W., Davis, S.M., and Keller, M.B. Gender differences in chronic major and double depression. *Journal of Affective Disorders* 60(1):1–11, 2000.

Kovalesky, A. Factors affecting mother–child visiting identified by women with histories of substance abuse and child custody loss. *Child Welfare* 80(6):749–768, 2001.

Kreek, M.J. Opiate-ethanol interactions: Implications for the biological basis and treatment of combined addictive diseases. In: Harris, L.S., ed. *Problems of Drug Dependence, 1987: Proceedings of the 49th Annual Scientific Meeting, the Committee on Problems of Drug Dependence, Inc.* NIDA Research Monograph Series 81. Rockville, MD: National Institute on Drug Abuse, 1988. pp. 428–439.

Krieger, N. Embodying inequality: A review of concepts, measures, and methods for studying health consequences of discrimination. *International Journal of Health Services* 29(2):295–352, 1999.

Kuba, S.A., and Hanchey, S.G. Reclaiming women's bodies: A feminist perspective on eating disorders. In: Van Den Bergh, N., ed. *Feminist Perspectives on Addictions*. New York: Springer Publishing, 1991. pp. 125–137.

Kuehn, B.M. Despite benefit, physicians slow to offer brief advice on harmful alcohol use. *JAMA* 299(7):751–753, 2008.

Kumar, C., McIvor, R.J., Davies, T., Brown, N., Papadopoulos, A., Wieck, A., Checkley, S.A., Campbell, I.C., and Marks, M.N. Estrogen administration does not reduce the rate of recurrence of affective psychosis after childbirth. *Journal of Clinical Psychiatry* 64(2):112–118, 2003.

Kurdek, L.A., and Schmitt, J.P. Relationship quality of partners in heterosexual married, heterosexual cohabiting, and gay and lesbian relationships. *Journal of Personality and Social Psychology* 51(4):711–720, 1986.

Kuyken, W., Dalgleish, T., and Holden, E.R. Advances in cognitive–behavioural therapy for unipolar depression. *The Canadian Journal of Psychiatry / La Revue Canadienne De Psychiatrie* 52(1):5–13, 2007.

LaFromboise, T.D., Trimble, J.E., and Mohatt, G.V. Counseling intervention and American Indian tradition: An integrative approach. In: Atkinson, D.R., and Morten, G., eds. *Counseling American minorities.* 5th ed. New York: McGraw-Hill, 1998. pp. 159–182.

Lai, S., Lai, H., Page, J.B., and McCoy, C.B. The association between cigarette smoking and drug abuse in the United States. *Journal of Addictive Diseases* 19(4):11–24, 2000.

Lando, H.A., Pirie, P.L., Hellerstedt, W.L., and McGovern, P.G. Survey of smoking patterns, attitudes, and interest in quitting. *American Journal of Preventive Medicine* 7(1):18–23, 1991.

Larson, M.J., Miller, L., Becker, M., Richardson, E., Kammerer, N., Thom, J., Gampel, J., and Savage, A. Physical health burdens of women with trauma histories and co-occurring substance abuse and mental disorders. *Journal of Behavior Health Services & Research* 32(2):128–140, 2005.

Larsson, S.C., Giovannucci, E., and Wolk, A. Alcoholic beverage consumption and gastric cancer risk: A prospective population-based study in women. *International Journal of Cancer* 120(2):373–377, 2007.

Laudet, A., Magura, S., Furst, R.T., Kumar, N., and Whitney, S. Male partners of substance-abusing women in treatment: An exploratory study. *American Journal of Drug and Alcohol Abuse* 25(4):607–627, 1999.

Laumann, E.O., Gagnon, J.H., Michael, R.T., and Michaels, S. *The social organization of sexuality: Sexual practices in the United States.* Chicago: University of Chicago Press, 1994.

Leech, S.L., Richardson, G.A., Goldschmidt, L., and Day, N.L. Prenatal substance exposure: Effects on attention and impulsivity of 6-year-olds. *Neurotoxicology and Teratology* 21(2):109–118, 1999.

Legal Action Center. *Steps to Success: Helping Women with Alcohol and Drug Problems Move from Welfare to Work.* Washington, DC: Legal Action Center, 1999.

Lehmann, E.R., Kass, P.H., Drake, C.M., and Nichols, S.B. Risk factors for first-time homelessness in low-income women. *American Journal of Orthopsychiatry* 77(1):20–28, 2007.

Leigh, W.A. Women of color health data book: Adolescents to seniors. (3rd): Bethesda, MD: Office of Research on Women's Health, Office of the Director, National Institutes of Health 2006.

Lenz, S.K., Goldberg, M.S., Labreche, F., Parent, M.E., and Valois, M.F. Association between alcohol consumption and postmenopausal breast cancer: Results of a case-control study in Montreal, Quebec, Canada. *Cancer Causes and Control* 13(8):701–710, 2002.

Leong, F.T., and Lee, S.H. A cultural accommodation model for cross-cultural psychotherapy: Illustrated with the case of Asian Americans. *Psychotherapy: Theory, Research, Practice, Training* 43(4):410-423, 2006.

Leong, F.T.L. Cultural accommodation as method and metaphor. *American Psychologist* 62(8):916-927, 2007.

Leong, F.T.L., Leach, M.M., Yeh, C., and Chou, E. Suicide among Asian Americans: What do we know? What do we need to know? *Death Studies* 31(5):417-434, 2007.

Leong, P. Religion, flesh, and blood: Re-creating religious culture in the context of HIV/AIDS. *Sociology of Religion: A Quarterly Review* 67(3): 2006.

Leserman, J. Sexual Abuse History: Prevalence, Health Effects, Mediators, and Psychological Treatment. *Psychosomatic Medicine* 67(6):906–915, 2005.

Lessler, J.T., and O'Reilly, J.M. Mode of interview and reporting of sensitive issues: Design and implementation of audio computer-assisted self-interviewing. In: Harrison, L., and Hughes, A., eds. *The Validity of Self-Reported Drug Use: Improving the Accuracy of Survey Estimates*. NIDA Research Monograph 167. Rockville, MD: National Institute on Drug Abuse, 1997. pp. 366–382.

Leukefeld, C., Godlaski, T., Clark, J., Brown, C., and Hays, L. *Behavioral Therapy for Rural Substance Abusers: A Treatment Intervention for Substance Abusers*. Lexington, KY: University Press of Kentucky, 2000.

Levin, R., McKean, L., and Raphael, J. Pathways to and from homelessness: Women and children in Chicago shelters. Chicago: Center for Impact Research 2004.

Levine, M.D., and Marcus, M.D. Do changes in mood and concerns about weight relate to smoking relapse in the postpartum period? *Archives of Women's Mental Health* 7(3):155–166, 2004.

Lewis, L.M. Culturally appropriate substance abuse treatment for parenting African American women. *Issues in Mental Health Nursing* 25(5):451–472, 2004*a*.

Lewis, M.W., Misra, S., Johnson, H.L., and Rosen, T.S. Neurological and developmental outcomes of prenatally cocaine-exposed offspring from 12 to 36 months. *American Journal of Drug & Alcohol Abuse* 30(2):299–320, 2004*b*.

Lewis, R.A., Haller, D.L., Branch, D., and Ingersoll, K.S. Retention issues involving drug-abusing women in treatment research. In: Rahdert, E.R., ed. *Treatment for Drug-Exposed Women and Their Children: Advances in Research Methodology*. NIDA Research Monograph 166. NIH Publication No. 96-3632. Rockville, MD: National Institute on Drug Abuse, 1996. pp. 110–122.

Lex, B. Gender differences and substance abuse. *Advances in Substance Abuse* 4:225–296, 1991.

Lex, B.W. Alcohol and other psychoactive substance dependence in women and men. In: Seeman, M.V., ed. *Gender and Psychopathology*. Washington, DC: American Psychiatric Press, 1995. pp. 311–358.

Lex, B.W., Mendelson, J.H., Bavli, S., Harvey, K., and Mello, N.K. Effects of acute marijuana smoking on pulse rate and mood states in women. *Psychopharmacology (Berl)* 84(2):178–187, 1984.

Li, C.I., Malone, K.E., Porter, P.L., Weiss, N.S., Tang, M.T., and Daling, J.R. The relationship between alcohol use and risk of breast cancer by histology and hormone receptor status among women 65–79 years of age. *Cancer Epidemiology Biomarkers Prevention* 12(10):1061–1066, 2003.

Li, L., and Ford, J.A. Illicit drug use by women with disabilities. *American Journal of Drug and Alcohol Abuse* 24(3):405–418, 1998.

Lieber, C. S. (2000). Ethnic and gender differences in ethanol metabolism. *Alcoholism: Clinical & Experimental Research* 24, 417-418.

Liechti, M.E., Gamma, A., and Vollenweider, F.X. Gender differences in the subjective effects of MDMA. *Psychopharmacology* 154(2):161–168, 2001.

Liepman, M., Goldman, R., Monroe, A., Green, K., Sattler, A., Broadhurst, J., and Gomberg, E. Substance abuse by special populations of women. In: Gomberg, E., and Nirenberg, T., eds. *Women and Substance Abuse*. Norwood, NJ: Ablex Press, 1993.

Lifschitz, M.H., Wilson, G.S., Smith, E.O., and Desmond, M.M. Factors affecting head growth and intellectual function in children of drug addicts. *Pediatrics* 75(2):269–274, 1985.

Lincoln, A.K., Liebschutz, J.M., Chernoff, M., Nguyen, D., and Amaro, H. Brief screening for co-occurring disorders among women entering substance abuse treatment. *Substance Abuse Treatment, Prevention and Policy* 1:26, 2006.

Longshore, D., Grills, C., Annon, K., and Grady, R. Promoting recovery from drug abuse: An Afrocentric intervention. *Journal of Black Studies* 28(3):319–332, 1998.

Longshore, D., Hsieh, S.C., Anglin, M.D., and Annon, T.A. Ethnic patterns in drug abuse treatment utilization. *Journal of Mental Health Administration* 19(3):268–277, 1992.

Lopez, F. *Confidentiality of Patient Records for Alcohol and Other Drug Treatment.* Technical Assistance Publication Series 13. HHS Publication No. (SMA) 99-3321. Rockville, MD: Center for Substance Abuse Treatment, 1994.

Loring, M., and Powell, B. Gender, race, and DSM-III: A study of the objectivity of psychiatric diagnostic behavior. *Journal of Health and Social Behavior* 29(1):1–22, 1988.

Louisiana Department of Health and Hospitals. News Release: New Screening Project Assists Pregnant Women Seeking to Quit Using Alcohol, Tobacco, Other Drugs. Baton Rouge, LA, 2007.

Lucas, G.M., Griswold, M., Gebo, K.A., Keruly, J., Chaisson, R.E., and Moore, R.D. Illicit drug use and HIV-1 disease progression: a longitudinal study in the era of highly active antiretroviral therapy. *American Journal of Epidemiology* 163(5):412–420, 2006.

Lundgren, L.M., Amaro, H., and Ben-Ami, L. Factors associated with drug treatment entry patterns among hispanic women injection drug users seeking treatment. *Journal of Social Work Practice in the Addictions* 5(1-2):157–174, 2005.

Lundgren, L.M., Schilling, R.F., Fitzgerald, T., Davis, K., and Amodeo, M. Parental Status of Women Injection Drug Users and Entry to Methadone Maintenance. *Substance Use & Misuse* 38(8):1109–1131, 2003.

Luty, S.E., Carter, J.D., McKenzie, J.M., Rae, A.M., Frampton, C.M.A., Mulder, R.T., and Joyce, P.R. Randomised controlled trial of interpersonal psychotherapy and cognitive–behavioural therapy for depression. *British Journal of Psychiatry* 190:496–502, 2007.

Lynch, W.J., Roth, M.E., and Carroll, M.E. Biological basis of sex differences in drug abuse: preclinical and clinical studies. *Psychopharmacology (Berl)* 164(2):121–137, 2002.

Maguire, K., and Pastore, A.L. Sourcebook of Criminal Justice Statistics [Online]. Albany, NY: University at Albany 2001.

Maharaj, R.G., Rampersad, J., Henry, J., Khan, K.V., Koonj-Beharry, B., Mohammed, J., Rajhbeharrysingh, U., Ramkissoon, F., Sriranganathan, M., Brathwaite, B., and Barclay, S. Critical incidents contributing to the initiation of substance use and abuse among women attending drug rehabilitation centres in Trinidad and Tobago. *West Indian Medical Journal* 54(1):51–58, 2005.

Malcolm, B.P., Hesselbrock, M.N., and Segal, B. Multiple substance dependence and course of alcoholism among Alaska native men and women. *Substance Use & Misuse* 41(5):729–741, 2006.

Mangrum, L.F., Spence, R.T., and Steinley-Bumgarner, M.D. Gender differences in substance-abuse treatment clients with co-occurring psychiatric and substance-use disorders. *Brief Treatment and Crisis Intervention* 6(3):255–267, 2006.

Mann, K., Ackermann, K., Croissant, B., Mundle, G., Nakovics, H., and Diehl, A. Neuroimaging of gender differences in alcohol dependence: Are women more vulnerable? *Alcoholism: Clinical and Experimental Research* 29(5):896–901, 2005.

Marcus, R.N., and Katz, J.L. Inpatient care of the substance-abusing patient with a concomitant eating disorder. *Hospital and Community Psychiatry* 41(1):59–63, 1990.

Marin, G., and Marin, B.V. *Research with Hispanic Populations.* Newbury Park, CA: Sage Publications, 1991.

Marin, G., Otero-Sabogal, R., and Perez-Stable, E. MARIN Short Scale. *Hispanic Journal of Behavioral Sciences* 9:183–205, 1987.

Markides, K.S., Krause, N., and Mendes de Leon, C.F. Acculturation and alcohol consumption among Mexican Americans: A three-generation study. *American Journal of Public Health* 78(9):1178–1181, 1988.

Markides, K.S., Ray, L.A., Stroup-Benham, C.A., and Trevino, F.M. Acculturation and alcohol consumption in the Mexican American population of the southwestern United States: Findings from HHANES 1982–84. *American Journal of Public Health* 80(Supplement):42–46, 1990.

Markoff, L.S., Finkelstein, N., Kammerer, N., Kreiner, P.e., and Prost, C.A. Relational systems change: Implementaing a model of change in integrating services for women with substance abuse and mental health disorders and histories of trauma. *Journal of Behavior Health Services & Research* 32(2):227–240, 2005a.

Markoff, L.S., Reed, B.G., Fallot, R.D., Elliott, D.E., and Bjelajac, P. Implementing trauma-informed alcohol and other drug and mental health services for women: lessons learned in a multisite demonstration project. *American Journal of Orthopsychiatry* 75(4):525–539, 2005b.

Markowitz, J.C. Interpersonal psychotherapy. In: Hales, R.E., and Yudofsky, S.C., eds. *The American Psychiatric Publishing Textbook of Clinical Psychiatry (4th ed.).* 1-58562-032-7 (hardcover). American Psychiatric Publishing, 2003. pp. 1207–1223.

Marks, M.N., Wieck, A., Checkley, S.A., and Kumar, R. Life stress and post-partum psychosis: A preliminary report. *British Journal of Psychiatry Supplement* May (10):45–49, 1991.

Marlatt, G.A., Baer, J.S., Donovan, D.M., and Kivlahan, D.R. Addictive behaviors: Etiology and treatment. *Annual Review of Psychology* 39:223–252, 1988.

Marr, D.D., and Wenner, A. Gender specific treatment for chemically dependent women: A rationale for inclusion of vocational services. *Alcoholism Treatment Quarterly* 14(1):21–31, 1996.

Martin, V., Cayla, J.A., Bolea, A., and Castilla, J. Mycobacterium tuberculosis and human immunodeficiency virus co-infection in intravenous drug users on admission to prison. *International Journal of Tuberculosis and Lung Disease* 4(1):41–46, 2000.

Matthews, A.K., and Hughes, T.L. Mental health service use by African American women: Exploration of subpopulation differences. *Cultural Diversity and Ethnic Minority Psychology* 7(1):75–87, 2001.

Matthews, D.A., McCullough, M.E., Larson, D.B., Koenig, H.G., Swyers, J.P., and Milano, M.G. Religious Commitment and Health Status: A Review of the Research and Implications for Family Medicine. *Archives of Family Medicine* 7(2):118–124, 1998.

Mayes, L.C., Grillon, C., Granger, R., and Schottenfeld, R. Regulation of arousal and attention in preschool children exposed to cocaine prenatally. *Annals of the New York Academy of Sciences* 846:126–143, 1998.

Mayfield, D., McLeod, G., and Hall, P. The CAGE questionnaire: Validation of a new alcoholism screening instrument. *American Journal of Psychiatry* 131(10):1121–1123, 1974.

Mays, V.M., Beckman, L.J., Oranchak, E., and Harper, B. Perceived social support for help-seeking behaviors of Black heterosexual and homosexually active women alcoholics. *Psychology of Addictive Behaviors* 8(4):235–242, 1994.

Mays, V.M., Cochran, S.D., and Barnes, N.W. Race, race-based discrimination, and health outcomes among African Americans. *Annual Review of Psychology* 58(1):201–225, 2007.

Mazure, C.M., Keita, G.P., and Blehar, M.C. Summit on Women and Depression: Proceedings and Recommendations. Washington, DC: American Psychological Association 2002.

McCance-Katz, E.F., Hart, C.L., Boyarsky, B., Kosten, T., and Jatlow, P. Gender effects following repeated administration of cocaine and alcohol in humans. *Substance Use & Misuse* 40(4):511–528, 2005.

McCoy, C.B., Comerford, M., and Metsch, L.R. Employment among chronic drug users at baseline and 6-month follow-up. *Substance Use and Misuse* 42(7):1055–1067, 2007.

McCrady, B.S., and Raytek, H.S. Women and substance abuse: Treatment modalities and outcomes. In: Gomberg, E.S., and Nirenberg, T.D., eds. *Women and Substance Abuse*. Stamford, CT: Ablex Publishing, 1993. pp. 314–338.

McCusker, J., Bigelow, C., Servigon, C., and Zorn, M. Test–retest reliability of the Addiction Severity Index composite scores among clients in residential treatment. *American Journal on Addictions* 3:254–262, 1994.

McElhatton, P.R. Heart and circulatory system drugs. In: Schaefer, C.H., ed. *Drugs During Pregnancy and Lactation: Handbook of Prescription Drugs and Comparative Risk Assessment: With Updated Information on Recreational Drugs*. Amsterdam: Elsevier, 2001. pp. 116–131.

McGee, G., Johnson, L., and Bell, P. *Black, Beautiful, and Recovering*. Center City, MN: Hazelden, 1985.

McGoldrick, M., Giordano, J., and Pearce, J.K. Families of African origin: An overview. In: *Ethnicity and Family Therapy*. 2nd ed. New York: Guilford Press, 1996. pp. 57–84.

McKay, J.R., Rutherford, M.J., Cacciola, J.S., Kabasakalian-McKay, R., and Alterman, A.I. Gender differences in the relapse experiences of cocaine patients. *Journal of Nervous and Mental Disease* 184(10):616–622, 1996.

McKirnan, D.J., and Peterson, P.L. Psychosocial and cultural factors in alcohol and drug abuse: An analysis of a homosexual community. *Addictive Behaviors* 14(5):555–563, 1989.

McKirnan, D.J., and Peterson, P.L. Gay and lesbian alcohol use: Epidemiological and psychosocial perspectives. In: Kelly, J., ed. *The Research Symposium on Alcohol and Other Drug Problem Prevention Among Lesbians and Gay Men*. Sacramento, CA: EMT Group, Inc., 1992. pp. 61-84.

McLellan, A.T., Grissom, G.R., Zanis, D., Randall, M., Brill, P., and O'Brien, C.P. Problem-service 'matching' in addiction treatment: A prospective study in 4 programs. *Archives of General Psychiatry* 54(8):730–735, 1997.

McLellan, A.T., Gutman, M., Lynch, K., McKay, J.R., Ketterlinus, R., Morgenstern, J., and Woolis, D. One-year outcomes from the CASAWORKS for families intervention for substance-abusing women on welfare. *Evaluation Review* 27(6):656–680, 2003.

McLellan, A.T., Luborsky, L., Cacciola, J., Griffith, J., Evans, F., Barr, H.L., and O'Brien, C.P. New data from the Addiction Severity Index: Reliability and validity in three centers. *Journal of Nervous and Mental Disease* 173(7):412–423, 1985.

McLellan, A.T., Luborsky, L., Woody, G.E., and O'Brien, C.P. An improved diagnostic evaluation instrument for substance abuse patients: The Addiction Severity Index. *Journal of Nervous and Mental Disease* 168(1):26–33, 1980.

McMahon, T.J., and Luthar, S.S. Bridging the gap for children as their parents enter substance abuse treatment. In: Hampton, R.L., Senatore, V., and Gullotta, T.P., eds. *Substance Abuse, Family Violence, and Child Welfare: Bridging Perspectives.* Issues in children's and families' lives, Vol. 10. 0-7619-1457-9 (hardcover); 0-7619-1458-7 (paperback). Sage Publications, 1998. pp. 143-187.

McMurtrie, C., Rosenberg, K.D., Kerker, B.D., Kan, J., and Graham, E.H. A unique drug treatment program for pregnant and post-partum substance-using women in New York City: Results of a pilot project, 1990–1995. *American Journal of Drug and Alcohol Abuse* 25(4):701–713, 1999.

McNeece, C.A., and DiNitto, D.M. *Chemical Dependency: A Systems Approach.* Englewood Cliffs, N.J: Prentice Hall, 1994.

Meara, E. Welfare reform, employment, and drug and alcohol use among low-income women. *Harvard Review of Psychiatry* 14(4):223–232, 2006.

Medina, C. Toward an understanding of Puerto Rican ethnicity and substance abuse. In: Straussner, S.L.A., ed. *Ethnocultural Factors in Substance Abuse Treatment.* New York: Guilford Press, 2001. pp. 137–163.

Mejta, C.L., and Lavin, R. Facilitating healthy parenting among mothers with substance abuse or dependence problems: Some considerations. *Alcoholism Treatment Quarterly* 14(1):33–46, 1996.

Melchior, L.A., Huba, G.J., Brown, V.B., and Slaughter, R. Evaluation of the effects of outreach to women with multiple vulnerabilities on entry into substance abuse treatment. *Evaluation & Program Planning* 22(3):269–277, 1999.

Mello, N.K., Mendelson, J.H., and Teoh, S.K. Overview of the effects of alcohol on the neuroendocrine function in women. In: Zakhari, S., ed. *Alcohol and the Endocrine System.* NIAAA Research Monograph No. 23. Bethesda, MD: National Institute on Alcohol Abuse and Alcoholism, 1993. pp. 139–169.

Melnick, S.M., and Bassuk, E.L. Identifying and responding to violence among poor and homeless women. Nashville, TN: National Health Care for the Homeless Council 2000.

Menninger, J.A. Assessment and treatment of alcoholism and substance-related disorders in the elderly. *Bulletin of the Menninger Clinic* 66(2):166–183, 2002.

Merikangas, K.R., and Stevens, D.E. Substance abuse among women: Familial factors and comorbidity. In: Wetherington, C.L., and Roman, A.B., eds. *Drug Addiction Research and the Health of Women.* NIH Publication No. 98-4290. Rockville, MD: National Institute on Drug Abuse, 1998. pp. 245–269.

Messinger, D.S., Bauer, C.R., Das, A., Seifer, R., Lester, B.M., LaGasse, L.L., Wright, L.L., Shankaran, S., Bada, H.S., Smeriglio, V.L., Langer, J.C., Beeghly, M., and Poole, W.K. The maternal lifestyle study: Cognitive, motor, and behavioral outcomes of cocaine-exposed and opiate-exposed infants through three years of age. *Pediatrics* 113(6):1677–1685, 2004.

Metsch, L.R., McCoy, C.B., Miller, M., McAnany, H., and Pereyra, M. Moving substance-abusing women from welfare to work. *Journal of Public Health Policy* 20(1):36–55, 1999.

Metsch, L.R., Pereyra, M., Miles, C.C., and McCoy, C.B. Welfare and work outcomes after substance abuse treatment. *Social Service Review*. 77(2):237–254, 2003.

Metsch, L.R., Rivers, J.E., Miller, M., Bohs, R., McCoy, C.B., Morrow, C.J., Bandstra, E.S., Jackson, V., and Gissen, M. Implementation of a family-centered treatment program for substance-abusing women and their children: Barriers and resolutions. *Journal of Psychoactive Drugs* 27(1):73–83, 1995.

Metsch, L.R., Wolfe, H.P., Fewell, R., McCoy, C.B., Elwood, W.N., Wohler-Torres, B., Petersen-Baston, P., and Haskins, H.V. Treating substance-using women and their children in public housing: Preliminary evaluation findings. *Child Welfare Journal* 80(2):199–220, 2001.

Michaels, S. The prevalence of homosexuality in the United States. In: Cabaj, R.P., and Stein, T.S., eds. *Textbook of Homosexuality and Mental Health*. Washington, DC: American Psychiatric Press, 1996. pp. 43–63.

Midanik, L.T., Zahnd, E.G., and Klein, D. Alcohol and drug CAGE screeners for pregnant, low-income women: The California perinatal needs assessment. *Alcoholism: Clinical and Experimental Research* 22(1):121–125, 1998.

Miller, B.A., Downs, W.R., and Testa, M. Interrelationships between victimization experiences and women's alcohol use. *Journal of Studies on Alcohol Supplement* 11(9):109–117, 1993.

Miller, D. *Women Who Hurt Themselves: A Book of Hope and Understanding*. New York: Basic Books, 1994.

Miller, D., and Guidry, L. *Addictions and Trauma Recovery: Healing the Body, Mind, and Spirit*. New York: W.W. Norton, 2001.

Miller, J.B. *Toward a New Psychology of Women*. Boston: Beacon Press, 1976.

Miller, J.B. *The Development of Women's Sense of Self*. Work in Progress No. 12. Wellesley, MA: Stone Center for Developmental Services and Studies, 1984.

Miller, S.D., Duncan, B.L., and Hubble, M.A. *Escape from Babel: Toward a Unifying Language for Psychotherapy Practice*. W W Norton & Co: New York, 1997.

Miller, W.R. Rediscovering fire: Small interventions, large effects. *Psychology of Addictive Behaviors* 14(1):6–18, 2000.

Miller, W.R., and Rollnick, S. *Motivational Interviewing: Preparing People to Change Addictive Behavior*. New York: Guilford Press, 1991.

Miller, W.R., and Rollnick, S. *Motivational Interviewing: Preparing People for Change*. 2nd ed. New York: Guilford Press, 2002.

Miller, W.R., Tonigan, J.S., and Longabaugh, R. *The Drinker Inventory of Consequences (DrInC): An Instrument For Assessing Adverse Consequences of Alcohol Abuse*. Project MATCH Monograph Series Vol. 4. Rockville, MD: National Institute on Alcohol Abuse and Alcoholism, 1995.

Minino, A.M., Arias, E., Kochanek, K.D., Murphy, S.L., and Smith, B.L. *Deaths: Final Data for 2000*. National Vital Statistics Reports: Vol. 50, no. 15. Hyattsville, MD: National Center for Health Statistics, 2002.

Mokuau, N. Health and well-being for Pacific Islanders: Status, barriers, and resolutions. In: Mokuau, N., Epstein, L.G., Pacheco, G., and Quinlan, J.W., eds. *Responding to Pacific Islanders: Culturally Competent Perspectives For Substance Abuse Prevention*. CSAP Cultural Competence Series 8. HHS Publication No. (SMA)98-3195. Rockville, MD: Center for Substance Abuse Prevention, 1998a. pp. 1–24.

Mokuau, N. Reality and vision: A cultural perspective in addressing alcohol and drug abuse among Pacific Islanders. In: Mokuau, N., Epstein, L.G., Pacheco, G., and Quinlan, J.W., eds. *Responding to Pacific Islanders: Culturally Competent Perspectives For Substance Abuse Prevention.* CSAP Cultural Competence Series 8. HHS Publication No. (SMA)98-3195. Rockville, MD: Center for Substance Abuse Prevention, 1998*b*. pp. 25–47.

Moncrieff, J., and Farmer, R. Sexual abuse and the subsequent development of alcohol problems. *Alcohol and Alcoholism* 33(6):592–601, 1998.

Mondanaro, J. Medical services for drug dependent women. In: Beschner, G.M., Reed, B.G., and Mondanaro, J., eds. *Treatment Services for Drug Dependent Women: Vol. 1.* HHS Publication No. (ADM) 81–1177. Rockville, MD: National Institute on Drug Abuse, 1981. pp. 208–257.

Moore, J., and Finkelstein, N. Parenting services for families affected by substance abuse. *Child Welfare* 80(2):221–238, 2001.

Moore, R.D., Bone, L.R., Geller, G., Mamon, J.A., Stokes, E.J., and Levine, D.M. Prevalence, detection, and treatment of alcoholism in hospitalized patients. *JAMA* 261(3):403–407, 1989.

Moos, R.H., Moos, B.S., and Timko, C. Gender, treatment and self-help in remission from alcohol use disorders. *Clinical Medicine & Research* 4(3):163–174, 2006.

Moos, R.H., Schutte, K., Brennan, P., and Moos, B.S. Ten-year patterns of alcohol consumption and drinking problems among older women and men. *Addiction* 99(7):829–838, 2004.

Mora, J. The treatment of alcohol dependency among Latinas: A feminist, cultural and community perspective. *Alcoholism Treatment Quarterly* 16(1-2):163–177, 1998.

Mora, J. Latinas in cultural transition: Addiction, treatment and recovery. In: Straussner, S.L.A., and Brown, S., eds. *The Handbook of Addiction Treatment for Women: Theory and Practice.* San Francisco: Jossey Bass, 2002. pp. 323–347.

Morgen, C.S., Bove, K.B., Larsen, K.S., Kjaer, S.K., and Gronbaek, M. Association Between Smoking and the Risk of Heavy Drinking Among Young Women: A Prospective Study. *Alcohol and Alcoholism*, 2008.

Morgenstern, J., Blanchard, K.A., McCrady, B.S., McVeigh, K.H., Morgan, T.J., and Pandina, R.J. Effectiveness of intensive case management for substance-dependent women receiving temporary assistance for needy families. *American Journal of Public Health* 96(11):2016–2023, 2006.

Morgenstern, J., McCrady, B.S., Blanchard, K.A., McVeigh, K.H., Riordan, A., and Irwin, T.W. Barriers to employability among substance dependent and nonsubstance-affected women on federal welfare: implications for program design. *Journal of Studies on Alcohol* 64(2):239–246, 2003.

Morrissey, J.P., Ellis, A.R., Gatz, M., Amaro, H., Reed, B.G., Savage, A., Finkelstein, N., Mazelis, R., Brown, V., Jackson, E.W., and Banks, S. Outcomes for women with co-occurring disorders and trauma: program and person-level effects. *Journal of Substance Abuse Treatment* 28(2):121–133, 2005*a*.

Morrissey, J.P., Jackson, E.W., Ellis, A.R., Amaro, H., Brown, V.B., and Najavits, L.M. Twelve-month outcomes of trauma-informed interventions for women with co-occurring disorders. *Psychiatric Services* 56(10):1213–1222, 2005*b*.

Morse, B., Gehshan, S., and Hutchins, E. *Screening for Substance Abuse During Pregnancy: Improving Care, Improving Health.* Arlington, VA: National Center for Education in Maternal and Child Health, 1997.

Moscato, B.S., Russell, M., Zielezny, M., Bromet, E., Egri, G., Mudar, P., and Marshall, J.R. Gender differences in the relation between depressive symptoms and alcohol problems: A longitudinal perspective. *American Journal of Epidemiology* 146(11):966–974, 1997.

Moses, D.J., Huntington, N., and D'Ambrosio, B. *Developing Integrated Services for Women with Co-Occurring Disorders and Trauma Histories: Lessons from the SAMHSA Women with Alcohol, Drug Abuse and Mental Health Disorders Who Have Histories of Violence Study.* Rockville, MD: Substance Abuse and Mental Health Services Administration, 2004.

Moses, D.J., Reed, B.G., Mazelis, R., and D'Ambrosio, B. *Creating Trauma Services for Women With Co-Occurring Disorders: Experiences from the SAMHSA Women with Alcohol, Drug Abuse and Mental Health Disorders Who Have Histories of Violence Study.* Women, Co-Occurring Disorders & Violence Study. Rockville, MD: Substance Abuse And Mental Health Services Administration, 2003.

Mrazek, P.B., Haggerty, R.J., Institute of Medicine, Committee on Prevention of Mental Disorders, United States, and Congress. *Reducing Risks For Mental Disorders: Frontiers For Preventive Intervention Research.* Washington, D.C: National Academy Press, 1994.

Mucha, L., Stephenson, J., Morandi, N., and Dirani, R. Meta-analysis of disease risk associated with smoking, by gender and intensity of smoking. *Gender Medicine* 3(4):279–291, 2006.

Mullen, P.D. How can more smoking suspension during pregnancy become lifelong abstinence? Lessons learned about predictors, interventions, and gaps in our accumulated knowledge. *Nicotine & Tobacco Research* 6(Suppl2):S217–S238, 2004.

Mumenthaler, M.S., Taylor, J.L., O'Hara, R., and Yesavage, J.A. Gender differences in moderate drinking effects. *Alcohol Research and Health* 23(1):55–64, 1999.

Mumola, C.J. Incarcerated Parents and Their Children. *Bureau of Justice Statistics Special Report* Washington, DC: Bureau of Justice Statistics, 2000.

Mumola, C.J., and Karberg, J.C. Drug use and dependence, State and Federal prisoners, 2004. *Bureau of Justice Statistics Special Report* Washington, DC: U.S. Department of Justice, 2007.

Musgrave, C.F., Allen, C.E., and Allen, G.J. Spirituality and health for women of color. *American Journal of Public Health* 92(4):557–560, 2002.

Najavits, L.M. Training clinicians in the Seeking Safety treatment protocol for posttraumatic stress disorder and substance abuse. *Alcoholism Treatment Quarterly* 18(3):83–98, 2000.

Najavits, L.M. *A woman's addiction workbook: Your guide to in-depth healing.* Oakland, CA: New Harbinger, 2002a.

Najavits, L.M. *Seeking safety: A treatment manual for PTSD and substance abuse.* New York: Guilford Press, 2002b.

Najavits, L.M. Treatment of posttraumatic stress disorder and substance abuse: clinical guidelines for implementing "Seeking Safety" therapy. *Alcoholism Treatment Quarterly* 22(1):43–62, 2004.

Najavits, L.M. Managing trauma reactions in intensive addiction treatment environments. *Journal of Chemical Dependency Treatment* 8:153–161, 2006.

Najavits, L.M. Seeking safety: An evidence-based model for substance abuse and trauma/PTSD. In: Witkiewitz, K.A., and Marlatt, G.A., eds. *Therapist's Guide to Evidence-Based Relapse Prevention*. Practical Resources for the Mental Health Professional. Boston, MA: Elsevier Academic Press, 2007. pp. 141–168.

Najavits, L.M., Gallop, R.J., and Weiss, R.D. Seeking safety therapy for adolescent girls with PTSD and substance use disorder: a randomized controlled trial. *Journal of Behavior Health Services Research* 33(4):453–463, 2006.

Najavits, L.M., Runkel, R., Neuner, C., Frank, A.F., Thase, M.E., Crits-Christoph, P., and Elaine, J. Rates and Symptoms of PTSD among cocaine-dependent patients. *Journal of Studies on Alcohol* 64(5):601–606, 2003.

Najavits, L.M., Schmitz, M., Gotthardt, S., and Weiss, R.D. Seeking safety plus exposure therapy: An outcome study on dual diagnosis men. *Journal of Psychoactive Drugs* 37(4):425–435, 2005.

Najavits, L.M., Weiss, R.D., and Liese, B. Group cognitive–behavioral therapy for women with PTSD and substance use disorder. *Journal of Substance Abuse Treatment* 13(1):13–22, 1996.

Najavits, L.M., Weiss, R.D., and Shaw, S.R. The link between substance abuse and posttraumatic stress disorder in women: A research review. *American Journal on Addictions* 6(4):273–283, 1997.

Najavits, L.M., Weiss, R.D., Shaw, S.R., and Muenz, L.R. "Seeking Safety": Outcome of a new cognitive–behavioral psychotherapy for women with posttraumatic stress disorder and substance dependence. *Journal of Traumatic Stress* 11(3):437–456, 1998.

Nanchahal, K., Ashton, W.D., and Wood, D.A. Alcohol consumption, metabolic cardiovascular risk factors and hypertension in women. *International Journal of Epidemiology* 29(1):57–64, 2000.

Nardi, D. Addiction recovery for low-income pregnant and parenting women: A process of becoming. *Archives of Psychiatric Nursing* 12(2):81–89, 1998.

National Alliance for Caregiving and AARP, Caregiving in the U.S. Bethesda, MD: National Alliance for Caregiving 2004.

National Association for Children of Alcoholics. Celebrating Families Model. 2007. Available on-line at: http://www.celebratingfamilies.net/CFmodel.htm

National Center on Addiction and Substance Abuse. Substance abuse and the American woman. New York: National Center on Addiction and Substance Abuse, 1996.

National Center on Addiction and Substance Abuse. *Depression, Substance Abuse and College Student Engagement: A Review of the Literature Report to the Charles Engelhard Foundation and the Bringing Theory to Practice Planning Group*. New York, NY: National Center on Addiction and Substance Abuse at Columbia University 2003.

National Coalition of Anti-Violence Programs. *Lesbian, Gay, Bisexual and Transgender Domestic Violence in the United States in 2006: A Report Of The National Coalition Of Anti-Violence Programs*. New York, NY: National Coalition of Anti-Violence Programs, 2007.

National Institute of Diabetes and Digestive and Kidney Diseases. *Binge Eating Disorders*. Bethesda, MD: National Institute of Diabetes and Digestive and Kidney Diseases, 2001.

National Institute of Mental Health. *Anxiety Disorders*. NIH Publication No. 06-3879 Bethesda, MD: National Institutes of Health, 2007.

National Institute on Drug Abuse. *Principles Of Drug Addiction Treatment: A Research-Based Guide*. NIH Publication No. 00-4180. Bethesda, MD: National Institutes of Health, 1999.

National Institute on Drug Abuse. Heroin: Abuse and Addiction. *National Institute on Drug Abuse Research Report Series* Rockville, MD: National Institute on Drug Abuse, 2000.

National Institute on Drug Abuse. Prescription drugs: Abuse and addiction. *National Institute on Drug Abuse Research Report Series* Rockville, MD: National Institute on Drug Abuse 2001.

National Institute on Drug Abuse. Behavioral problems related to maternal smoking during pregnancy manifest early in childhood. *NIDA Notes* 21(6):7–8, 2008.

National Institutes of Health - Office of Research on Women's Health. *Women of Color Health Data Book: Adolescents to Seniors*. Bethesda, MD: National Institutes of Health, Office of Research on Women's Health, 1999.

National Poverty Center. *Poverty in the United States: Frequently Asked Questions*. Ann Arbor, MI: University of Michigan 2006.

Neff, J.A., and Mantz, R.J. Marital status transition, alcohol consumption, and number of sex partners over time in a tri-ethnic sample. *Journal of Divorce and Remarriage* 29(1-2):19–42, 1998.

Nelson-Zlupko, L., Kauffman, E., and Dore, M.M. Gender differences in drug addiction and treatment: implications for social work intervention with substance-abusing women. *Soc Work* 40(1):45–54, 1995.

Nelson-Zlupko, L., Dore, M.M., Kauffman, E., and Kaltenbach, K. Women in recovery: Their perceptions of treatment effectiveness. *Journal of Substance Abuse Treatment* 13(1):51–59, 1996.

Neumarker, K.J. Mortality and sudden death in anorexia nervosa. *International Journal of Eating Disorders* 21(3):205–212, 1997.

Neuspiel, D.R. Racism and perinatal addiction. *Ethnicity and Disease* 6(1-2):47–55, 1996.

New York State Education Department -- Office of Bilingual Education. *Directory of Languages*. Albany, NY: New York State Education Department, Office of Bilingual Education, 1997.

Newmann, J.P., and Sallmann, J. Women, trauma histories, and co-occurring disorders: Assessing the scope of the problem. *Social Service Review* 78(3):446–499, 2004.

Niccols, A., and Sword, W. "New Choices" for substance-using mothers and their children: Preliminary evaluation. *Journal of Substance Use* 10(4):239–251, 2005.

Nicoloff, L.K., and Stiglitz, E.A. Lesbian alcoholism: Etiology, treatment, and recovery. In: Boston Lesbian Psychologies Collective, ed. *Lesbian psychologies: Explorations and challenges*. Urbana, IL: University of Illinois Press, 1987. pp. 283–293.

Nielsen Forman, D., Videbech, P., Hedegaard, M., Dalby, S.J., and Secher, N.J. Postpartum depression: Identification of women at risk. *BJOG: An International Journal of Obstetrics and Gynaecology* 107(10):1210–1217, 2000.

Nikolopoulou, G.B., Nowicki, M.J., Du, W., Homans, J., Stek, A., Kramer, F., and Kovacs, A. HCV viremia is associated with drug use in young HIV-1 and HCV coinfected pregnant and non-pregnant women. *Addiction* 100(5):626–635, 2005.

Nishimoto, R.H., and Roberts, A.C. Coercion and drug treatment for postpartum women. *American Journal of Drug Alcohol Abuse* 27(1):161–181, 2001.

Nishith, P., Resick, P.A., and Mueser, K.T. Sleep difficulties and alcohol use motives in female rape victims with posttraumatic stress disorder. *Journal of Traumatic Stress* 14(3):469–479, 2001.

Niv, N., and Hser, Y.I. Women-only and mixed-gender drug abuse treatment programs: service needs, utilization and outcomes. *Drug and Alcohol Dependence* 87(2-3):194–201, 2007.

Niv, N., Wong, E.C., and Hser, Y.I. Asian Americans in community-based substance abuse treatment: service needs, utilization, and outcomes. *Journal of Substance Abuse Treatment* 33(3):313–319, 2007.

Norris, J., and Hughes, T.L. Alcohol consumption and female sexuality: A review. In: Howard, J.M., Martin, S.E., Mail, P.D., Hilton, M.E., and Taylor, E.D., eds. *Women and Alcohol: Issues for Prevention Research.* NIAAA Research Monograph No. 32. Bethesda, MD: National Institute on Alcohol Abuse and Alcoholism, 1996. pp. 315–345.

North, C.S., Eyrich, K.M., Pollio, D.E., and Spitznagel, E.L. Are rates of psychiatric disorders in the homeless population changing? *American Journal of Public Health* 94(1):103–108, 2004a.

North, C.S., Eyrich, K.M., Pollio, D.E., Foster, D.A., Cottler, L.B., and Spitznagel, E.L. The Homeless Supplement to the Diagnostic Interview Schedule: test-retest analyses. *International Journal of Methods in Psychiatric Research* 13(3):184–191, 2004b.

Oates, M. Management of major mental illness in pregnancy and the puerperium. *Baillieres Best Practice and Research: Clinical Obstetrics and Gynaecology* 3(4):905–920, 1989.

Oetjen, H., and Rothblum, E.D. When lesbians aren't gay: Factors affecting depression among lesbians. *Journal of Homosexuality* 39(1):49–73, 2000.

Oetzel, J., Duran, B., Jiang, Y., and Lucero, J. Social support and social undermining as correlates for alcohol, drug, and mental disorders in American Indian women presenting for primary care at an Indian Health Service hospital. *Journal of Health Communication* 12(2):187–206, 2007.

Office of Applied Studies. *Results from the 2001 National Household Survey on Drug Abuse: Vol.1. Summary of National Findings.* National Household Survey on Drug Abuse Series: H-17. HHS Publication No. (SMA) 02-3758. Rockville, MD: Substance Abuse and Mental Health Services Administration, 2002a.

Office of Applied Studies. *Results from the 2001 National Household Survey on Drug Abuse: Volume III. Detailed Tables.* Rockville, MD: Substance Abuse and Mental Health Services Administration, 2002b.

Office of Applied Studies. Characteristics of homeless female admissions to substance abuse treatment: 2002. *The DASIS Report* (October 8, 2004): Rockville, M.D.: Substance Abuse and Mental Health Services Administration 2004a.

Office of Applied Studies. Gender differences in substance dependence and abuse. *The NSDUH Report* (October 29, 2004): Rockville, MD: Substance Abuse and Mental Health Services Administration 2004b.

Office of Applied Studies. Women with co-occurring serious mental illness and a substance use disorder. *The NSDUH Report* (August 20, 2004):1-3. Rockville, MD: Substance Abuse and Mental Health Services Administration 2004*c*.

Office of Applied Studies. *Results from the 2004 National Survey on Drug Use and Health: National Findings.* HHS Publication No. SMA 05-4062 Rockville, MD: Substance Abuse and Mental Health Services Administration 2005.

Office of Applied Studies. Facilities offering special programs or groups for women: 2005. *The DASIS Report* Issue 35 Rockville, MD: Substance Abuse and Mental Health Services Administration, 2006.

Office of Management and Budget. Recommendations from the Interagency Committee for the review of the racial and ethnic standards to the Office of Management and Budget Concerning Changes to the Standards for the Classification of Federal Data on Race and Ethnicity. *Federal Register* 62(13):36873-36946, 1997.

Office of National Drug Control Policy. *National Drug Control Strategy.* Washington, DC: Office of National Drug Control Policy, 2007.

Office of the Surgeon General. Fact Sheets: Asian Americans/Pacific Islanders. *Mental Health: Culture, Race, and Ethnicity A Supplement to Mental Health: A Report of the Surgeon General* Rockville, MD: U.S. Public Health Service 2001*a*.

Office of the Surgeon General. *Women and Smoking: A Report of the Surgeon General.* Atlanta, GA: Centers for Disease Control and Prevention, Office on Smoking and Health 2001*b*.

O'Hara, M.W., Stuart, S., Gorman, L.L., and Wenzel, A. Efficacy of interpersonal psychotherapy for postpartum depression. *Archives of General Psychiatry* 57(11):1039–1045, 2000.

Okazaki, S. Psychological assessment of Asian Americans: Research agenda for cultural competency. *Journal of Personality Assessment* 70(1):54–70, 1998.

Oklahoma Department of Mental Health and Substance Abuse Services. Title 450. Department of Mental Health and Substance Abuse Services. chapter 18. *Standards and Criteria for Alcohol and Drug Treatment Programs.* Oklahoma City, OK: Oklahoma Department of Mental Health and Substance Abuse Services, 2008.

Oncology Nursing Society 31st Annual Congress Podium and Poster Abstracts. *Oncology Nursing Forum* 33(2):394–491, 2006.

Onland-Moret, N.C., Peeters, P.H., Van Der Schouw, Y.T., Grobbee, D.E., and van Gils, C.H. Alcohol and endogenous sex steroid levels in postmenopausal women: a cross-sectional study. *Journal of Clinical Endocrinology and Metabolism* 90(3):1414–1419, 2005.

Oregon Secretary of State, and Department of Human Services, A.S. *Standards for Outpatient and Residential Alcohol and Drug Treatment Programs.* Salem, OR: Oregon Secretary of State, 2008.

Orenstein, R., and Tsogas, N. Hepatitis C virus and human immunodeficiency virus co-infection in women. *Journal of the American Osteopathic Association* 101(12 Suppl Pt 2):S1–S6, 2001.

Ouimette, P.C., Kimerling, R., Shaw, J., and Moos, R.H. Physical and sexual abuse among women and men with substance use disorders. *Alcoholism Treatment Quarterly* 18(3):7–17, 2000.

Page, R.M. Perceived physical attractiveness and frequency of substance use among male and female adolescents. *Journal of Alcohol and Drug Education* 38(2):81-91, 1993.

Paniagua, F.A. *Assessing and Treating Culturally Diverse Clients: A Practical Guide.* 2d ed. Thousand Oaks, CA: Sage Publications, 1998.

Paranjape, A., and Liebschutz, J. STaT: a three-question screen for intimate partner violence. *Journal of Women's Health (Larchment)* 12(3):233–239, 2003.

Parelman, A. *Emotional Intimacy in Marriage: A Sex-Roles Perspective. Research in Clinical Psychology.* Ann Arbor, Mich: UMI Research Press, 1983.

Parks, C.A. Lesbian identity development: An examination of differences across generations. *American Journal of Orthopsychiatry* 69(3):347–361, 1999*a*.

Parks, C.A. Lesbian social drinking: The role of alcohol in growing up and living as a lesbian. *Contemporary Drug Problems* 26(1):75–129, 1999*b*.

Parks, C.A., and Hughes, T.L. Alcohol use and alcohol-related problems in self-identified lesbians: age and racial/ethnic comparisons. *Journal of Lesbian Studies* 9(3):31–44, 2005.

Parks, C.A., Hesselbrock, M.N., Hesselbrock, V.M., and Segal, B. Factors affecting entry into substance abuse treatment: Gender differences among alcohol-dependent Alaska Natives. *Social Work Research* 27(3):151–161, 2003.

Passaro, K.T., and Little, R.E. Childbearing and alcohol use. In: Wilsnack, R.W., and Wilsnack, S.C., eds. *Gender and Alcohol: Individual and Social Perspectives.* New Brunswick, NJ: Rutgers Center of Alcohol Studies, 1997. pp. 90–113.

Patkar, A.A., Sterling, R.C., Gottheil, E., and Weinstein, S.P. A comparison of medical symptoms reported by cocaine-, opiate-, and alcohol-dependent patients. *Substance Abuse* 20(4):227–235, 1999.

Pedersen, P.B., Fukuyama, M., and Heath, A. Client, counselor, and contextual variables in multicultural counseling. In: Pedersen, P.B., Draguns, J.G., Lonner, W.J., and Trimble, J.E., eds. *Counseling Across Cultures.* 3d ed. Honolulu, HI: University of Hawaii Press, 1989. pp. 23–52.

Pelissier, B. Gender differences in substance use treatment entry and retention among prisoners with substance use histories. *American Journal of Public Health* 94(8):1418–1424, 2004.

Peluso, E., and Peluso, L.S. *Women and Drugs: Getting Hooked, Getting Clean.* Minneapolis, MN: CompCare Publishers, 1988.

Penn, P.E., Brooks, A.J., and Worsham, B.D. Treatment concerns of women with co-occurring serious mental illness and substance abuse disorders. *Journal of Psychoactive Drugs* 34(4):355–362, 2002.

Peters, T.J., Millward, L.M., and Foster, J. Quality of life in alcohol misuse: Comparison of men and women. *Archives of Women's Mental Health* 6(4):239–243, 2003.

Pettinati, H.M., Rukstalis, M.R., Luck, G.J., Volpicelli, J.R., and O'Brien, C.P. Gender and psychiatric comorbidity: Impact on clinical presentation of alcohol dependence. *American Journal on Addictions* 9(3):242–252, 2000.

Piazza, N.J., Vrbka, J.L., and Yeager, R.D. Telescoping of alcoholism in women alcoholics. *International Journal of the Addictions* 24(1):19–28, 1989.

Pickens, R.W., Svikis, D.S., McGue, M., Lykken, D.T., Heston, L.L., and Clayton, P.J. Heterogeneity in the inheritance of alcoholism: A study of male and female twins. *Archives of General Psychiatry* 48(1):19–28, 1991.

Piran, N., and Robinson, S.R. Associations between disordered eating behaviors and licit and illicit substance use and abuse in a university sample. *Addictive Behaviors* 31(10):1761–1775, 2006.

Pomerleau, C.S., Zucker, A.N., and Stewart, A.J. Characterizing concerns about postcessation weight gain: results from a national survey of women smokers. *Nicotine and Tobacco Research* 3(1):51–60, 2001.

Poole, N., and Dell, C.A. *Girls, Women and Substance Use*. 1–16. Ottawa, ON: Canadian Centre on Substance Abuse 2005.

Porter, L. *Women and HCV: Treatment. HCSP Factsheet* June version 1.0 San Francisco, CA: Hepatitis C Support Project, 2005.

Porter, L.K. *Women and Hepatitis C: An HCSP Guide*. San Francisco, CA: Hepatits C Support Project, 2008.

Poundstone, K.E., Chaisson, R.E., and Moore, R.D. Differences in HIV disease progression by injection drug use and by sex in the era of highly active antiretroviral therapy. *AIDS* 15(9):1115–1123, 2001.

Power, C., Rodgers, B., and Hope, S. Heavy alcohol consumption and marital status: Disentangling the relationship in a national study of young adults. *Addiction* 94(10):1477–1487, 1999.

Prescott, C.A. Sex differences in the genetic risk for alcoholism. *Alcohol Research & Health* 26(4):264–273, 2002.

Prescott, L. *Consumer/Survivor/Recovering Women: A Guide for Partnerships in Collaboration*. Delmar, NY: Policy Research Associates, 2001.

Price, A., and Simmel, C. *Partners' Influence on Women's Addiction and Recovery: The Connection Between Substance Abuse, Trauma, and Intimate Relationships*. Berkeley, CA: University of California at Berkeley, School of Social Welfare, National Abandoned Infants Assistance Resource Center, 2002.

Prochaska, J.J., Delucchi, K., and Hall, S.M. A meta-analysis of smoking cessation interventions with individuals in substance abuse treatment or recovery. *Journal of Consulting & Clinical Psychology* 72(6):1144–1156, 2004.

Project MATCH Research Group. Project MATCH secondary a priori hypotheses. *Addiction* 92(12):1671–1698, 1997.

Pugatch, D., Ramratmanm M., Strong, L., Feller, A., and Levesque, B. Gender differences in HIV risk behaviors among young adults and adolescents entering a Massachusetts detoxification center. *Substance Abuse* 21(2):79–86, 2000.

Quinlivan, J.A., and Evans, S.F. The impact of continuing illegal drug use on teenage pregnancy outcomes--a prospective cohort study. *BJOG : An International Journal of Obstetrics and Gynaecology* 109(10):1148–1153, 2002.

Radloff, L.S. The CES-D Scale: A self-report depression scale for research in the general population. *Applied Psychological Measurement* 1(3):385–401, 1977.

Raeburn, S.D. Women and eating disorders. In: Straussner, S.L.A., and Brown, S., eds. *The Handbook of Addiction Treatment for Women: Theory and Practice*. San Francisco: Jossey-Bass, 2002. pp. 127–153.

Randall, C.L. Alcohol and pregnancy: Highlights from three decades of research. *Journal of Studies on Alcohol* 62(5):554–561, 2001.

Randolph, W.M., Stroup-Benham, C., Black, S.A., and Markides, K.S. Alcohol use among Cuban-Americans, Mexican-Americans, and Puerto Ricans. *Alcohol Health and Research World* 22(4):265–269, 1998.

Ratner, P.A., Johnson, J.L., Bottorff, J.L., Dahinten, S., and Hall, W. Twelve-month follow-up of a smoking relapse prevention intervention for postpartum women. *Addictive Behaviors* 25(1):81–92, 2000.

Ravndal, E., and Vaglum, P. Treatment of female addicts: the importance of relationships to parents, partners, and peers for the outcome. *International Journal of Addictions* 29(1):115–125, 1994.

Rayburn, W.F., and Bogenschutz, M.P. Pharmacotherapy for pregnant women with addictions. *American Journal of Obstetrics and Gynecology* 191(6):1885–1897, 2004.

Reed, B.G., and Mowbray, C.T. Mental illness and substance abuse: Implications for women's health and health care access. *Journal of the American Medical Women's Association* 54(2):71–78, 1999.

Reeves, T., and Bennett, C. The Asian and Pacific Islander population in the United States: March 2002. *Current Psychiatry Reports* Washington, DC: U. S. Census Bureau 2003.

Register, T.C., Cline, J.M., and Shively, C.A. Health issues in postmenopausal women who drink. *Alcohol Research & Health* 26(4):299–307, 2002.

Register, T.C., Cline, J.M., and Shively, C.A. *Health Issues in Postmenopausal Women Who Drink*. Bethesda, MD: National Institute on Alcohol Abuse and Alcoholism, 2003.

Reid, D.J. Addiction, African Americans, and a Christian recovery. In: Krestan, J.A., ed. *Bridges to Recovery: Addiction, Family Therapy, and Multicultural Treatment*. New York: The Free Press, 2000. pp. 145–172.

Renzetti, C.M. Violence in lesbian relationships. In: Hansen, M., and Harway, M., eds. *Battering and Family Therapy: A Feminist Perspective*. Thousand Oaks, CA: Sage Publications, 1993. pp. 188–199.

Renzetti, C.M. On dancing with a bear: Reflections on some of the current debates among domestic violence theorists. *Violence and Victims* 9(2):195–200, 1994.

Reyes, M. Latina lesbians and alcohol and other drugs: Social work implications. *Alcoholism Treatment Quarterly* 16(1/2):179–192, 1998.

Reynolds, E.W., and Bada, H.S. Pharmacology of drugs of abuse. *Obstetrics and Gynecology Clinics of North America* 30(3):501–522, 2003.

Rhoades, J.A., and Chu, M.C. Health insurance status of the civilian noninstitutionalized population: 1999. Rockville, MD: Agency for Healthcare Research and Quality 2000.

Rhodes, R., and Johnson, A. A feminist approach to treating alcohol and drug-addicted African-American women. *Women & Therapy* 20(3):23–37, 1997.

Rice, C., Mohr, C.D., Del Boca, F.K., Mattson, M.E., Young, L., Brady, K., and Nickless, C. Self-reports of physical, sexual and emotional abuse in an alcoholism treatment sample. *Journal of Studies on Alcohol* 62(1):114–123, 2001.

Richardson, G.A., Goldschmidt, L., and Larkby, C. Effects of prenatal cocaine exposure on growth: a longitudinal analysis. *Pediatrics* 120(4):e1017–e1027, 2007.

Ridenour, T.A., Maldonado-Molina, M., Compton, W.M., Spitznagel, E.L., and Cottler, L.B. Factors associated with the transition from abuse to dependence among substance abusers: implications for a measure of addictive liability. *Drug and Alcohol Dependence* 80(1):1–14, 2005.

Riehman, K.S., Hser, Y.I., and Zeller, M. Gender differences in how intimate partners influence drug treatment motivation. *Journal of Drug Issues* 30(4):823–838, 2000.

Riehman, K.S., Iguchi, M.Y., Zeller, M., and Morral, A.R. The influence of partner drug use and relationship power on treatment engagement. *Drug and Alcohol Dependence* 70(1):1–10, 2003.

Rinehart, D.J., Becker, M.A., Buckley, P.R., Dailey, K., Reichardt, c.S., Graeber, C., VanDeMark, N.R., and Brown, E. The relationship between mothers' child abuse potential and current metal health symptoms: Implications for screening and referral. *Journal of Behavior Health Services & Research* 32(2):155–166, 2005.

Roberts, A., Jackson, M.S., and Carlton-LaNey, I. Revisiting the need for feminism and afrocentric theory when treating African-American female substance abusers. *Journal of Drug Issues* 30(4):901–918, 2000.

Roberts, A.C., and Nishimoto, R. Barriers to engaging and retaining African American post-partum women in drug treatment. *Journal of Drug Issues* 36(1):53–76, 2006.

Roberts, A.C., and Nishimoto, R.H. Predicting treatment retention of women dependent on cocaine. *American Journal of Drug and Alcohol Abuse* 22(3):313–333, 1996.

Robertson, M.J., Zlotnick, C., and Westerfelt, A. Drug use disorders and treatment contact among homeless adults in Alameda County, California. *American Journal of Public Health* 87(2):221–228, 1997.

Robin, R.W., Chester, B., Rasmussen, J.K., and Jaranson, J.M. Factors influencing utilization of mental health and substance abuse services by American Indian men and women. *Psychiatric Services* 48(6):826–832, 1997.

Rodriguez-Andrew, S. Alcohol use and abuse among Latinos: Issues and examples of culturally competent services. *Alcoholism Treatment Quarterly* 16(1-2):55–70, 1998.

Rogers, C. Older women and poverty in rural America. *Rural Population and Migration: Trend 6-Challenges From an Aging Population* Washington, DC: U.S. Department of Agriculture, 2005.

Rohan, T.E., Jain, M., Howe, G.R., and Miller, A.B. Alcohol consumption and risk of breast cancer: A cohort study. *Cancer Causes and Control* 11(3):239–247, 2000.

Romach, M.K., and Sellers, E.M. Alcohol dependence: Women, biology, and pharmacotherapy. In: McCance-Katz, E.F., and Kosten, T.R., eds. *New Treatments for Chemical Addictions*. Washington, DC: American Psychiatric Press, 1998. pp. 35–73.

Rome, E.S. Eating disorders. *Obstetrics and Gynecology Clinics of North America* 30(2):353–377, 2003.

Root, M.P. Treatment failures: The role of sexual victimization in women's addictive behavior. *American Journal of Orthopsychiatry* 59(4):542–549, 1989.

Rosenberg, L., Palmer, J.R., Rao, R.S., and Adams-Campbell, L.L. Patterns and correlates of alcohol consumption among African-American women. *Ethnicity and Disease* 12(4):548–554, 2002.

Ross, J. Food addiction: A new look at the nature of craving. *Addiction and Recovery* 13(5):17–19, 1993.

Ross-Durow, P.L., and Boyd, C.J. Sexual abuse, depression, and eating disorders in African American women who smoke cocaine. *Journal of Substance Abuse Treatment* 18(1):79–81, 2000.

Rotgers, F. Clinically useful, research validated assessment of persons with alcohol problems. *Behaviour Research and Therapy* 40(12):1425–1441, 2002.

Rotter, J.C., and Casado, M. Promoting strengths and celebrating culture: Working with Hispanic families. *Family Journal* 6(2):132-137, 1998.

Rouse, B.A., Carter, J.H., and Rodriguez-Andrew, S. Race/ethnicity and other sociocultural influences on alcoholism treatment for women. In: Galanter, M., ed. *Recent Developments in Alcoholism, Vol. 12: Alcoholism and Women.* New York: Plenum Press, 1995. pp. 343–367.

Rubin, A., Stout, R.L., and Longabaugh, R. Gender differences in relapse situations. *Addiction* 91(Suppl):S111–S120, 1996.

Rush, M.M. Perceived social support: Dimensions of social interaction among sober female participants in Alcoholics Anonymous. *Journal of the American Psychiatric Nurses Association* 8(4):114–119, 2002.

Russell, M. New assessment tools for risk drinking during pregnancy: T-ACE, TWEAK, and others. *Alcohol Health and Research World* 18(1):55–61, 1994.

Russell, M., Czarnecki, D.M., Cowan, R., McPherson, E., and Mudar, P.J. Measures of maternal alcohol use as predictors of development in early childhood. *Alcoholism: Clinical & Experimental Research* 15(6):991–1000, 1991.

Russell, M., Martier, S.S., Sokol, R.J., Mudar, P., Jacobson, S., and Jacobson, J. Detecting risk drinking during pregnancy: A comparison of four screening questionnaires. *American Journal of Public Health* 86(10):1435–1439, 1996.

Russell, P.L. Trauma and the cognitive function of affects. In: Teicholz, J.G., and Kriegman, D., eds. *Trauma, Repetition, and Affect Regulation: The Work of Paul Russell.* New York: The Other Press, 1998. pp. 23–47.

Ryland, S.A., and Lucas, L. A rural collaborative model of treatment and recovery services for pregnant and parenting women with dual disorders. *Journal of Psychoactive Drugs* 28(4):389–395, 1996.

Sabol, W.J., Couture, H., and Harrison, P.M. Prisoners in 2006. *Bureau of Justice Statistics Bulletin* Washington, DC: U.S. Department of Justice 2007.

Safer, D.L., Telch, C.F., and Agras, W.S. Dialectical behavior therapy adapted for bulimia: A case report. *International Journal of Eating Disorders* 30(1):101–106, 2001.

Salasin, S.E. Evolution of women's trauma-integrated services at the Substance Abuse and Mental Health Services Administration. *Journal of Community Psychology* 33(4):379–393, 2005.

Sale, E., Sambrano, S., Springer, J.F., Pena, C., Pan, W., and Kasim, R. Family protection and prevention of alcohol use among Hispanic youth at high risk. *American Journal of Community Psychology* 36(3-4):195-205, 2005.

Salmon, M.M., Joseph, B.M., Saylor, C., and Mann, R.J. Women's perception of provider, social, and program support in an outpatient drug treatment program. *Journal of Substance Abuse Treatment* 19(3):239–246, 2000.

Sampson, H.W. Alcohol's harmful effects on bone. *Alcohol Health and Research World* 22(3):190–194, 1998.

Sampson, H.W. Alcohol and other factors affecting osteoporosis risk in women. *Alcohol Research & Health* 26(4):292–298, 2002.

Sandfort, T.G., de Graaf, R., Bijl, R.V., and Schnabel, P. Same-sex sexual behavior and psychiatric disorders: Findings from the Netherlands Mental Health Survey and Incidence Study (NEMESIS). *Archives of General Psychiatry* 58(1):85–91, 2001.

Santen, F.J., Sofsky, J., Bilic, N., and Lippert, R. Mechanism of action of narcotics in the production of menstrual dysfunction in women. *Fertility and Sterility* 26(6):538–548, 1975.

Sartor, C.E., Lynskey, M.T., Bucholz, K.K., McCutcheon, V.V., Nelson, E.C., Waldron, M., and Heath, A.C. Childhood sexual abuse and the course of alcohol dependence development: Findings from a female twin sample. *Drug and Alcohol Dependence* 89(2–3):139–144, 2007.

Satre, D.D., Mertens, J.R., and Weisner, C. Gender differences in treatment outcomes for alcohol dependence among older adults. *Journal of Studies on Alcohol* 65(5):638–642, 2004.

Saunders, E.J. A new model of residential care for substance-abusing women and their children. *Adult Residential Care Journal* 7(2):104–117, 1993.

Saylors, K., and Daliparthy, N. Violence against Native women in substance abuse treatment. *American Indian and Alaska Native Mental Health Research* 13(1):32–51, 2006.

Schauer, C., Everett, A., del, V.P., and Anderson, L. Promoting the value and practice of shared decision-making in mental health care. *Psychiatric Rehabilitation Journal* 31(1):54–61, 2007.

Schilit, R., Lie, G.Y., and Montagne, M. Substance use as a correlate of violence in intimate lesbian relationships. *Journal of Homosexuality* 19(3):51–65, 1990.

Schnoll, R.A., Patterson, F., and Lerman, C. Treating tobacco dependence in women. *Journal of Women's Health (Larchmt.)* 16(8):1211–1218, 2007.

Schuck, A.M., and Widom, C.S. Childhood victimization and alcohol symptoms in females: causal inferences and hypothesized mediators. *Child Abuse and Neglect* 25(8):1069–1092, 2001.

Schweinsburg, B.C., Alhassoon, O.M., Taylor, M.J., Gonzalez, R., Videen, J.S., Brown, G.G., Patterson, T.L., and Grant, I. Effects of alcoholism and gender on brain metabolism. *American Journal of Psychiatry* 160(6):1180–1183, 2003.

Scogin, F., Morthland, M., Kaufman, A., Burgio, L., Chaplin, W., Kong, G., and `. Improving quality of life in diverse rural older adults: A randomized trial of a psychological treatment. *Psychology and Aging* 22(4):657–665, 2007.

Scott-Lennox, J., Rose, R., Bohlig, A., and Lennox, R. The impact of women's family status on completion of substance abuse treatment. *Journal of Behavioral Health Services and Research* 27(4):366–379, 2000.

Setiawan, V.W., Monroe, K.R., Goodman, M.T., Kolonel, L.N., Pike, M.C., and Henderson, B.E. Alcohol consumption and endometrial cancer risk: the multiethnic cohort. *International Journal of Cancer* 122(3):634–638, 2008.

Severance, T.A. Concerns and coping strategies of women inmates concerning release: "It's going to take somebody in my corner." *Journal of Offender Rehabilitation* 38(4):73–97, 2004.

Sheehan, D., Janavs, J., Baker, R., Harnett-Sheehan, K., Knapp, E., Sheehan, M., Lecrubier, Y., Weiller, E., Hergueta, T., Amorim, P., Bonora, L.I., and Lepine, J.P. *M.I.N.I.: Mini International Neuropsychiatric Interview*. English Version 5.0.0. n.p.: Medical Outcome Systems 2002.

Sherman, C. Drugs Affect Men's and Women's Brains Differently. NIDA Notes vol. 20:6 2006.

Shieh, C., and Kravitz, M. Severity of drug use, initiation of prenatal care, and maternal-fetal attachment in pregnant marijuana and cocaine/heroin users. *Journal of Obstetric, Gynecologic, & Neonatal Nursing: Clinical Scholarship for the Care of Women, Childbearing Families, & Newborns* 35(4):499–508, 2006.

Shiffman, S., and Balabanis, M. Associations between alcohol and tobacco. In: Fertig, J.B., and Allen, J.P., eds. *Alcohol and Tobacco: From Basic Science to Clinical Practice*. NIAAA Research Monograph No. 30. Bethesda, MD: National Institute on Alcohol Abuse and Alcoholism, 1995. pp. 17–36.

Silverman, J.G., Raj, A., and Clements, K. Dating violence and associated sexual risk and pregnancy among adolescent girls in the United States. *Pediatrics* 114(2):e220–e225, 2004.

Silverman, J.G., Raj, A., Mucci, L.A., and Hathaway, J.E. Dating violence against adolescent girls and associated substance use, unhealthy weight control, sexual risk behavior, pregnancy, and suicidality. *Journal of the American Medical Association* 286(5):572–579, 2001.

Silverstein, B. Women show higher rates of anxious somatic depression but maybe not "pure" depression. *Clinician's Research Digest* 20(10):3, 2002.

Simoni, J.M., Sehgal, S., and Walters, K.L. Triangle of risk: urban American Indian women's sexual trauma, injection drug use, and HIV sexual risk behaviors. *AIDS and Behavior* 8(1):33–45, 2004.

Simoni-Wastila, L. The use of abusable prescription drugs: The role of gender. *Journal of Women's Health and Gender-Based Medicine* 9(3):289–297, 2000.

Simpson, D.D. *Patient Engagement and Duration of Treatment*. Bethesda, MD: National Institute on Drug Abuse, 1997.

Simpson, D.D., and Knight, D.K. TCU Data Collection Forms for Women and Children Residential Treatment: Intake. Fort Worth, TX: Texas Christian University, Institute of Behavioral Research, 1997.

Simpson, T.L. Childhood sexual abuse, PTSD and the functional roles of alcohol use among women drinkers. *Substance Use & Misuse* 38(2):249–270, 2003.

Singer, L.T., Arendt, R., Minnes, S., Farkas, K., and Salvator, A. Neurobehavioral outcomes of cocaine-exposed infants. *Neurotoxicology and Teratology* 22(5):653–666, 2000.

Singer, L.T., Minnes, S., Short, E., Arendt, R., Farkas, K., Lewis, B., Klein, N., Russ, S., Min, M.O., and Kirchner, H.L. Cognitive outcomes of preschool children with prenatal cocaine exposure. *JAMA* 291(20):2448–2456, 2004.

Singletary, K.W., and Gapstur, S.M. Alcohol and breast cancer: Review of epidemiologic and experimental evidence and potential mechanisms. *Journal of the American Medical Association* 286(17):2143–2151, 2001.

Slade, A., and Cohen, L.J. The process of parenting and the remembrance of things past. *Infant Mental Health Journal* 17(3):217–238, 1996.

Slaymaker, V.J., and Owen, P.L. Employed men and women substance abusers: Job troubles and treatment outcomes. *Journal of Substance Abuse Treatment* 31(4):347–354, 2006.

Smith, C., and Erford, B.T. *Test Review: Beck Depression Inventory - II.* Greensboro, NC: Association for Assessment in Counseling, 2001.

Smith, D.E., Moser, C., Wesson, D.R., Apter, M., Buxton, M.E., Davison, J.V., Orgel, M., and Buffum, J. A clinical guide to the diagnosis and treatment of heroin-related sexual dysfunction. *Journal of Psychoactive Drugs* 14(1-2):91–99, 1982.

Smith, J.W. Medical manifestations of alcoholism in the elderly. *International Journal of the Addictions* 30(13-14):1749–1798, 1995.

Smith, L.M., LaGasse, L.L., Derauf, C., Grant, P., Shah, R., Arria, A., Huestis, M., Haning, W., Strauss, A., Della, G.S., Liu, J., and Lester, B.M. The infant development, environment, and lifestyle study: Effects of prenatal methamphetamine exposure, polydrug exposure, and poverty on intrauterine growth. *Pediatrics* 118(3):1149–1156, 2006.

Smith, S.S., Jorenby, D.E., Leischow, S.J., Nides, M.A., Rennard, S.I., Johnston, J.A., Jamerson, B., Fiore, M.C., and Baker, T.B. Targeting smokers at increased risk for relapse: treating women and those with a history of depression. *Nicotine and Tobacco Research* 5(1):99–109, 2003.

Smolak, L., and Murnen, S.K. Gender and eating problems. In: Striegel-Moore, R.H., and Smolak, L., eds. *Eating Disorders: Innovative Directions in Research and Practice.* 1-55798-778-5 (hardcover). American Psychological Association: Washington, 2001. pp. 91–110.

Sobell, L.C., Cunningham, J.A., and Sobell, M.B. Recovery from alcohol problems with and without treatment: Prevalence in two population surveys. *American Journal of Public Health* 86(7):966–972, 1996.

Sohrabji, F. Neurodegeneration in women. *Alcohol Research & Health* 26(4):316–318, 2002.

Sokol, R.J., and Clarren, S.K. Guidelines for use of terminology describing the impact of prenatal alcohol on the offspring. *Alcoholism: Clinical and Experimental Research* 13(4):597–598, 1989.

Sokol, R.J., Martier, S.S., and Ager, J.W. The T-ACE questions: practical prenatal detection of risk-drinking. *American Journal of Obstetrics and Gynecology* 160(4):863–868, 1989.

Solarz, A.L. (Ed.) *Lesbian Health: Current Assessment And Directions For The Future.* Washington, D.C.: National Academy Press, 1999.

Solomon, S.D., and Johnson, D.M. Psychosocial treatment of posttraumatic stress disorder: A practice-friendly review of outcome research. *Journal of Clinical Psychology* 58(8):947–959, 2002.

Sorensen, J.L., Masson, C.L., Delucchi, K., Sporer, K., Barnett, P.G., Mitsuishi, F., Lin, C., Song, Y., Chen, T., and Hall, S.M. Randomized trial of drug abuse treatment-linkage strategies. *Journal of Consulting & Clinical Psychology* 73(6):1026–1035, 2005.

Specker, S., Westermeyer, J., and Thuras, P. Course and severity of substance abuse in women with comorbid eating disorders. *Substance Abuse* 21(3):137–147, 2000.

Stahler, G.J., Shipley, T.E., Kirby, K.C., Godboldte, C., Kerwin, M.E., Shandler, I., and Simons, L. Development and initial demonstration of a community-based intervention for homeless, cocaine-using, African-American Women. *Journal of Substance Abuse Treatment* 28(2):171–179, 2005.

Stamler, V.L., Christiansen, M.D., Staley, K.H., and agno-Shang, L. Client preference for counselor gender. *Psychology of Women Quarterly* 15(2):317–321, 1991.

Steele, C.T. Providing clinical treatment to substance abusing trauma survivors. *Alcoholism Treatment Quarterly* 18(3):71–82, 2000.

Steer, R.A., Beck, A.T., and Brown, G. Sex differences on the revised Beck Depression Inventory for outpatients with affective disorders. *Journal of Personality Assessment* 53(4):693–702, 1989.

Steffens, A.A., Moreira, L.B., Fuchs, S.C., Wiehe, M., Gus, M., and Fuchs, F.D. Incidence of hypertension by alcohol consumption: is it modified by race? *Journal of Hypertension* 24(8):1489–1492, 2006.

Steinberg, M.B., Akincigil, A., Delnevo, C.D., Crystal, S., and Carson, J.L. Gender and age disparities for smoking-cessation treatment. *American Journal of Preventive Medicine* 30(5):405–412, 2006.

Steiner, M. Perinatal mood disorders: Position paper. *Psychopharmacology Bulletin* 34(3):301–306, 1998.

Steiner, M. Postnatal depression: A few simple questions. *Family Practice* 19(5):469–470, 2002.

Steinhausen, H.C. The outcome of anorexia nervosa in the 20th century. *American Journal of Psychiatry* 159(8):1284–1293, 2002.

Sterling, R.C., Gottheil, E., Weinstein, S.P., and Serota, R. Therapist/patient race and sex matching: Treatment retention and 9-month follow-up outcome. *Addiction* 93(7):1043–1050, 1998.

Stevens, S.J. American-Indian women and health. In: Wechsberg, W.M., ed. *Prevention issues for women's health in the new millennium*. Binghamton, NY: Haworth Press, 2001. pp. 97–109.

Stevens, S.J., and Estrada, B. *Substance involved women: Ethnic differences, contraceptive practices and HIV sex risk behaviors*. Presented at the Society for Menstrual Cycle Research Biennial Conference, Tucson, AZ, June, 1999.

Stevens, S.J., and Murphy, B.S. *Women's-Specific Health Assessment*. Tucson, AZ: University of Arizona, Southwest Institute for Research on Women, 1998.

Stevens, S.J., and Patton, T. Residential treatment for drug addicted women and their children: Effective treatment strategies. In: Stevens, S.J., and Wexler, H.K., eds. *Women and Substance Abuse: Gender Transparency*. New York: Haworth Press, 1998a. pp. 235–249.

Stevens, S.J., and Patton, T. Residential treatment for drug addicted women and their children: Effective treatment strategies. *Drugs & Society* 13(1/2):235–249, 1998b.

Stevens, S.J., Estrada, A.L., and Estrada, B.D. HIV sex and drug risk behavior and behavior change in a national sample of injection drug and crack cocaine using women. *Women & Health* 27(1-2):25–48, 1998.

Stewart, D.E. *Menopause: A Mental Health Practitioner's Guide*. 1st ed ed. Washington, DC: American Psychiatric Pub, 2005.

Stewart, S.H., Conrod, P.J., Samoluk, S.B., Pihl, R.O., and Dongier, M. Posttraumatic stress disorder symptoms and situation-specific drinking in women substance abusers. *Alcoholism Treatment Quarterly* 18(3):31–47, 2000.

Strantz, I.H., and Welch, S.P. Postpartum women in outpatient drug abuse treatment: Correlates of retention/completion. *Journal of Psychoactive Drugs* 27(4):357–373, 1995.

Stratton, K., Howe, C., and Battaglia, F. (Eds.) *Fetal Alcohol Syndrome: Diagnosis, Epidemiology, Prevention, and Treatment*. Washington, DC: National Academy Press, 1996.

Stromwall, L.K., and Larson, N.C. Women's experience of co-occurring substance abuse and mental health conditions. *Journal of Social Work Practice in the Addictions* 4(1):81–96, 2004.

Substance Abuse and Mental Health Administration. Blueprint for change: Ending chronic homelessness for persons with serious mental illnesses and co-occurring substance use disorders. HHS Pub. No. SMA-04-3870 Rockville, MD: Center for Mental Health Services, Substance Abuse and Mental Health Services Administration, 2003*a*.

Substance Abuse and Mental Health Services Administration. *Questions About Sexual Abuse*. Women, Violence and Co-Occurring Disorders Grant. TI 98-004. Unpublished instrument, 2003*b*.

Substance Abuse and Mental Health Services Administration. *Results from the 2003 National Survey on Drug Use and Health: National Findings*. (Office of Applied Studies, NSDUH Series: H-25, HHS Publication No. SMA 04-3964). Rockville, MD, 2004.

Substance Abuse and Mental Health Services Administration. *Recovery Community Services Program*. Rockville, MD: Center for Substance Abuse Treatment, Substance Abuse and Mental Health Services Administration, 2006*a*.

Substance Abuse and Mental Health Services Administration. *Results from the 2005 National Survey on Drug Use and Health: National Findings*. HHS Publication No. SMA 06-4194 Rockville, MD: Office of Applied Studies, 2006*b*.

Substance Abuse and Mental Health Services Administration. *Results from the 2006 National Survey on Drug Use and Health: National Findings*. HHS Publication No. SMA SMA 07-4293 Rockville, MD: Office of Applied Studies, 2007.

Substance Abuse and Mental Health Services Administration. *Results from the 2007 National Survey on Drug Use and Health: National Findings*. (Office of Applied Studies, NSDUH Series H-34, HHS Publication No.SMA 08-4343) 2008.

Substance Abuse and Mental Health Services Administration, and Office of Applied Studies. *Treatment Episode Data Set (TEDS): 1992–2000. National Admissions to Substance Abuse Treatment Services*. Drug and Alcohol Services Information System Series: S-17. Rockville, MD: Substance Abuse and Mental Health Services Administration, 2002.

Substance Abuse and Mental Health Services Administration, and Office of Applied Studies. *Overview of Findings from the 2002 National Survey on Drug Use and Health*. (Office of Applied Studies, NHSDA Series H-21, HHS Publication No. SMA 03-3774). Rockville, MD: Substance Abuse and Mental Health Services Administration, 2003.

Substance Abuse and Mental Health Services Administration, and Office of Applied Studies. Table 4.11b. Facility services offered, by facility operation: March 31, 2003. *National Survey of Substance Abuse Treatment Services (N-SSATS): 2003 Data on Substance Abuse Treatment Facilities* Rockville, MD, 2004*a*.

Substance Abuse and Mental Health Services Administration and Office of Applied Studies. *Treatment Episode Data Set (TEDS). Highlights - 2002. National Admissions to Substance Abuse Treatment Services, DASIS Series: S-22* HHS Publication No. (SMA) 04-3946 Rockville, MD: Substance Abuse and Mental Health Services Administration, 2004*b*.

Substance Abuse and Mental Health Services Administration, Office of Applied Studies. Treatment Episode Data Set (TEDS): 1992-2002. National Admissions to Substance Abuse Treatment Services. HHS Publication No. (SMA) 04-3965 Rockville, MD: Substance Abuse and Mental Health Services Administration, 2004*c*.

Substance Abuse and Mental Health Services Administration, Office of Applied Studies. *The National Survey of Substance Abuse Treatment Services: 2003. The DASIS Report* (March 11, 2005): Rockville, MD: Substance Abuse and Mental Health Services Administration 2005*a*.

Substance Abuse and Mental Health Services Administration, Office of Applied Studies. Treatment Episode Data Set (TEDS). Highlights - 2003. *National Admissions to Substance Abuse Treatment Services, DASIS Series: S-27* HHS Publication No. (SMA) 05-4043 Rockville, MD: Substance Abuse and Mental Health Services Administration 2005*b*.

Substance Abuse and Mental Health Services Administration, Office of Applied Studies. *National Survey of Substance Abuse Treatment Services (N-SSATS): 2005. Data on Substance Abuse Treatment Facilities.* DASIS Series: S-34. HHS Publication No. (SMA) 06-4206. Rockville, MD: Substance Abuse and Mental Health Services Administration, 2006.

Substance Abuse and Mental Health Services Administration and Office of Applied Studies. Gender differences in alcohol use and alcohol dependence or abuse: 2004 and 2005. *The NSDUH Report* April 2, 2007*a*.

Substance Abuse and Mental Health Services Administration, Office of Applied Studies. Hispanic female admissions in substance abuse treatment: 2005. *The DASIS Report* April 13 Rockville, MD, 2007*b*.

Substance Abuse and Mental Health Services Administration, Office of Applied Studies. Treatment Admissions with Medicaid as the Primary expected or Actual Payment source: 2005. *The DASIS Report* July 12 Rockville, MD: Substance Abuse and Mental Health Services Administration 2007*c*.

Substance Abuse and Mental Health Services Administration, Office of Applied Studies. *Results from the 2007 National Survey on Drug Use and Health: National Findings.* (Office of Applied Studies, NSDUH Series H-34, HHS Publication No. SMA 08-4343) Rockville, MD: Office of Applied Studies, 2008.

Suchman, N., Mayes, L., Conti, J., Slade, A., and Rounsaville, B. Rethinking parenting interventions for drug-dependent mothers: From behavior management to fostering emotional bonds. *Journal of Substance Abuse Treatment* 27(3):179–185, 2004.

Suchman, N., Pajulo, M., DeCoste, C., and Mayes, L. Parenting interventions for drug-dependent mothers and their young children: The case for an attachment-based approach. *Family Relations* 55(2):211–226, 2006.

Suchman, N.E., Rounsaville, B., DeCoste, C., and Luthar, S. Parental control, parental warmth, and psychosocial adjustment in a sample of substance-abusing mothers and their school-aged and adolescent children. *Journal of Substance Abuse Treatment* 32(1):1–10, 2007.

Sue, D.W., and Sue, D. *Counseling the Culturally Different: Theory and Practice.* 3d ed. New York: John Wiley and Sons, 1999.

Sue, D.W., and Sue, D. *Counseling the Culturally Diverse: Theory and Practice.* 4th ed. New York: John Wiley and Sons, 2003.

Sullivan, E.V., Fama, R., Rosenbloom, M.J., and Pfefferbaum, A. A profile of neuropsychological deficits in alcoholic women. *Neuropsychology* 16(1):74–83, 2002.

Sullivan, J.M., and Evans, K. Integrated treatment for the survivor of childhood trauma who is chemically dependent. *Journal of Psychoactive Drugs* 26(4):369–378, 1994.

Sullivan, J.T., Sykora, K., Schneiderman, J., Naranjo, C.A., and Sellers, E.M. Assessment of alcohol withdrawal: The revised Clinical Institute Withdrawal Assessment for alcohol scale (CIWA-Ar). *British Journal of Addiction* 84(11):1353–1357, 1989.

Sun, A.P. Helping substance-abusing mothers in the child-welfare system: Turning crisis into opportunity. *Families in Society* 81(2):142–151, 2000.

Sun, A.P. Program factors related to women's substance abuse treatment retention and other outcomes: A review and critique. *Journal of Substance Abuse Treatment* 30(1):1–20, 2006.

Sun, A.P. Relapse among substance-abusing women: Components and processes. *Substance Use and Misuse* 42(1):1–21, 2007.

Sussman, S. Smoking cessation among persons in recovery. *Substance Use & Misuse* 37(8–10):1275–1298, 2002.

Swan, G.E., and Denk, C.E. Dynamic models for the maintenance of smoking cessation: event history analysis of late relapse. *Journal of Behavioral Medicine* 10(6):527–554, 1987.

Swan, S., Farber, S., and Campbell, D. Violence in the lives of women in substance abuse treatment: Service and policy implications. *Report to the New York State Office of the Prevention of Domestic Violence.* Rensselear, NY: Author, 2000.

Sylvestre, D.L., and Zweben, J.E. Integrating HCV services for drug users: a model to improve engagement and outcomes. *International Journal of Drug Policy* 18(5):406–410, 2007.

Szuster, R.R., Rich, L.L., Chung, A., and Bisconer, S.W. Treatment retention in women's residential chemical dependency treatment: The effect of admission with children. *Substance Use and Misuse* 31(8):1001–1013, 1996.

Tafoya, T., and Roeder, K.R. Spiritual exiles in their own homelands: Gays, lesbians and Native Americans. *Journal of Chemical Dependency Treatment* 5(2):179–197, 1995.

Tatum, T. Rural women's recovery program and women's outreach: Serving rural Appalachian women and families in Ohio. In: Center for Substance Abuse Treatment, ed. *Treating Alcohol and Other Drug Abusers in Rural and Frontier Areas.* Technical Assistance Publication Series 17. HHS Publication No. (SMA) 99-3339. Rockville, MD: Center for Substance Abuse Treatment, 1995. pp. 13–20.

Taylor, T.R., Williams, C.D., Makambi, K.H., Mouton, C., Harrell, J.P., Cozier, Y., Palmer, J.R., Rosenberg, L., and dams-Campbell, L.L. Racial discrimination and breast cancer incidence in us black women: The black women's health study. *American Journal of Epidemiology* 166(1):46–54, 2007.

Terner, J.M., and de Wit, H. Menstrual cycle phase and responses to drugs of abuse in humans. *Drug and Alcohol Dependence* 84(1):1–13, 2006.

Testa, M., Livingston, J.A., and Leonard, K.E. Women's substance use and experiences of intimate partner violence: A longitudinal investigation among a community sample. *Addictive Behaviors* 28(9):1649–1664, 2003.

Teusch, R. Substance-abusing women and sexual abuse. In: Straussner, S.L.A., and Zelvin, E., eds. *Gender and Addictions: Men and Women in Treatment*. Northvale, NJ: Jason Aronson, 1997. pp. 97–122.

Thaithumyanon, P., Limpongsanurak, S., Praisuwanna, P., and Punnahitanon, S. Perinatal effects of amphetamine and heroin use during pregnancy on the mother and infant. *Journal of the Medical Association of Thailand* 88(11):1506–1513, 2005.

The C. Everett Koop Institute. High risk Groups - United States. *Hepatitis C: An Epidemic for Anyone* Hanover, NH: Dartmouth Medical School, 2008.

Theall, K.P., Sterk, C.E., and Elifson, K. Illicit drug use and women's sexual and reproductive health. In: Wingood, G.M., and DiClemente, R.J., eds. *Handbook of Women's Sexual and Reproductive Health*. New York, NY: Kluwer Academic/Plenum Publishers, 2002. pp. 129–152.

Thevos, A.K., Roberts, J.S., Thomas, S.E., and Randall, C.L. Cognitive behavioral therapy delays relapse in female socially phobic alcoholics. *Addictive Behaviors* 25(3):333–345, 2000.

Thom, B. Sex differences in help-seeking for alcohol problems: I. The barriers to help-seeking. *British Journal of Addiction* 81(6):777-788, 1986.

Thom, B. Sex differences in help-seeking for alcohol problems: II. Entry into treatment. *British Journal of Addiction* 82(9):989-997, 1987.

Thomasson, H. Alcohol elimination: Faster in women? *Alcoholism: Clinical and Experimental Research* 24(4):419–420, 2000.

Thompson, R.S., Bonomi, A.E., Anderson, M., Reid, R.J., Dimer, J.A., Carrell, D., and Rivara, F.P. Intimate partner violence: prevalence, types, and chronicity in adult women. *American Journal of Preventive Medicine* 30(6):447–457, 2006.

Thornberry, J., Bhaskar, B., Krulewitch, C.J., Wesley, B., Hubbard, M.L., Das, A., Foudin, L., and Adamson, M. Audio computerized self-report interview use in prenatal clinics: Audio computer-assisted self interview with touch screen to detect alcohol consumption in pregnant women. Application of a new technology to an old problem. *Computers, Informatics, Nursing* 20(2):46–52, 2002.

Thorpe, L.E., Frederick, M., Pitt, J., Cheng, I., Watts, D.H., Buschur, S., Green, K., Zorrilla, C., Landesman, S.H., and Hershow, R.C. Effect of hard-drug use on CD4 cell percentage, HIV RNA level, and progression to AIDS-defining class C events among HIV-infected women. *Journal of Acquired Immune Deficiency Syndromes* 37(3):1423–1430, 2004.

Tiemersma, E.W., Wark, P.A., Ocke, M.C., Bunschoten, A., Otten, M.H., Kok, F.J., and Kampman, E. Alcohol Consumption, Alcohol Dehydrogenase 3 Polymorphism, and Colorectal Adenomas. *Cancer Epidemiology Biomarkers Prevention* 12(5):419–425, 2003.

Timko, C., Moos, R.H., Finney, J.W., and Connell, E.G. Gender differences in help-utilization and the 8-year course of alcohol abuse. *Addiction* 97(7):877–889, 2002.

Timko, C., Sutkowi, A., Pavao, J., and Kimerling, R. Women's childhood and adult adverse experiences, mental health, and binge drinking: The California Women's Health Survey. *Substance Abuse Treatment, Prevention and Policy* 3(1):15, 2008.

Tjaden, P., and Thoennes, N. Prevalence, Incidence, and Consequences of Violence Against Women: Findings from the National Violence Against Women Survey. *National Institute of Justice / Centers for Disease Control Prevention Research in Brief* Washington, DC: National Institute of Justice, 1998.

Tjaden, P., and Thoennes, N. Extent, nature, and consequences of intimate partner violence. *Findings From the National Violence Against Women Survey* (July):NCJ 181867 Washington, D.C.: U.S. Department of Justice, 2000.

Tjaden, P., and Thoennes, N. Extent, nature, and consequences of rape victimization: Findings from the National Violence Against Women Survey. *Findings From the National Violence Against Women Survey* Washington, DC: U.S. Department of Justice, National Institute of Justice, 2006.

Tolin, D.F., and Foa, E.B. Sex differences in trauma and posttraumatic stress disorder: A quantitative review of 25 years of research. *Psychological Bulletin* 132(6):959–992, 2006.

Tolstrup, J.S., Kjaer, S.K., Holst, C., Sharif, H., Munk, C., Osler, M., Schmidt, L., Andersen, A.M., and Gronbaek, M. Alcohol use as predictor for infertility in a representative population of Danish women. *Acta Obstetricia Et Gynecologica Scandinavica* 82(8):744–749, 2003.

Tonigan, J.S., and Miller, W.R. The inventory of drug use consequences (InDUC): test-retest stability and sensitivity to detect change. *Psychology of Addictive Behaviors* 16(2):165–168, 2002.

Torabi, M.R., Bailey, W.J., and Majd-Jabbari, M. Cigarette smoking as a predictor of alcohol and other drug use by children and adolescents: Evidence of the "gateway drug effect." *Journal of School Health* 63(7):302–306, 1993.

Torsch, V.L., and Xueqin Ma, G. Cross-cultural comparison of health perceptions, concerns, and coping strategies among Asian and Pacific Islander American elders. *Qualitative Health Research* 10(4):471–489, 2000.

Tough, S., Tofflemire, K., Clarke, M., and Newburn-Cook, C. Do women change their drinking behaviors while trying to conceive? An opportunity for preconception counseling. *Clinical Medicine and Research* 4(2):97–105, 2006.

Tourangeau, R., and Smith, T.W. Asking sensitive questions: The impact of data collection mode, question format, and question context. *Public Opinion Quarterly* 60(2):275–304, 1996.

Towle, L.H. Japanese-American drinking: Some results from the Joint Japanese-U.S. Alcohol Epidemiology Project. *Alcohol Health and Research World* 12(3):216–223, 1988.

Tracy, E.M., and Martin, T.C. Children's roles in the social networks of women in substance abuse treatment. *Journal of Substance Abuse Treatment* 32(1):81–88, 2007.

Trepper, T.S., McCollum, E.E., Dankoski, M.E., Davis, S.K., and LaFazia, M.A. Couples therapy for drug abusing women in an inpatient setting: A pilot study. *Contemporary Family Therapy* 22(2):201–221, 2000.

Triffleman, E. Gender differences in a controlled pilot study of psychosocial treatment in substance dependent patients with posttraumatic stress disorder: Design considerations and outcomes. *Alcoholism Treatment Quarterly* 18(3):113–126, 2000.

Triffleman, E. Issues in implementing posttraumatic stress disorder treatment outcome research in community-based treatment programs. In: Sorensen, J.L., Rawson, R.A., Guydish, J., and Zweben, J.E., eds. *Drug Abuse Treatment Through Collaboration: Practice and Research Partnerships that Work.* 1-55798-985-0 (hardcover). American Psychological Association: Washington, 2003. pp. 227–247.

Trimble, J.E., and Jumper Thurman, P. Ethnocultural considerations and strategies for providing counseling services to Native American Indians. In: Pedersen, P.B., Draguns, J.G., Lonner, W.J., and Trimble, J.E., eds. *Counseling Across Cultures.* Thousand Oaks, CA: Sage, 2002. pp. 53–91.

Tronick, E.Z., and Beeghly, M. Prenatal cocaine exposure, child development, and the compromising effects of cumulative risk. *Clinics in Perinatology* 26(1):151–171, 1999.

Tuten, M., and Jones, H.E. A partner's drug-using status impacts women's drug treatment outcome. *Drug and Alcohol Dependence* 70(3):327–330, 2003.

Tuten, M., Jones, H.E., Tran, G., and Svikis, D.S. Partner violence impacts the psychosocial and psychiatric status of pregnant, drug-dependent women. *Addictive Behaviors* 29(5):1029–1034, 2004.

Ullman, S.E., Filipas, H.H., Townsend, S.M., and Starzynski, L.L. Trauma exposure, posttraumatic stress disorder and problem drinking in sexual assault survivors. *Journal of Studies on Alcohol* 66(5):610–619, 2005.

Underhill, B.L., and Ostermann, S.E. The pain of invisibility: Issues for lesbians. In: Roth, P., ed. *Alcohol and Drugs Are Women's Issues: Vol. 1. A Review of the Issues.* Metuchen, NJ: Scarecrow Press, 1991. pp. 71–77.

United Nations General Assembly. *Declaration on the Elimination of Violence Against Women. A/RES/48/104* New York: United Nations, 1993.

Urbano-Marquez, A., Estruch, R., Fernandez-Sola, J., Nicolas, J.M., Pare, J.C., and Rubin, E. The greater risk of alcoholic cardiomyopathy and myopathy in women compared with men. *Journal of the American Medical Association* 274(2):149–154, 1995.

U.S. Census Bureau. *Census Bureau Projects Doubling of Nation's Population by 2100.* Washington, DC: U.S. Census Bureau, 2000a.

U.S. Census Bureau. *Projections of the Total Resident Population by 5-Year Age Groups, Race, and Hispanic Origin, with Special Age Categories: Middle Series, 2050 to 2070.* Washington, DC: U.S. Census Bureau, 2000b.

U.S. Census Bureau. *Census 2000 PHC-T-10: Hispanic or Latino Origin for the United States, Regions, Divisions, States, and for Puerto Rico..* Washington, DC: U.S. Census Bureau, 2001a.

U.S. Census Bureau. *Profile of General Demographic Characteristics for the United States: 2000.* Washington, DC: U.S. Census Bureau, 2001b.

U.S. Census Bureau. *Statistical Abstract of the United States, 2001: The National Data Book*. Washington, DC: U.S. Census Bureau, 2001c.

U.S. Census Bureau. Table 1: Male-female ratio by race alone or in combination and Hispanic or Latino origin for the United States. 2000. Washington, DC: U.S. Census Bureau, 2001d.

U.S. Census Bureau. Table 1: Population by race and Hispanic or Latino origin, for all ages and for 18 years and over, for the United States. 2000. Washington, DC: U.S. Census Bureau, 2001e.

U.S. Census Bureau. Table 2: Percent of population by race and Hispanic or Latino origin, for the United States, Regions, divisions, and states, and for Puerto Rico. 2000. Washington, DC: U.S. Census Bureau, 2001f.

U.S. Census Bureau. Table 4: Difference in population by race and Hispanic or Latino origin, for the United States. 1990 to 2000. *Census 2000: PHC-T-1* Washington, DC: U.S. Census Bureau, 2001g.

U.S. Census Bureau. DP-2: Profile of selected social characteristics. 2000. Census 2000 Summary File 3 (SF-3) Sample data. United States. Washington, DC: U.S. Census Bureau, 2002.

U.S. Census Bureau. Table 8. Foreign-born population by sex, citizenship status, and year of entry, for Asian alone and White alone, not Hispanic: March 2004. Current Population Survey, 2004 2004.

U.S. Census Bureau. *The American Community—Asians: 2004*. U.S. Department of Commerce, U.S. Census Bureau 2007a.

U.S. Census Bureau. *The American Community—Hispanics: 2004*. American Community Survey Reports Washington, DC: U.S. Census Bureau, 2007b.

U.S. Census Bureau. U.S. Hispanic Population Surpasses 45 Million Now 15 Percent of Total. *U.S. Census Bureau News* May 1, 2008 Washington, DC: U.S. Census Bureau, 2008.

U.S. Department of Agriculture, Economic Research Service. Rural population and migration. *ERS/USDA Briefing Room* Washington, DC: U.S. Department of Agriculture, 2007.

U.S. Department of Health and Human Services. Center for Substance Abuse Treatment comprehensive treatment model for alcohol and other drug abusing women and their children. *Blending Perspectives and Building Common Ground: A Report to Congress on Substance Abuse and Child Protection*: Appendix B. Washington, D.C.: U.S. Government Printing Office, 1999.

U.S. Department of Health and Human Services - Office on Women's Health. *Eating Disorders*. Washington, DC, 2000.

U.S. Department of Health and Human Services - Office for Civil Rights. *Standards of Privacy for Individually Identifiable Health Information: Unofficial Version, 45 CFR Parts 160 and 164*. Washington, DC: U.S. Department of Health and Human Services, Office for Civil Rights, 2002.

U.S. Department of Health and Human Services, Substance Abuse and Mental Health Services Administration, Office of Applied Studies, and Prepared by Synetics for Management Decisions Incorporated. *Treatment Episode Data Set (TEDS), 2006*. Ann Arbor, MI: Consortium for Political and Social Research, 2008a.

U.S. Department of Health and Human Services, Substance Abuse and Mental Health Services Administration, and Office of Applied Studies. *Treatment Episode Data Set (TEDS), 2006* [Computer file]. Prepared by Synectics for Management Decisions, Incorporated. ICPSR21540-V2 Ann Arbor, MI: Inter-university Consortium for Political and Social Research [producer and distributor], 2008-05-07, 2008*b*.

U.S. Department of Health and Human Services, and Office of Women's Health. Depression during and after pregnancy, 2009. http://www.womenshealth.gov/publications/ our-publications/fact-sheet/depression-pregnancy.html

U.S. Department of Health and Human Services, National Institute on Drug Abuse, and Center for Substance Abuse Treatment. DRAFT---*CSAT's Comprehensive Substance Abuse Treatment Model for Women and Their Children*. Unpublished manuscript.

U.S. Department of Housing and Urban Development. The annual homeless assessment report to Congress. Washington, DC: U.S. Department of Housing and Urban Development, 2007.

U.S. Department of Housing and Urban Development. The second annual homeless assessment report to Congress. Washington, DC: Office of Community Planning and Development, 2008.

U.S. Department of Labor. *Women in the Labor Force: A Databook*. 2006. Available on-line: http://www.bls.gov/cps/wlf-databook-2006.pdf

U.S. Preventive Services Task Force. Screening for depression: Recommendations and rationale. *Annals of Internal Medicine* 136(10):760–764, 2002.

van der Kolk, B.A., McFarlane, A.C., and Van der Hart, O. A general approach to treatment of posttraumatic stress disorder. In: van der Kolk, B.A., McFarlane, A.C., and Weisaeth, L., eds. *Traumatic Stress: The Effects of Overwhelming Experience on Mind, Body, and Society*. New York: Guilford Press, 1996. pp. 417–440.

van Etten, M.L., and Anthony, J.C. Male–female differences in transitions from first drug opportunity to first use: Searching for subgroup variation by age, race, region, and urban status. *Journal of Women's Health & Gender-Based Medicine* 10(8):797–804, 2001.

van Etten, M.L., and Neumark, Y.D. Male-female differences in the earliest stages of drug involvement. *Addiction* 94(9):1413–1419, 1999.

Van Gundy, K. Substance abuse in rural and small town America. *Reports on Rural America Volume 1, Number 2* Durham, New Hampshire: Carsey Institute, 2006.

Van Thiel, D.H., Gavaler, J.S., Rosenblum, E., and Tarter, R.E. Ethanol, its metabolism and hepatotoxicity as well as its gonadal effects: Effects of sex. *Pharmacology and Therapeutics* 41(1-2):27–48, 1989.

van Wormer, K., and Askew, E. Substance-abusing women and eating disorders. In: Straussner, S.L.A., and Zelvin, E., eds. *Gender and Addictions: Men and Women in Treatment*. Northvale, NJ: Jason Aronson, 1997. pp. 243–262.

VanDeMark, N.R., Russell, L.A., O'Keefe, M., Finkelstein, N., Noether, C.D., and Gampel, J.C. Children of mothers with histories of substance abuse, mental illness, and trauma. *Journal of Community Psychology* 33(4):445–459, 2005.

Vannicelli, M. Treatment outcome of alcoholic women: The state of the art in relation to sex bias and expectancy effects. In: Wilsnack, S.C., and Beckman, L., eds. *Alcohol Problems in Women: Antecedents, Consequences, and Intervention.* New York: Guilford, 1984. pp. 369–412.

VanZile-Tamsen, C., Testa, M., Harlow, L.L., and Livingston, J.A. A measurement model of women's behavioral risk taking. *Health Psychology* 25(2):249–254, 2006.

Varan, L.R., Gillieson, M.S., Skene, D.S., and Sarwer-Foner, G.J. ECT in an acutely psychotic pregnant woman with actively aggressive (homicidal) impulses. *Canadian Journal of Psychiatry* 30(5):363–367, 1985.

Vega, W.A., Alderete, E., Kolody, B., and Aguilar-Gaxiola, S. Illicit drug use among Mexicans and Mexican Americans in California: The effects of gender and acculturation. *Addiction* 93(12):1839–1850, 1998.

Vega, W.A., Sribney, W.M., and Achara-Abrahams, I. Co-Occurring alcohol, drug and other psychiatric disorders among Mexican-Origin people in the United States. *American Journal of Public Health* 93(7):1057–1064, 2003.

Velez, M.L., Jansson, L.M., Montoya, I.D., Schweitzer, W., Golden, A., and Svikis, D. Parenting knowledge among substance abusing women in treatment. *Journal of Substance Abuse Treatment* 27(3):215–222, 2004.

Velez, M.L., Montoya, I.D., Jansson, L.M., Walters, V., Svikis, D., Jones, H.E., Chilcoat, H., and Campbell, J. Exposure to violence among substance-dependent pregnant women and their children. *Journal of Substance Abuse Treatment* 30(1):31–38, 2006.

Vernon, I., and Jumper Thurman, P. The changing face of HIV/AIDS among native populations. *Journal of Psychoactive Drugs* 37(3):247–255, 2005.

Vernon, I.S. American Indian women, HIV/AIDS, and health disparity. *Substance Use & Misuse* 42(4):741–752, 2007.

Visscher, W.A., Feder, M., Burns, A.M., Brady, T.M., and Bray, R.M. The impact of smoking and other substance use by urban women on the birthweight of their infants. *Substance Use & Misuse* 38(8):1063–1093, 2003.

Vogel, L.C., and Marshall, L.L. PTSD symptoms and partner abuse: low income women at risk. *Journal of Traumatic Stress* 14(3):569–584, 2001.

Volk, R.J., Steinbauer, J.R., and Cantor, SB. Patient factors influencing variation in the use of preventive interventions for alcohol abuse by primary care physicians. *Journal of Studies on Alcohol* 57(2):203–209, 1996.

Volkman, S. Music therapy and the treatment of trauma-induced dissociative disorders. *Arts in Psychotherapy* 20(3):243–251, 1993.

Volpicelli, J.R., Markman, I., Monterosso, J., Filing, J., and O'Brien, C.P. Psychosocially enhanced treatment for cocaine-dependent mothers: Evidence of efficacy. *Journal of Substance Abuse Treatment* 18(1):41–49, 2000.

Wagner, C.L., Katikaneni, L.D., Cox, T.H., and Ryan, R.M. The impact of prenatal drug exposure on the neonate. *Obstetrics and Gynecology Clinics of North America* 25(1):169–194, 1998.

Wakabayashi, C., and Donato, K.M. Does caregiving increase poverty among women in later life? Evidence from the health and retirement survey. *Journal of Health and Social Behavior* 47(3):258–274, 2006.

Wakschlag, L.S., Leventhal, B.L., Pine, D.S., Pickett, K.E., and Carter, A.S. Elucidating early mechanisms of developmental psychopathology: the case of prenatal smoking and disruptive behavior. *Child Development* 77(4):893–906, 2006.

Wakschlag, L.S., Pickett, K.E., Cook E Jr, Benowitz, N.L., and Leventhal, B.L. Maternal smoking during pregnancy and severe antisocial behavior in offspring: a review. *American Journal of Public Health* 92(6):966–974, 2002.

Walitzer, K.S., and Dearing, R.L. Gender differences in alcohol and substance use relapse. *Clinical Psychology Review* 26(2):128–148, 2006.

Wallace, B.C. Crack cocaine smokers as adult children of alcoholics: The dysfunctional family link. *Journal of Substance Abuse Treatment* 7(2):89–100, 1990.

Walton-Moss, B., and McCaul, M.E. Factors associated with lifetime history of drug treatment among substance dependent women. *Addictive Behaviors* 31(2):246–253, 2006.

Wampold, B.E. *The Great Psychotherapy Debate: Models, Methods, and Findings.* Mahwah, NJ: Lawrence Erlbaum Associates, Publishers, 2001.

Wang, J., and Patten, S.B. Prospective study of frequent heavy alcohol use and the risk of major depression in the Canadian general population. *Depression and Anxiety* 15(1):42–45, 2002.

Warren, M., Frost-Pineda, K., and Gold, M. Body mass index and marijuana use. *Journal of Addictive Diseases* 24(3):95–100, 2005.

Washington, O.G., and Moxley, D.P. Group interventions with low-income African American women recovering from chemical dependency. *Health and Social Work* 28(2):146–156, 2003.

Waterson, E.J., and Murray-Lyon, I.M. Are the CAGE question outdated? *British Journal of Addiction* 83(9):1113–1115, 1988.

Waxman, B.F. Hatred: The unacknowledged dimension in violence against disabled people. *Sexuality and Disability* 9(3):185–199, 1991.

Wayment, H.A., and Peplau, L.A. Social support and well-being among lesbian and heterosexual women: A structural modeling approach. *Personality & Social Psychology Bulletin* 21(11):1189–1199, 1995.

Weathers, F.W., Litz, B.T., Herman, D.S., Huska, J.A., and Keane, T.M. *The PTSD Checklist: Reliability, Validity, & Diagnostic Utility. Paper presented at the Annual Meeting of the International Society for Traumatic Stress Studies*, San Antonio, TX, October. 1993.

Weatherspoon, A.J., Park, J.Y., and Johnson, R.C. A family study of homeland Korean alcohol use. *Addictive Behaviors* 26(1):101–113, 2001.

Webster, J., Linnane, J.W., Dibley, L.M., and Pritchard, M. Improving antenatal recognition of women at risk for postnatal depression. *Australian and New Zealand Journal of Obstetrics and Gynaecology* 40(4):409–412, 2000.

Wechsberg, W.M., Zule, W.A., Riehman, K.S., Luseno, W.K., and Lam, W.K. African-American crack abusers and drug treatment initiation: Barriers and effects of a pretreatment intervention. *Substance Abuse Treatment, Prevention and Policy* 2:10, 2007.

Weiderpass, E., Ye, W., Tamimi, R., Trichopolous, D., Nyren, O., Vainio, H., and Adami, H.O. Alcoholism and risk for cancer of the cervix uteri, vagina, and vulva. *Cancer Epidemiology, Biomarkers and Prevention* 10(8):899–901, 2001.

Weir, B.W., Stark, M.J., Fleming, D.W., He, H., and Tesselaar, H. Revealing drug use to prenatal providers: Who tells or who is asked? In: Stevens, S.J., and Wexler, H.K., eds. *Women and Substance Abuse: Gender Transparency.* New York: Haworth Press, 1998. pp. 161–176.

Weisner, C., Delucchi, K., Matzger, H., and Schmidt, L. The role of community services and informal support on five-year drinking trajectories of alcohol dependent and problem drinkers. *Journal of Studies on Alcohol* 64(6):862–873, 2003a.

Weisner, C., Matzger, H., and Kaskutas, L.A. How important is treatment? One-year outcomes of treated and untreated alcohol-dependent individuals. *Addiction* 98(7):901–911, 2003b.

Weisner, C., Mertens, J., Tam, T., and Moore, C. Factors affecting the initiation of substance abuse treatment in managed care. *Addiction* 96(5):705–716, 2001.

Weiss, R.D., Martinez-Raga, J., Griffin, M.L., Greenfield, S.F., and Hufford, C. Gender differences in cocaine dependent patients: A 6 month follow-up study. *Drug and Alcohol Dependence* 44(1):35–40, 1997.

Welch, S.S. A review of the literature on the epidemiology of parasuicide in the general population. *Psychiatric Services* 52(3):368–375, 2001.

Welle, D., Falkin, G.P., and Jainchill, N. Current approaches to drug treatment for women offenders: Project WORTH, Women's Options for Recovery, Treatment, and Health. *Journal of Substance Abuse Treatment* 15(2):151–163, 1998.

Wellisch, J., Prendergast, M.L., and Anglin, M.D. Needs assessment and services for drug-abusing women offenders: Results from a national survey of community-based treatment programs. *Women and Criminal Justice* 8(1):27–60, 1996.

West, C., and Zimmerman, D.H. Doing gender. *Gender and Society* 1:125–151, 1987.

Wetter, D.W., Fiore, M.C., Jorenby, D.E., Kenford, S.L., Smith, S.S., and Baker, T.B. Gender differences in smoking cessation. *Journal of Consulting and Clinical Psychology* 67(4):555–562, 1999.

Wexler, H.K., Cuadrado, M., and Stevens, S.J. Residential treatment for women: Behavioral and psychological outcomes. In: Stevens, S.J., and Wexler, H.K., eds. *Women and Substance Abuse: Gender Transparency.* New York: Haworth Press, 1998. pp. 213–233.

White, W.L. Recovery across the life cycle from alcohol/other drug problems: Pathways, styles, developmental stages. *Alcoholism Treatment Quarterly* 24(1–2):185–201, 2006.

White, W.L., and Whiters, D.L. Faith-based recovery: Its historical roots. *Counselor Magazine* 6(5):58–62, 2005.

Wilcox, S., Evenson, K.R., Aragaki, A., Wassertheil-Smoller, S., Mouton, C.P., and Loevinger, B.L. The effects of widowhood on physical and mental health, health behaviors, and health outcomes: The Women's Health Initiative. *Health Psychology* 22(5):513–522, 2003.

Wilkins, A. Substance Abuse and TANF. *Welfare Reform*: 1-12. Denver, CO: National Conference of State Legislators 2003.

Williams, D.R. Race and health: Basic questions, emerging directions. *Annals of Epidemiology* 7(5):322–333, 1997.

Williams, D. R. Racial/ethnic variations in women's health: the social embeddedness of health. *American Journal of Public Health*, 92, 588–597, 2002.

Wilsnack, R.W., and Cheloha, R. Women's roles and problem drinking across the lifespan. *Social Problems* 34(3):231–248, 1987.

Wilsnack, R.W., Wilsnack, S.C., Kristjanson, A.F., and Harris, T.B. Ten-year prediction of women's drinking behavior in a nationally representative sample. *Women's Health* 4(3):199–230, 1998a.

Wilsnack, R.W., Wilsnack, S.C., Kristjanson, A.F., Harris, T.R., and Vogeltanz, N.D. *"Drinking in couples: How is partners' consumption connected?"* Paper presented at the Annual Scientific Meeting of the Research Society on Alcoholism, Hilton Head, SC, June, 1998b.

Wilsnack, S.C. Barriers to treatment for alcoholic women. *Addiction and Recovery* 11(4):10–12, 1991.

Wilson, D.J. Drug Use, Testing, and Treatment in Jails. Washington, DC: Bureau of Justice Statistics 2000.

Wilt, S., and Olson, S. Prevalence of domestic violence in the United States. *Journal of the American Medical Women's Association* 51(3):77–82, 1996.

Winhusen, T., Kropp, F., Babcock, D., Hague, D., Erickson, S.J., Renz, C., Rau, L., Lewis, D., Leimberger, J., and Somoza, E. Motivational enhancement therapy to improve treatment utilization and outcome in pregnant substance users. *Journal of Substance Abuse Treatment* 2007.

Winslow, B.T., Voorhees, K.I., and Pehl, K.A. Methamphetamine abuse. *American Family Physician* 76(8):1169–1174, 2007.

Winters, J., Fals-Stewart, W., O'Farrell, T.J., Birchler, G.R., and Kelley, M.L. Behavioral couples therapy for female substance-abusing patients: Effects on substance use and relationship adjustment. *Journal of Consulting and Clinical Psychology* 70(2):344–355, 2002.

Wise, L., and Correia, A. A review of nonpharmacologic and pharmacologic therapies for smoking cessation. (cover story). *Formulary* 43(2):44–64, 2008.

Wobie, K., Eyler, F.D., Conlon, M., Clarke, L., and Behnke, M. Women and children in residential treatment: Outcomes for mothers and their infants. *Journal of Drug Issues* 27(3):585–606, 1997.

Wolpe, J. *The practice of behavior therapy.* 1st ed. ed. New York: Pergamon Press, 1969.

Wright, N.M., Tompkins, C.N., and Sheard, L. Is peer injecting a form of intimate partner abuse? A qualitative study of the experiences of women drug users. *Health & Social Care in the Community* 15(5):417–425, 2007.

Young, A.M., and Boyd, C. Sexual trauma, substance abuse, and treatment success in a sample of African American women who smoke crack cocaine. *Substance Abuse* 21(1):9–19, 2000.

Young, N.K., and Gardner, S.L. *Implementing Welfare Reform: Solutions to the Substance Abuse Problem.* Irvine, CA: Children and Family Futures, 1997.

Young, N.K., Gardner, S.L., and Dennis, K. *Responding to Alcohol and Other Drug Problems in Child Welfare: Weaving Together Practice and Policy.* Washington, DC: Child Welfare League of America, 1998.

Young, R.M., Friedman, S.R., and Case, P. Exploring an HIV paradox: an ethnography of sexual minority women injectors. *Journal of Lesbian Studies.* 9(3):103–116, 2005.

Zambrana, R.E., Ell, K., Dorrington, C., Wachsman, L., and Hodge, D. The relationship between psychosocial status of immigrant Latino mothers and use of emergency pediatric services. *Health and Social Work* 19(2):93–102, 1994.

Zanis, D.A., McLellan, A.T., Cnaan, R.A., and Randall, M. Reliability and validity of the Addiction Severity Index with a homeless sample. *Journal of Substance Abuse Treatment* 11(6):541–548, 1994.

Zerbe, K.J. *The Body Betrayed: Women, Eating Disorders, and Treatment.* Washington, DC: American Psychiatric Press, 1993.

Zhang, S.M., Lee, I.M., Manson, J.E., Cook, N.R., Willett, W.C., and Buring, J.E. Alcohol consumption and breast cancer risk in the Women's Health Study. *American Journal of Epidemiology* 165(6):667–676, 2007.

Zilberman, M.L., Tavares, H., Andrade, A.G., and el-Guebaly, N. The impact of an outpatient program for women with substance use-related disorders on retention. *Substance Use and Misuse* 38(14):2109–2124, 2003.

Zilm, D.H., and Sellers, E.M. The quantitative assessment of physical dependence on opiates. *Drug and Alcohol Dependence* 3(6):419–428, 1978.

Zlotnick, C., Franchino, K., St Claire, N., Cox, K., and St John, M. The impact of outpatient drug services on abstinence among pregnant and parenting women. *Journal of Substance Abuse Treatment* 13(3):195–202, 1996.

Zlotnick, C., Najavits, L.M., Rohsenow, D.J., and Johnson, D.M. A cognitive–behavioral treatment for incarcerated women with substance abuse disorder and posttraumatic stress disorder: findings from a pilot study. *Journal of Substance Abuse Treatment* 25(2):99–105, 2003.

Zolopa, A.R., Hahn, J.A., Gorter, R., Miranda, J., Wlodarczyk, D., Peterson, J., Pilote, L., and Moss, A.R. HIV and tuberculosis infection in San Francisco's homeless adults. Prevalence and risk factors in a representative sample. *JAMA: The Journal of the American Medical Association* 272(6):455–461, 1994.

Zuckerman, B., Frank, D., and Brown, E. Overview of the effects of abuse and drugs on pregnancy and offspring. In: Chiang, C.N., and Finnegan, L.P., eds. *Medications Development for the Treatment of Pregnant Addicts and Their Infants.* NIDA Research Monograph 149. NIH Publication No. 95-3891. Rockville, MD: National Institute on Drug Abuse, 1995. pp. 16–38.

Zule, W.A., Flannery, B.A., Wechsberg, W.M., and Lam, W.K. Alcohol use among out-of-treatment crack using African -American women. *American Journal of Drug & Alcohol Abuse* 28(3):525, 2002.

Zule, W.A., Lam, W.K., and Wechsberg, W.M. Treatment readiness among out-of-treatment African-American crack users. *Journal of Psychoactive Drugs* 35(4):503–510, 2003.

Zweben, J.E. Psychiatric problems among alcohol and other drug dependent women. *Journal of Psychoactive Drugs* 28(4):345–366, 1996.

Zywiak, W.H., Stout, R.L., Trefry, W.B., Glasser, I., Connors, G.J., Maisto, S.A., and Westerberg, V.S. Alcohol relapse repetition, gender, and predictive validity. *Journal of Substance Abuse Treatment* 30(4):349–353, 2006.

Appendix B: CSAT's Comprehensive Substance Abuse Treatment Model for Women and Their Children

By the CSAT Women, Youth and Families Task Force

Background

In the early 1990s, Congress appropriated funds to the newly created Substance Abuse and Mental Health Services Administration (SAMHSA), Center for Substance Abuse Treatment (CSAT) to support long-term residential substance abuse treatment programs for women with children. Two separate demonstration programs were funded, including the Residential Women and Children's (RWC) program, and the Pregnant and Postpartum Women and Children's (PPW) program. Based in part on the experiences of the RWC and PPW programs, CSAT published a "Comprehensive Treatment Model for Alcohol and Other Drug-Abusing Women and Their Children" in order to help substance abuse treatment providers develop program services to meet the comprehensive needs of the women and children served by these and other programs. The model was included in a 1994 CSAT publication, *Practical Approaches in the Treatment of Women Who Abuse Alcohol and Other Drugs*.

This model recognized that there was an important difference between "treatment that addresses alcohol and other drug abuse only" and "treatment that addresses the full range of women's needs." As stated in the model

> Treatment that addresses the full range of a woman's needs is associated with increasing abstinence and improvement in other measures of recovery, including parenting skills and overall emotional health. Treatment that addresses alcohol and other drug abuse only may well fail and contribute to a higher potential for relapse (CSAT 1994*f*).

CSAT's model remains an important contribution toward describing an approach to working with women that recognizes the importance of gender in the design and delivery of services for women and their families.

Since 1994, the field has gained additional insights about critical needs of women and children and the role that partners and fathers play regarding these needs. The knowledge gained in the past decade should drive the delivery of services to women. These insights include the following:

- Psychological differences between men and women and, in particular, the heightened importance that women place on relationships have a great impact on both women's gateways into addiction and relapse once in recovery. A woman's focus within relationships is often to serve as "caretaker," a role that can result in a woman not attending to her own needs. Positive, therapeutic relationships, on the other hand, can also act as powerful tools for supporting a woman's recovery.
- Women self-medicate with addictive substances to mask pain associated with underlying trauma, including past and ongoing domestic violence as well as childhood abuse and neglect. The high prevalence of a history of trauma among women receiving substance abuse treatment heightens the need for substance abuse treatment to recognize the critical impact of trauma on the woman's recovery.
- The prevalence of co-occurring mental health disorders among women receiving substance abuse treatment has also come to light over the past decade and raises the need for providing coordinated services to address both substance use and mental health disorders.
- Women appear to be significantly affected by the service systems they depend on, including welfare agencies and child welfare agencies, which tend to operate independently, with different timetables and perspectives on the purposes of recovery.
- A new understanding has arisen about the benefits of women's economic self-sufficiency

in the process of long-term recovery. This is partly a result of the pressures of society, exemplified by welfare reform and data indicating that gainful employment can be a protective influence for preventing relapse.

- The field has also come to appreciate that children of women in treatment have many of their own needs that cannot simply be addressed by the provision of child care and residential living space. These needs are addressed when children are provided services directly, as well as when the needs of their parents are met.
- Both mothers and fathers should receive the education and support necessary to prepare them for the responsibility of parenthood, understanding that the roles fathers play in families are diverse and related to cultural and community norms, the health and well-being of the father, and the viability of the parents' relationship to one another.
- Changes in family composition play a role in supporting women and recovery. In 1960, fewer than 10 million children did not live with their fathers (U.S. Bureau of Labor Statistics n.d.). By the turn of the century, the number had risen to nearly 25 million. More than one-third of these children will not see their fathers at all during the course of a year. Studies show that children who grow up without responsible fathers are significantly more likely to experience poverty, perform poorly in school, engage in criminal activity, and abuse drugs and alcohol (U.S. Department of Health and Human Services 2000a).

This update to the model considers the needs of women, their children, and their families in the context of their community and culture.

An Evolving Paradigm

As was the case with the earlier version, the purpose of this model is to

Foster the development of state-of-the-art recovery for women with alcohol and other drug dependence and to foster the healthy development of the children of substance abusing women. The model is a guide that can be adapted by communities and used to build comprehensive programs over time (CSAT 1994*f*, p. 267).

CSAT's Comprehensive Treatment Model continues to reinforce that confidentiality and informed consent, as well as the establishment of universal precautions against the spread of sexually transmitted and other infectious diseases, are essential throughout all aspects of treatment (CSAT 1994*e*, 2000*d*).

In addition to incorporating the new knowledge about the common histories and service needs of women and their children, this model goes a step further by delineating the relational elements of the service continuum that have an impact on treatment for women. These elements shown in Figure B-1 below and are categorized as

- Clinical treatment services: those services necessary to address the medical and biopsychosocial issues of addiction
- Clinical support services: services that assist clients in their recovery
- Community support services: those services and community resources outside of treatment but within a community that serve as an underpinning or support system for the recovering individual

In parallel, the model also describes clinical treatment and clinical support services for children of women in treatment.

Research has established that there are many paths to recovery from alcohol and drug problems. Some women resolve their alcohol and drug problems with individual and family supports and without any outside intervention. Others recover with support from self-help groups such as Alcoholics Anonymous and/ or the faith community. Still others have found recovery through formal treatment interventions. A variety of factors can influence which of these paths is successful, including the severity of the problems and the support systems available to women with substance use disorders.

To achieve the best outcomes at the lowest cost, SAMHSA encourages the establishment of a comprehensive continuum of recovery. The full complement of these services is appropriate for many women who meet the Diagnostic and Statistical Manual of Mental Disorders, Fourth Edition (DSM-IV) diagnostic criteria for substance use disorders. However, not all services and/or interventions are needed by every woman in treatment or recovery for substance dependence, and those who meet the diagnostic criteria for substance abuse may require a less comprehensive range of services than those who are substance dependent. Similarly, women with a range of family, social, and economic supports may not require a full complement of services while those who have fewer naturally occurring supports may require more services from the formal health, social, and economic supportive systems.

The array of services described below does not need to be provided by a single entity, but in most instances will be provided by a consortium of addiction treatment, health, and human service providers. The continuum is not specific to philosophies of treatment and recovery, modality, or setting. It is a generic framework within which providers can conceptualize service arrays, service capabilities, and appropriate managerial and administrative processes.

Methods of implementing each service, the manner and setting in which different services are delivered, and other ingredients of the model should be based upon an assessment and patient placement determination that considers (1) the needs of the individual, and (2) the extent to which the continuum of services is available in the community.

To better understand the model, it is helpful to view services as a series of interwoven and interdependent circles of care that are necessary to support the recovery process for women.

> In the Navajo Nation, the woven basket is actually a series of concentric rings, one lying within the other, expanding outward and upward until the entire basket is shaped. By itself, one ring can hold nothing and bear no load. When

Interrelated Elements in the Comprehensive Treatment Model

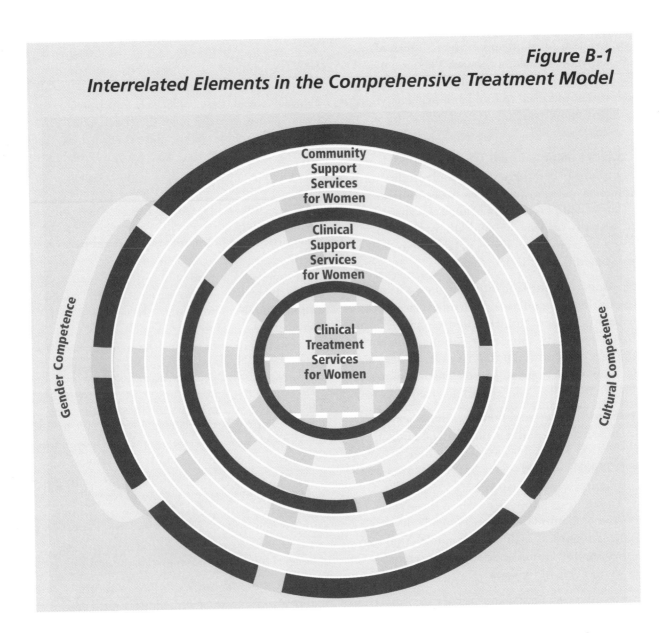

bound together, the circles join, gain strength, and what before could hold nothing now holds stones for building nations and water for building bodies.

The concept of interdependence is critical to understanding the model. Each circle requires the existence of the other two and yet they are depicted as dotted lines to illustrate their permeability. The three circles together comprise comprehensive treatment, and any provider seeking to emulate the model must also ensure that there is an interdependent relationship among the three systems.

Borrowing again from the basket metaphor, the circles are also three-dimensional as a basket must be and, as such, have binders that interweave and hold the circles together. Likewise, in treatment, there are activities that weave through each circle, helping to bind the service continuum together. Housing is a good example. Some people with substance use disorders are functionally homeless and, thus, the issue of housing permeates clinical treatment, clinical support, and community support.

A final and critical aspect of how the circles are interrelated requires the inclusion of two concepts that provide the foundational support to the network of comprehensive care: cultural competence and gender competence. These concepts are graphically displayed as the handles to pick up and use the basket. For a system of care to be comprehensive in nature, it must have cultural and gender competence at all levels of treatment and support. The terms cultural competence and gender competence mean more than knowledge about culture or gender. The terms require practitioners to be knowledgeable, understanding, and sensitive to the milieu from which the woman comes regarding the issues and concerns she may bring to treatment. These include the socioeconomic context of her background; her sexual identity; the sources of potential anger, hurt, and fear;

and disconnection from family, friends, and community. Both cultural competence and gender competence require recognition of the biases that may exist within the programs and practitioner that will impact treatment and relationships with clients.

Clinical Treatment Services

As shown in Figure B-2, the fabric of the basket is interwoven with a range of clinical treatment services. These services include the following elements: outreach and engagement, screening, detoxification, crisis intervention, assessment, treatment planning, case management, substance abuse counseling and education,

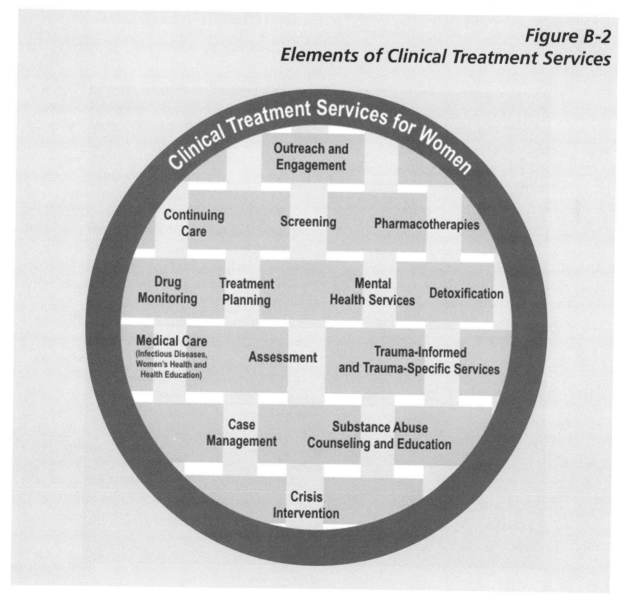

Figure B-2
Elements of Clinical Treatment Services

trauma-informed and trauma-specific services and psychoeducational therapies, medical care (including treatment for infectious diseases, women's health, and health education), pharmacotherapies, mental health services, drug monitoring, and continuing care (these services are defined and further explained in the last section of this appendix). While arguments could be made to support the addition of other core services to this continuum, experience has shown that these elements of service are typical of those that are under the core umbrella of treatment programs.

For most women in treatment, particularly those burdened with issues such as intergenerational poverty, violence, and homelessness, time-limited clinical treatment services alone will not likely result in sustained recovery. Women with multiple needs will need support from other systems, designated clinical support, and community support to achieve success in recovery.

Addiction affects women's connections and relationships, causing them to leave or abandon many of the relational systems upon which they formerly depended—family, friends, and roots in the community. Thus, for a woman to succeed in treatment, deliberate steps must connect her with the support structures that allow her to reverse the isolation and fragmentation often synonymous with addiction and reconnect with these important relationships. While some of that occurs within the context of clinical treatment itself, other aspects of the reconnection process occur as a result of clinical support and community support services.

Clinical Support Services

Within this circle is an array of services that, by themselves, are not necessarily part of the treatment modality but, like ball bearings to machinery, make the treatment modality work. These support services (shown in Figure B-3) include primary healthcare services, life skills, parenting and child development education, family programs, educational remediation

and support, employment readiness services, linkages with the legal and child welfare systems, housing support, advocacy, and recovery support services. Elsewhere in this appendix, similar circles are identified that relate to the special needs of children. While introduced separately, they are inextricably intertwined with those of the parenting woman.

Clinical support services are not ancillary services, they are a critical part of treatment designed to prevent relapse. This model suggests that these services are not enhancements of treatment but, rather, critical elements of treatment designed to promote overall well-being and prevent relapse.

Community Support Services

Community support services are those that must be available in the community to ensure long-term recovery. These services, as shown in Figure B-4, include recovery management, recovery community support services, housing services, family strengthening, child care, transportation, Temporary Assistance for Needy Families (TANF) linkages, employer support services, vocational and academic education services, and faith-based organization support. This ring represents some areas that are not typically included in the service array for women, but women's treatment program staff and policy analysts increasingly view these elements as critical to long-term recovery.

Over the last decade, the concept of relapse prevention and aftercare evolved into the approach known as continuing care. This approach recognizes both the need to provide continuing support to a person in recovery and that treatment providers share some of the responsibility for providing this support. The concept of community support operationalizes continuing care by recognizing the systems and services that must exist in the community in order to make continuing care a meaningful reality.

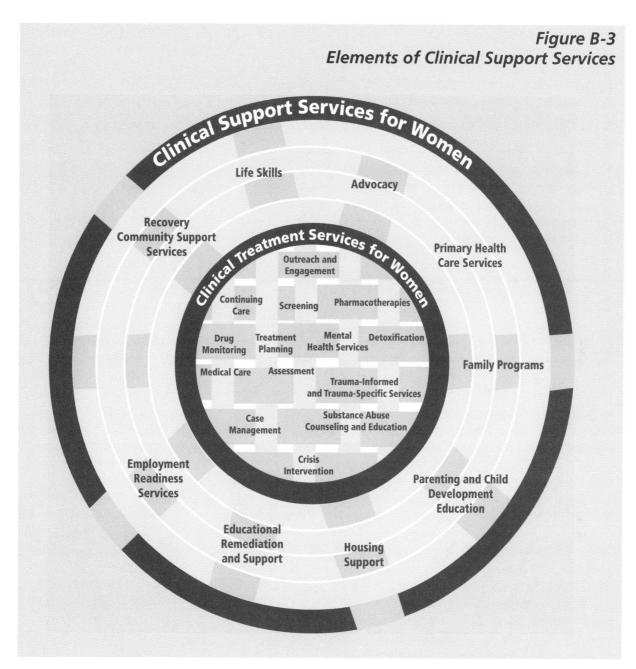

Figure B-3
Elements of Clinical Support Services

Clinical Support Services for Women

Life Skills

Advocacy

Recovery Community Support Services

Clinical Treatment Services for Women

Outreach and Engagement

Primary Health Care Services

Continuing Care

Screening

Pharmacotherapies

Drug Monitoring

Treatment Planning

Mental Health Services

Detoxification

Medical Care

Assessment

Family Programs

Trauma-Informed and Trauma-Specific Services

Case Management

Substance Abuse Counseling and Education

Crisis Intervention

Parenting and Child Development Education

Employment Readiness Services

Educational Remediation and Support

Housing Support

Taken together, as shown in Figure B-4, clinical treatment, clinical supports, and community supports complete the basket and provide the comprehensive services needed by many women in substance abuse treatment. Implicit in the model is the responsibility of providers to look inward to their own resources as well as outward to community partners' resources to ensure that the elements of comprehensive services are made available in the community.

The Next Generation: Services for Children of Women in Substance Abuse Treatment

While it is important to provide the comprehensive array of services and supports to all women, women who are also mothers demand increased attention to their unique roles as parents and their children require additional services and supports. Treatment agencies

Elements of Community Support Services

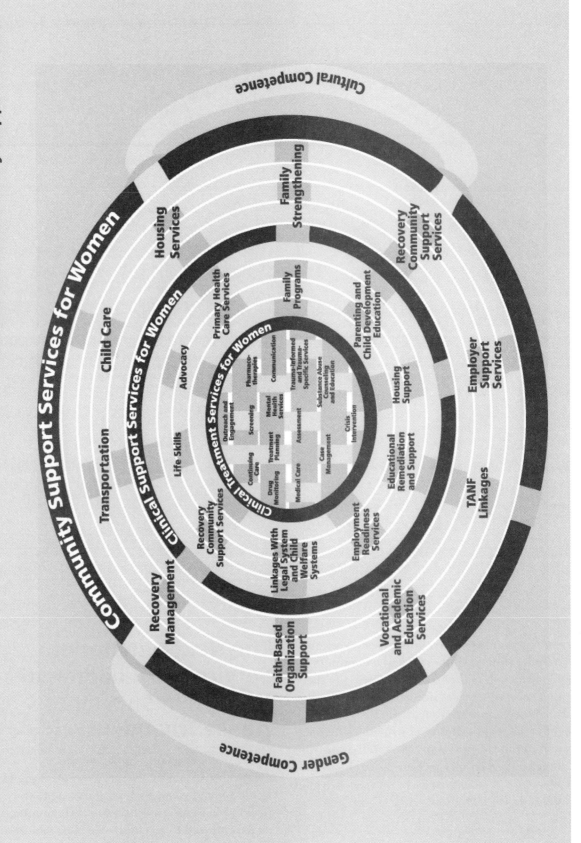

have come to understand that, for women who are mothers, their children are a major factor influencing why they enter, complete, and/or leave treatment. Mothers in treatment are, in most instances, the custodial parent who carries out the tasks of parenting and child-rearing. In some cases, the mother in treatment may not currently have custody and the daily responsibility for the care of her children. Those cases require special considerations by treatment providers to assist the woman in her efforts to regain custody if appropriate, and, when regaining custody is not an option, assist the mother as she transitions in the loss of her children.

Among mothers in treatment with custody of their children, the experience of the RWC and PPW programs is clear: Providing child care alone is an insufficient response to the needs of children whose mothers abuse alcohol and/or drugs. In many cases, the children themselves need services ranging from interventions for fetal alcohol spectrum disorders, to intervention services for childhood mental health disorders and developmental delays. Treatment programs have responded to the needs of children and have reported that treatment for women and their children requires a whole-family perspective in service delivery and in clinical practice.

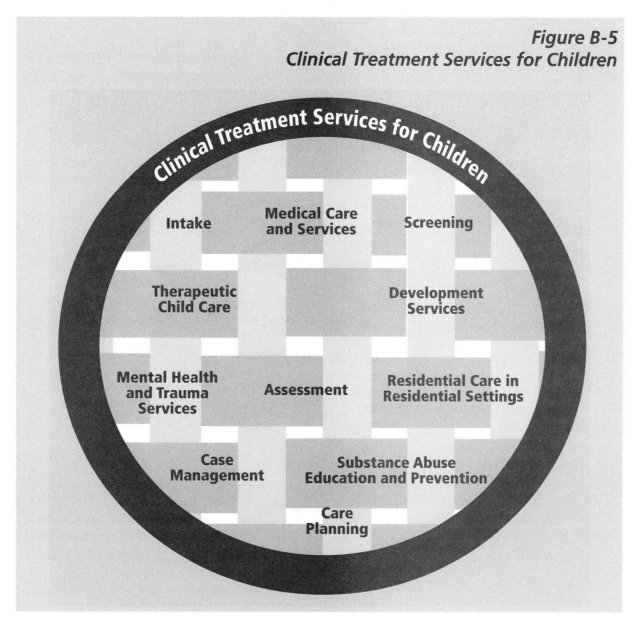

Figure B-5
Clinical Treatment Services for Children

Clinical Treatment Services for Children

Intake

Medical Care and Services

Screening

Therapeutic Child Care

Development Services

Mental Health and Trauma Services

Assessment

Residential Care in Residential Settings

Case Management

Substance Abuse Education and Prevention

Care Planning

Children's clinical treatment needs are depicted in Figure B-5. Their clinical needs include intake; screening and assessment of the full range of medical, developmental, emotional-related factors; care planning; residential care; case management; therapeutic child care; substance abuse education and prevention; medical care and services; developmental services; and mental health and trauma services.

In addition, children need supports that reinforce their individual needs. These clinical support services are shown in Figure B-6 and include the concepts of cultural competence and developmentally appropriate services. As with the women's model, cultural competence is a critical aspect and is depicted as the handles

for using the service array in the model. Needs and services for young children must be tailored to their developmental status and cognition. Clinical support services include primary health care, onsite or nearby child care, mental health and remediation services, prevention services, recreational opportunities, educational services and advocacy, advocacy in other service arenas and with legal issues, and peer supports for recovery such as self-help and mutual support groups.

Regardless of the child's current custody status, services to address children's needs should be coordinated, and when appropriate, should be integrated with their primary caregivers' treatment and case plans to ensure that the whole

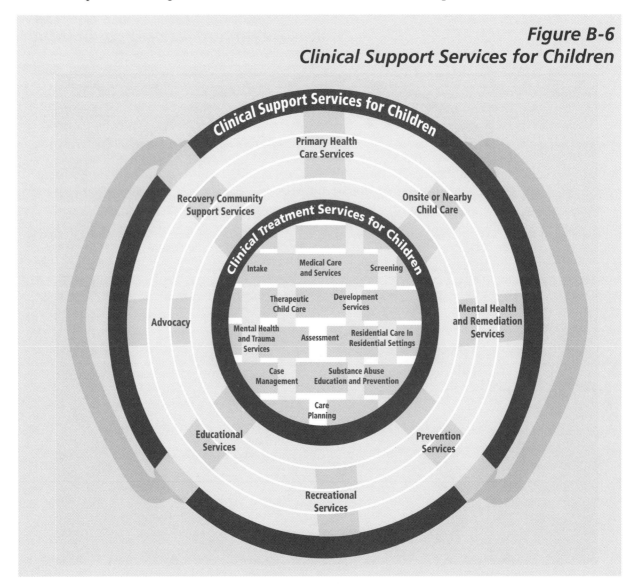

Figure B-6
Clinical Support Services for Children

Clinical Support Services for Children

Primary Health Care Services

Recovery Community Support Services

Onsite or Nearby Child Care

Clinical Treatment Services for Children

Intake   Medical Care and Services   Screening

Therapeutic Child Care   Development Services

Advocacy

Mental Health and Trauma Services   Assessment   Residential Care In Residential Settings

Mental Health and Remediation Services

Case Management   Substance Abuse Education and Prevention

Care Planning

Educational Services

Prevention Services

Recreational Services

family's needs are met. Ensuring that parents' and children's case plans are in harmony in terms of timing and strategies is imperative for family recovery. While children can be significant motivators for women to seek treatment, without proper planning, caring for children can also produce stress that may contribute to relapse.

Taken together, providing comprehensive services for women and their children (as shown in Figure B-7) requires treatment agencies to provide an array of direct services and to establish linkages to a wide range of supports and community resources. This is no easy feat. The need for coordination and collaborative relationships among agencies and service systems can tax scarce resources in staff time and expertise to establish those bonds. While it may seem overwhelming to consider all of the various linkages needed, treatment agencies can prioritize their most immediate need for collaboration by understanding the most immediate needs of their clients.

Putting the Elements Together

The elements of treatment for women, including those who are mothers, are described below. Together the elements make up the continuum of services that women and women who are mothers need to succeed in substance abuse treatment. The intensity, duration, and type of treatment will vary depending upon the assessment and diagnosis of the woman and the needs of her child or children. The manner in which services are delivered will also vary, depending on factors specific to the woman and the child, including culture, race, ethnicity, social class, age, and sexual orientation. Treatment intensity, philosophy, and methods will vary depending on the needs of the client, reimbursement policies, and treatment methods used by providers.

Clinical Treatment Services

Clinical treatment services are generally provided directly by the substance abuse treatment provider. As such, they are considered core services. Providers recognize that providing core services without support services is likely to result in less than optimum outcomes for women and children over the longer term; thus, support services are pivotal to the successful treatment of women and children.

Clinical treatment services for women

- *Outreach, engagement, and pretreatment.* Activities designed to assist clients in engaging in treatment are essential elements of service, falling into the broad category of outreach, engagement, and pretreatment services. For many women, these services break the ice and help them overcome the shame and denial that often serve as obstacles to treatment. Same-day services, visits to programs, and familiarization with program staff should be facilitated whenever possible. Identification of and attention to women's immediate needs (e.g., legal, health, safety) are important aspects of engagement, even if those problems cannot be resolved immediately. When a program slot is not immediately available, services should be offered to keep women connected to the treatment organization. Outreach for women must address barriers that keep women from treatment, such as fear of reprisal from significant others and family members, fear of not being able to care for children or the loss of custody, as well as language and/or cultural barriers. Outreach must also address systemic barriers such as lack of money or insurance, waiting lists, lack of treatment for pregnant women, absence of child care, lack of transportation, inability to find sustaining employment, and need for time to address demands of other systems, such as child welfare and TANF stipulations.
- *Screening.* Intake screening is part of the admissions process and can be an important strategy that assists in engaging a woman in treatment. As such, the interview should be relevant and sensitive to the woman's immediate needs, including the needs of her children. Intake screening should be

Figure B-7

Interrelated Elements of Clinical Treatment and Support Services for
Women and Their Children

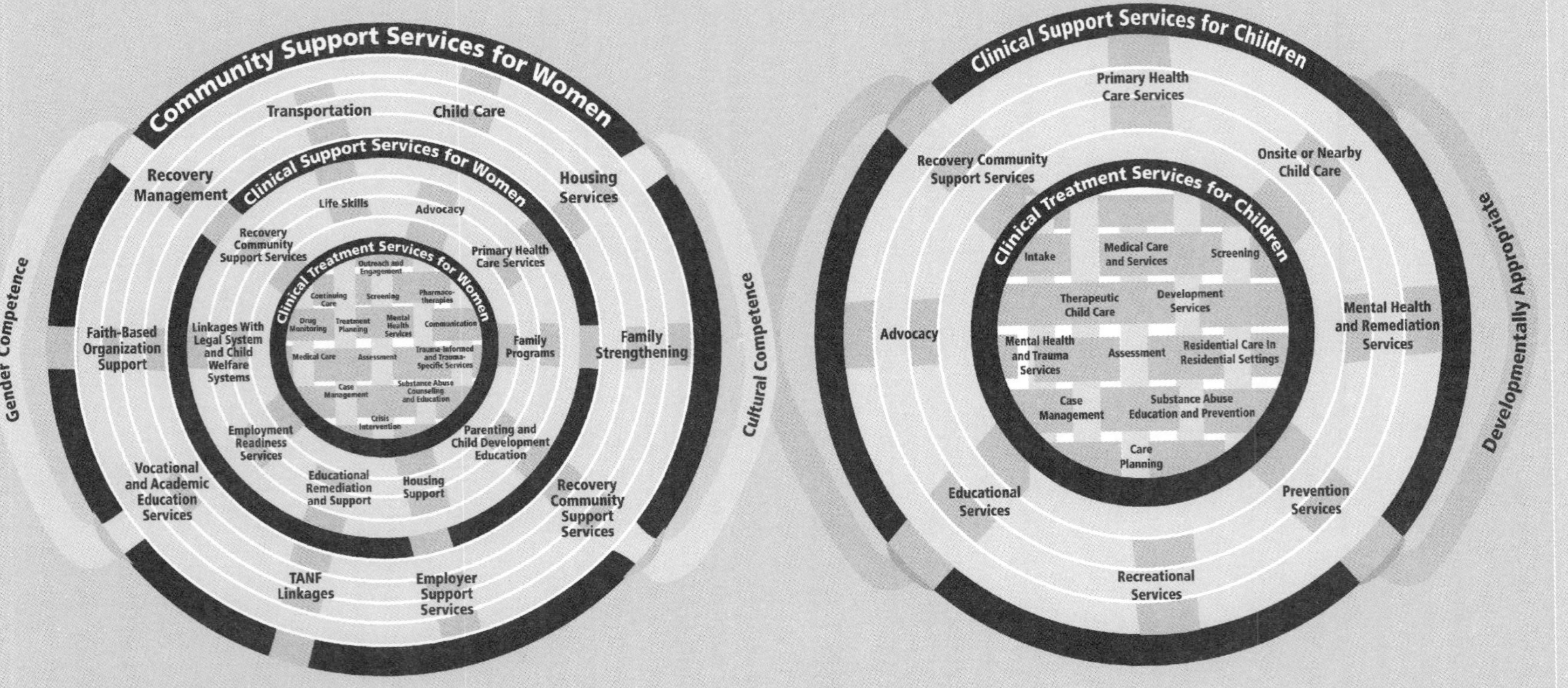

conducted by a staff person, preferably a female, who is respectful of the complex needs of women, who is nonjudgmental, and who can determine critical immediate needs, including medical, prenatal care, detoxification, housing, safety, food, clothing, urgent dental needs, and transportation. Screening is a good opportunity to provide a complete explanation of confidentiality and represents the beginning of the treatment engagement and case management process.

- *Detoxification.* Detoxification services are generally provided in an inpatient or residential setting and generally include close medical supervision. Although some treatment providers consider detoxification to be part of the continuum of care, others consider it a pretreatment activity. When needed, these services are critical to the comprehensive care model and offer another opportunity for a provider to engage a woman in longer-term treatment.

- *Crisis intervention.* Women coming into treatment are often victims of violence and may be experiencing crises warranting emergency intervention. Ideally, programs would have crisis intervention specialists available or they may have established strong linkages for immediate access to crisis services. While some crises may be evident at intake, others may arise during the course of the treatment and may affect the woman and her children.

- *Assessment.* Full assessment for women encompasses a wide range of concerns and includes a focus on her strengths; a comprehensive view of health-related needs; risks for HIV/AIDS and other infectious diseases; psychological status and screening and/or assessment for disorders that commonly co-occur in women with substance use disorders (e.g., depression and posttraumatic stress disorder [PTSD]); personal and community safety issues; understanding her significant current relationships and family-of-origin factors that may predispose her to abuse substances (such as sexual, emotional, and physical abuse, neglect, parental addiction, and parental

mental illness); her current parenting and caregiving roles; responsibility and issues such as custody of children, special needs of children living with the mother; options for care of children if the mother is to enter residential treatment without her children; her housing status and the safety of her housing; financial resources; vocational/educational/employment issues; legal issues; and involvement with other health, social, and/or criminal justice service systems. Using the information garnered in the assessment process, a recommendation on the level of care and treatment placement should be made. The placement decisions should follow those promulgated by the American Society for Addiction Medicine (ASAM). Known as Patient Placement Criteria, ASAM's criteria are increasingly the standard for determining the needed level of care.

- *Treatment planning.* Treatment planning is a collaborative process that should be done in the context of the unique needs and informed choices of women, and should be based on their individual strengths. Treatment planning should include any immediately needed services to help stabilize the family and assist the woman as she prepares for treatment. It needs to build on the internal and external resources available to the agency and should integrate the assistance offered and stipulations required by other health and social service systems. Treatment planning with women and their children requires attention to re-entry and continuing care planning as well.

- *Case management.* Case management addresses coordination of the myriad service elements that are needed by women and their families. Case management can occur as a pretreatment activity, during treatment, and posttreatment. Among services requiring coordination are medical, housing, child care, transportation, employment/vocational preparation, educational, and legal. Coordination with child protective services, welfare, and probation and parole offices must also be managed.

- *Substance abuse counseling and education.*

Substance abuse counseling and education for women needs to address the dynamics associated with addiction in women, as well as current behavioral issues in her addiction and the interrelationship between addiction and other co-occurring disorders. These include issues stemming from family-of-origin dynamics and the importance of relationships in the lives of women. It also needs to address the physical and social consequences of substance use disorders. Programs should ensure that all counseling activities are conducted in a respectful and caring manner and should not use counseling approaches that are contraindicated for trauma survivors, such as shaming, harsh confrontation, and intrusive monitoring. Staff should work with women in a manner that builds self-esteem, using nonaggressive and nonthreatening techniques so as not to revictimize clients. In addition, relapse prevention and recovery management are important components of substance abuse counseling and education.

- *Trauma-informed and trauma-specific services.* Given the high prevalence of histories of violence among women with substance use disorders, providing treatment in a trauma-informed environment is especially important. Staff should be trained to understand the multiple and complex links between violence, trauma, and addiction; to understand trauma-related symptoms as attempts to cope; to understand that violence and victimization play large and complex roles within the lives of most consumers in substance abuse and mental health services; and to behave in ways that are not retraumatizing to women. Trauma-specific services include individual and group services that directly address the impact of trauma and facilitate recovery and healing. A woman should not have to disclose her trauma history to receive trauma-specific services. The best practice is to enter into every treatment relationship as if the woman has experienced trauma, whether disclosed or not.

- *Medical care, including treatment for infectious diseases, women's health, and health education.* Medical assessments and subsequent care should be provided onsite or by referral by care providers who are sensitive to gender, addiction, mental health, and trauma issues. The types of services that may be needed include primary care; prenatal and postnatal care; emergency and hospital care; chronic diseases care (arthritis, diabetes, etc.) and testing, treatment, and counseling for HIV/AIDS, tuberculosis, and sexually transmitted diseases; and gynecological care. During pregnancy, special consideration should be given to the medical management of the pregnancy. Maternal education about and preparation for delivery and postpartum needs, including postpartum relapse prevention, should be included. Methadone maintenance and medication management of opioid dependence is particularly important during pregnancy. For women with a history of mood disorder, the postpartum period should include close monitoring for psychiatric symptoms.

- *Pharmacotherapies.* The use of methadone for treatment of opioid dependence is an accepted standard of care. Although usually provided on an outpatient basis, it should be available at all levels of care. Special attention may be needed when integrating patients on methadone and other phamacotherapies into treatment milieus with other clients who may not understand the utility of pharmacotherapies or who may have a negative attitude toward their use.

- *Mental health services.* Provision of or linkage to psychiatric and psychological care providers is often needed, given the high prevalence of co-occurring psychiatric disorders among female substance abuse treatment clients. It is not unusual for women to need services for affective disorders, anxiety disorders (including PTSD), and somatization disorders. Services for other mental illnesses (including severe mental illnesses such as bipolar disorder or major depression) are not as common but are also needed. Pharmacotherapy is sometimes part of mental health care, and onsite staff can provide medication education and monitoring.

- *Drug use monitoring.* Drug use monitoring, as part of ongoing assessment of the client's progress, is a component of treatment and can be used as a deterrent to relapse.
- *Continuing care.* Continuing care is a critical element of clinical treatment services for women. Trusting relationships formed among women, their peers, and their counselors continue to provide support to women once they have completed the formal treatment period. Planning for discharge is often anxiety-provoking and counselors should be prepared for a recurrence of presenting problems and possible resistance and procrastination by the client. Continuing care takes place, ideally, in all three domains— clinical treatment, clinical supports, and community supportive services. It addresses individual needs identified in a woman's relapse prevention plan, and builds a supportive network for the woman and her family to encourage and reinforce her recovery. When possible, a mother's schedule of continuing care services and her child's prevention services should be coordinated in order to encourage maximum attendance by both mother and child. A variety of self-help support programs can also promote the integration of the woman and her family into the community.

Clinical treatment services for children

- *Intake.* Substance abuse treatment agencies able to serve children should establish criteria that encourage enrollment of children in the program. In providing children with developmentally appropriate services, the agency's criteria might consider the child's age, as well as the number of children who may be involved for each mother. The child's safety and well-being, including bonding and attachment issues, are paramount and any threats to these must be evaluated and considered in the intake criteria.
- *Screening.* Screening of children is an important part of providing family-centered and family-supportive treatment. Screening

of children should be done in a supportive and friendly environment conducive to open dialog. There are advantages to having the same person conduct the screening who might later perform an assessment.
- *Assessment.* Medical, developmental, psychological, and trauma history should be assessed for all children participating in treatment with their mothers. Particular attention should be paid to issues that require immediate attention, such as methamphetamine lab exposure and physical abuse or severe neglect. As with screening, the assessment environment should be supportive, friendly, and conducive to open dialog. Determinations must be made as early as possible and should be continuously reviewed as to whether the child needs education, prevention services, intervention, treatment, or a combination of these. The child's own support system should be assessed, including the role that the child's father and extended family plays (or could play) in the child's life.
- *Care planning.* For children, care planning includes planning for education, prevention, and intervention services. Care planning should be conducted by professionals with particular experience in addressing the physical, psychological, and developmental needs of children whose mothers abuse alcohol and/or drugs. When age appropriate, it should include education about the treatment process that the mother will undergo and concerns about the transition that may be associated with that process.
- *Residential care in residential settings.* Providing safe and appropriate living space and adequate services for children whose mothers are in residential care is a powerful motivating factor for women to enter and continue in treatment. It enables children to either avoid separation or be reunited with the mother when treatment is made a condition of reunification by the courts.
- *Case management.* In addressing the service needs of children of mothers with substance use disorders, special attention should be paid to coordinating the child's services with those of the mother. Active

involvement of the mother will aid in the transition from treatment program to home. Of critical importance to care for children are the dual concepts of personal safety and environmental stability. When children are not in their birth mothers' custody, engagement of the foster or kin caregiver in care management is critical.

- *Therapeutic child care.* Children born to mothers who use substances are at high risk for poor developmental outcomes including neurological effects and alcohol-related spectrum disorders as well as consequences stemming from preterm delivery. Living with a parent with an addiction may also result in mental health issues for the children, particularly those associated with witnessing violence or separation from primary caregivers. Children with medical and mental health disabilities may need specialized child care provided by professionals with advanced training and in a setting where accommodations can be made to the physical environment that are responsive to these disabilities.

- *Substance abuse education and prevention.* Children whose mothers have substance use disorders need substance abuse education and prevention support at an early age, in part to correct their misconceptions of what is normal adult behavior. These programs should present information about the role of substances in the mother's role in caring for her children and to put the mother's treatment in the context of the child's view of reality.

- *Medical care and services.* In addition to a need for primary health care, attention must be given to the possibility of organic damage resulting from prenatal or early childhood substance exposure. This includes the physiological damage of alcohol-related spectrum disorders and exposure to drug production such as methamphetamine. Medical assessments and subsequent care should be provided onsite when possible or by referral when necessary. The types of services that may be needed include neonatal

and perinatal care; pediatric care; emergency and hospital care; and testing, treatment, and counseling for pediatric HIV/AIDS.

- *Developmental services.* Children who have been exposed to alcohol or drugs in utero or within their family environment may be at risk for physical and cognitive developmental delays. Physical, occupational, and speech therapy may be indicated for these children. Children experiencing developmental delays may also require behavior modification support, tutoring, and medication that will need to be managed.

- *Mental health and trauma services.* Children who grow up in the care of adults with substance use disorders can suffer psychological distress resulting from the experience of neglect as well as emotional, physical, or sexual abuse. Some children have witnessed domestic or other acts of violence. Children of mothers with substance use disorders often benefit from psychological counseling and therapy and from having their own trauma issues addressed through individual and group modalities.

Clinical Support Services

Clinical support services assist women in making the transition to independent and healthy alcohol- and drug-free living. They introduce or stabilize the woman's ability to care for herself and her family and to fulfill her role as a community and family member. For children, these services support healthy development and increase their capacity to reach their potential.

Clinical support services for women

- *Primary health care services.* Primary health care services, which are often provided at the beginning of the treatment episode, are clinical support services (as opposed to medical interventions such as detoxification and related triage services considered clinical treatment services). These clinical support medical services include obstetric and gynecologic services, HIV/AIDS counseling, general medical and dental care, nutrition counseling, eating behavior issues, family planning, reproductive health, health education, and physical and exercise therapy. Also critical to primary health care for women are medical self-awareness, personal hygiene, and self-advocacy for wellness.

- *Life skills*. Life skills include all of the activities that support independent, healthy lifestyles. They include budgeting and banking; negotiating access to services such as housing, English as a second language, income support including access to TANF, food stamps, and Medicaid; navigating legal services and commitments; setting up and running a household; grooming and clothing; recreation and leisure; nutrition; using public transportation; and arranging for child care.

- *Parenting and child development education.* Treatment for women with children is optimized and interaction between the mother and child is improved when the women's role as a mother is acknowledged and incorporated throughout treatment. Parenting skills are improved through education about child development and caretaking, skill building, and addressing shame and guilt over past parenting activities. Mothers who are being reunited with children will need support in preparation for and after the reunion. Fathers can also be important contributors to the well-being of their children, and when possible, should receive the education and support necessary to prepare them for the responsibility of parenthood.

- *Family programs.* The more psychologically and emotionally healthy a woman's significant others are, the more likely they are to help her remain engaged in treatment and recovery. Significant others should be involved in understanding family members' roles in the family and how those roles may have become maladaptive coping strategies while the woman was in active addiction. When significant others are directly involved in relapse prevention planning, they are more likely to become productively involved in supporting positive efforts at recovery

and intervening on relapse warning signs. Family-centered programs address all members in the family and include efforts to improve relationships with significant others, including partners, parents, siblings, children, and caretakers. These family interventions can be an important part of the woman's preparation for long-term recovery.

- *Educational remediation and support.* Educational deficiencies may be a consequence of a woman's addiction or may be a significant contributor to her addiction. A lack of education is reflected in poor reading skills, conduct issues, illiteracy, special education needs, low family income, and psychological barriers associated with poor performance and low self-esteem. Cognitive impairments due to alcohol-related spectrum disorders and other congenital or biological origins may require significant educational supports. Establishing linkages and/or services to address these educational issues may be significant motivators for women to remain in treatment and provide hope for her to establish economic independence.

- *Employment readiness services.* Given the relationship of meaningful employment to recovery success and societal pressures to move the unemployed to the workforce, employment readiness services are an essential element of treatment. These services include reading and numeric skills testing, literacy tutoring, GED classes, vocational assessments, pre-employment readiness training (soft skills), job referral, job retention services, and transitional employment placement. Treatment programs should establish as one of their goals the self-sufficiency of the client, seeking effective linkages with TANF and child welfare agencies.

- *Linkages with the legal and child welfare systems.* Many women in treatment have conditions set by the child welfare system to maintain their parenting role or for reunification with children who may have been removed from the mother's custody. These requirements often include reports that progress is being made toward treatment goals, completion of parenting and anger management programs, supervised visits, drug testing, and court appearances. Communication among treatment providers, child welfare workers, the mother's legal advocate, and the dependency court helps women move toward these goals. When mothers are also involved in the criminal justice system, linkages and communication with probation and parole staff are also critical. Criminal justice requirements may include drug testing, court appearances, and documentation regarding treatment progress toward goals. Often these communications require access to the community's legal aid services.

- *Housing support services.* For women, particularly women with children, housing represents more than just shelter. It is a crucial support for recovery. It represents safety both for her and for her children. Thus, a comprehensive care provider must address the issue of where the woman will reside when she completes treatment and make the provision for adequate housing a part of the program's continuum of care. Given the time involved in arranging for affordable, safe, drug-free housing, this service needs to be part of early planning.

- *Advocacy.* Women entering treatment often require advocates to assist them in negotiating the various systems they may need to interact with. Although direct advocacy services provide immediate access to remediation, the goal of this process is to transform women into empowered individuals who can effectively advocate for themselves and their families.

- *Recovery community support services.* Regardless of the treatment model or modality, women need to appreciate that they are not alone and that others have traveled the same road. It is critical for women to be supported in developing relationships with other women and persons in recovery who can be role models and provide support, friendships, and companionship in pursuing safe and sober leisure activities. Thus, early in the treatment process, providers must help women develop a gender-sensitive support

network within the recovery community.

- Clinical support services for children
- *Primary health care services.* Primary health care services are an ongoing need for children of mothers with substance use disorders. Monitoring medical conditions should include screening for a range of potential medical complications including effects resulting from prenatal substance exposure and risks of HIV/AIDS and other communicable diseases. Primary health care services should also focus on wellness and prevention, including immunizations and regular medical examinations.

- *Onsite or nearby child care.* Developmentally appropriate, quality child care is needed for children whose mothers participate in treatment. Child care should be onsite or proximate to the program and should include a full range of services, from therapeutic child care to developmentally appropriate interventions and recreational play.

- *Mental health and remediation services.* Children whose mothers abuse alcohol and/ or drugs often have developmental delays that require specific interventions. These children may experience higher rates of attention deficit disorder, attention deficit/ hyperactivity disorder, conduct disorder, speech and language delays, and learning disabilities.

- *Prevention services.* Children whose mothers have substance use disorders are at higher risk of developing a substance use disorder of their own as they enter preadolescence and adolescence. Evidence-based prevention services tailored to these children may be most appropriate when offered in the context of the parent's own history and recovery. Prevention programs that have demonstrated their effectiveness with a range of child and adolescent populations can be found at http://www.samhsa.gov/children

- *Recreational services.* Participation in pleasurable recreational activities helps children socialize, express themselves, relax, experience new activities, and become knowledgeable about healthful alcohol- and drug-free leisure activities. Participation in developmentally appropriate recreational activities is a critical learning experience for children. Participation in sports, hobbies, and creative outlets can also provide vehicles for enhanced self-image and self-esteem.

- *Educational services.* The needs of school-age children, including attention to academic progress, are a necessary part of each child's service plan. Often, children in treatment with their mothers experience disruption in their academic experience because of frequent moves or other family crises. Children who were prenatally exposed to substances may have ongoing learning disabilities that require advocacy to ensure special education services are available and to ensure children's academic success. When regular reviews of individual education plans are needed, the treatment agencies must recognize the critical role that the mother may play in attending such sessions.

- *Advocacy.* Mothers with substance use disorders may not be effective advocates for their children. Programs may need to provide direct advocacy services as well as assist mothers in developing appropriate advocacy skills to ensure that they are able to negotiate for the needs of their children. Children, as well, should be introduced to advocacy skills when developmentally appropriate.

- *Recovery community support services.* Because of the significant impact of peers and role modeling on the development of children, there is a marked need for age-appropriate recovery support activities. By building their own community of support, children can identify with peers and learn from those who have coped with similar experiences.

Community Support Services

Community support services are those services that extend beyond the treatment program and are found within the community. These services help to ensure that short-term treatment success can be sustained in long-term recovery. While

there are additional services that women, children, and other family members may need in order to support the recovery of the family, those included below represent the more common services used by families as they progress in their recovery.

- *Recovery management and recovery community support services.* Community-based recovery management services include activities that provide relapse prevention and continuing care. While these services may begin during treatment, they are part of the community-based network that supports recovery. Consistent with the importance of women's personal relationships, women will benefit from the availability of peer-driven recovery mutual support services, which can include Alcoholics Anonymous, Narcotics Anonymous, and Women for Sobriety.

- *Housing services.* Adequate housing is essential both for safety and for security. While housing services are often placed within clinical support services, in the context used here, housing services are also a community infrastructure issue. In this context, housing which encourages alcohol- and drug-free living can be a vital component for sustaining recovery.

- *Family strengthening.* Recognizing the family disruption that is common to addiction, women (particularly those who are heads of their households), need services that support the re-establishment of important family ties, including ongoing family therapy and family support services.

- *Child care.* This is both an immediate and short-term treatment support service as well as a broader community service. As a community support, quality preschool, child care, and after-school care programs are longer-term needs that enable mothers to work outside the home.

- *Transportation.* Accessible and reliable transportation is important given the complicated schedules of women caretakers who often have to balance the transportation needs of their children with the transportation needs of employment and ongoing participation in continuing care.

- *TANF linkages.* With some exceptions, women from lower socioeconomic strata who progress through treatment are either TANF eligible or may become TANF eligible. TANF agencies have a role to play in providing support for recovery by serving as a bridge between the three circles of clinical treatment, with an emphasis on work preparation and sustaining employment for women going through the recovery process.
- *Employer support services.* Communities need to create systems within employment settings that support recovery and combat workplace substance abuse. Larger employers may offer employee assistance programs and smaller employers may be able to coordinate needed job support services with treatment providers from their communities.
- *Vocational and academic education services.* Critical to recovery success is the continuation of educational and vocational services that are begun during treatment.
- *Faith-based organization support.* Recognizing that spirituality plays a crucial role in the recovery process, it is important that connections are established by treatment providers with faith-based institutions that can serve as appropriate resources for addressing the spiritual issues related to addiction and recovery. Faith-based organizations can play an important role in the community and can connect families in a supportive community network.

Funding Issues

Finally, in response to the needs of providers to understand funding options for this array of services, this revision to the model allows providers to identify discrete elements of the comprehensive model and to make their own assessments of how to finance the elements through available funding streams. For some elements, funding will be readily available and sufficient to cover the full cost of services delivery. Other elements, such as continuing care and many of the services for children, are not as easily supported; providers will have to use more flexible funding to cover these services while they continue to communicate to funders that unfunded and underfunded components are critical elements in the comprehensive model of care.

Providing comprehensive services through the separate agencies serving women and their children involves connecting the multiple funding streams that flow into the various health, human service, and educational agencies serving families. The more comprehensively a continuum of care is defined, the wider the array of funding streams that is needed. The more committed an agency is to family-centered services, the more mastery is needed of all the different funding streams that can support families. No single agency has adequate funding sources by itself to achieve comprehensive outcomes; interagency funding streams are therefore critical to converting hopes for new linkages into reality.

Fiscal context always matters, and in tight fiscal climates, tapping new sources of funding is both desired and resisted. It is desired for the obvious reason that hard-pressed agencies are anxious to find alternative funding streams to support their programs; it is resisted for the equally obvious reason that agencies seek to protect their own funding streams even more when funding is tight. The descriptions of funding and suggestions that follow are made in full awareness that in most States, fiscal constraints are very significant factors at present.

Several issues affect the ability of programs to provide the comprehensive services needed by women and children affected by substance use disorders. Some of these issues are based on the nature of the collaborative relationship between the agencies, some flow from categorical funding constraints, and some are based on other Federal or State policies. Understanding which of these barriers are affecting a State's or community's ability to provide comprehensive services is a critical first step in developing its response. These concerns may include the following:

- Existing categorical definitions of funding streams and eligibility restrictions can create barriers to interagency efforts, with agency officials sometimes resistant to what seems like "one more earmark" on funding streams.
- Decisions by agencies to provide services directly or to negotiate for services with outside agencies are critical choices, but at times they may be made based on limited understanding of other agencies' funding streams.
- Each system sees the other's funding streams as mysterious and difficult to access, and each sees its own as overcommitted and possibly threatened, leading to a debate over "your money, our money, or their money."
- A sustained, time-consuming effort is required to achieve new Federal, State, and local collaboration, which is needed to create financing responsive to the multiple needs of children and families.
- As the majority of funding flows through State-level government, State systems may need specific legislation to overcome categorical requirements.
- There are significant financial incentives to maintain the status quo in fragmented funding streams.
- Categorically funded programs that do not apply adequate "dosage" to ensure treatment effectiveness may require additional layers of funding from additional sources to get to scale and provide an adequate dosage of services. For example, programs that do not provide aftercare services to parents may be unable to respond to relapse issues, resulting in readmission to treatment that was underfunded but that ends up with a higher overall cost due to clients' readmission.

Unified Fiscal Planning

The concept of unified fiscal planning has been introduced recently. This approach includes a variety of strategies used by States and communities to create and sustain an integrated and flexible continuum of care for children and families (Crocker 2003). Some of the more commonly used strategies include decategorization, pooled funding, blended funding, braided funding, wraparound services, and refinancing. Often the terms are used interchangeably or without clear definition; however, the following are common definitions used for these concepts:

- *Decategorization* refers to State-level efforts to reduce or eliminate categorical requirements on how funds are spent. This reduction in requirements is often created in exchange for greater accountability for a set of negotiated outcomes.
- *Pooled or blended funding* is generally a local-level effort that is implemented among a group of agencies that formally integrates a set of funding streams into a single source of dollars. A new funding structure is often developed that administers and allocates the funds to the participating agencies based on negotiated contracts.
- *Braided funding* is generally implemented by an individual agency or program and refers to administrative efforts to obtain multiple funding sources to create more comprehensive services. This strategy typically works within the categorical system and administrative responsibilities for maintaining the various categorical requirements remain.
- *Wraparound services.* The term "wraparound" came into use in 1986, in an article by Lenore Behar, who defined it as a way to "surround multi-problem youngsters and families with services rather than with institutional walls, and to customize these services" (Behar 1986). The wraparound approach is more a process than a service, in which a child's or family's individual needs are addressed by the full range of services they need, with maximum flexibility in funding.
- *Refinancing.* "Refinancing entails aggressively pursuing monies from uncapped Federal appropriations such as entitlement funds, using these new Federal funds to pay for standard services, and then applying the freed-up local and State funds to pay

Specific Treatment-Related Funding Streams

While the Substance Abuse Prevention and Treatment Block Grant is still the largest source of publicly supported substance abuse treatment (approximately 40 percent), treatment providers should become familiar with the Medicaid-reimbursable services in their States and learn how to bill for these services. Medicaid is a joint Federal–State entitlement program and the third largest source of health insurance in the country. It makes up approximately one quarter of public funds available for treatment. Medicaid coverage varies from State to State. Nearly all States restrict services when paying for alcohol and drug abuse treatment. The types of restrictions include low payment rates for treatment providers, restrictions on the settings for treatment, low limits on the days of inpatient treatment, low limits on the number of outpatient visits, and restrictions on types of providers that can be reimbursed (Legal Action Center 2002).

The Medicaid codes published by the Centers for Medicare and Medicaid Services (CMS) are also known as the HCPCS codes (Health Care Financing Administration Common Procedure Coding System). With few exceptions, all of the services described here as clinical treatment services for women have applicable HCPCS codes. There are fewer applicable HCPCS codes for the clinical support services for women, and HCPCS codes do not apply to community support services. As noted earlier, the existence of a code does not necessarily mean that a State reimburses for a service (at any level). States are only responsible for a short list of mandatory services, whereas most services are optional reimbursable services. The CMS updates the HCPCS codes on an annual basis. Information on applicable alcohol, drug, and behavioral health HCPCS codes can be found on the Web site of the National Association of State Alcohol and Drug Abuse Directors (www.nasadad.org).

In addition to the mandatory and optional Medicaid alcohol and drug benefits, Medicaid includes a benefit known as Early and Periodic Screening, Diagnostic, and Treatment (EPSDT) to cover both prevention and treatment services for children and adolescents under age 21. All children enrolled in Medicaid are entitled to EPSDT. "Under EPSDT, States must screen and then furnish appropriate medically necessary treatment to 'correct or ameliorate defects and physical and mental illness and conditions discovered by the screening services'" (Legal Action Center 2002, p. 10). In practice, use of this resource has been limited by States' ability to pay for the services. An additional source of funding for uninsured, low-income children is the State Children's Health Insurance Program, which is allocated by block grant formula to the States.

TANF can fund a range of nonmedical clinical treatment services as well as clinical and community support services for both women and children. The extent to which this is used varies greatly from State to State. Other additional valuable funding sources are available for many of the services described, although many are time-limited and/or specialized, increasing the time demands on the provider to seek and manage multiple funding streams.

Closing Considerations

In designing a comprehensive substance abuse treatment model for women and their children, CSAT is not attempting to articulate every element of treatment for this population. Rather, CSAT wishes to provide a standard or goal to which programs should aspire as they design and plan services that will be characterized as holistic, wraparound, and/or comprehensive. Additionally, it is not CSAT's intention to see this model adopted without reference to the context of the community in which it is used. Thus, for the model to be truly comprehensive, it should be more than adopted; it should be adapted to its community and its consumers.

In adapting this model, different communities will emphasize different aspects. For example, the American Indian and Alaska Native communities have demonstrated the special role that spirituality, culture, and historical trauma play in treatment, and for these communities, a worthwhile adaptation requires an increased emphasis on these issues. For a community of older women, an emphasis on medication abuse may also be appropriate.

This model embodies the best practices known to CSAT, as well as the agency's experience in addressing this issue on a nationwide basis.

Appendix C: Screening and Assessment Instruments

Addiction Severity Index (ASI)

Purpose: The ASI is most useful as a general intake screening tool. It effectively assesses a client's status in several areas, and the composite score measures how a client's need for treatment changes over time.

Clinical utility: The ASI has been used extensively for treatment planning and outcome evaluation. Outcome evaluation packages for individual programs or for treatment systems are available.

Groups with whom this instrument has been used: Designed for adults of both sexes who are not intoxicated (drugs or alcohol) when interviewed.

Norms: The ASI has been used with males and females with drug and alcohol disorders in both inpatient and outpatient settings. Female version: ASI-F.

Format: Structured interview

Administration time: 50 minutes to 1 hour

Scoring time: 5 minutes for severity rating

Computer scoring? Yes

Administrator training and qualifications: A self-training packet is available as is onsite training by experienced trainers.

Available from:
A. Thomas McLellan, Ph.D.
Building 7
PVAMC
University Avenue
Philadelphia, PA 19104
Ph: (800) 238-2433

Clinical Institute Withdrawal Assessment (CIWA-Ar)

Purpose: To track severity of withdrawal and measure severity of alcohol withdrawal.

Clinical utility: Aid to adjustment of care related to withdrawal severity.

Groups with whom this instrument has been used: Adults

Norms: N/A

Format: A 10-item scale for clinical quantification of the severity of the alcohol withdrawal syndrome.

Administration time: 2 minutes

Scoring time: 4 to 5 minutes

Computer scoring? No

Administrator training and qualifications: Training is required, and the CIWA is administered by nurses, doctors, research associates/detoxification unit workers.

Fee for use: No

Available from:
Dr. E.M. Sellers
Ventana Clinical Research Corporation
340 College Street, Suite 400
Toronto, Canada
M5T 3A9
Phone: 416-963-9338
Fax: 416-963-9732
www.ventana-crc.com/

Level of Care Utilization System (LOCUS)

Purpose: To assess immediate service needs (e.g., for clients in crisis); to plan resource needs over time, as in assessing service requirements for defined populations; to monitor changes in status or placement at different points in time.

Clinical utility: LOCUS is divided into three sections. The first defines six evaluation parameters or dimensions: (1) Risk of Harm, (2) Functional Status, (3) Medical, Addictive, and Psychiatric Co-Morbidity, (4) Recovery Environment, (5) Treatment and Recovery History, and (6) Engagement. A five-point scale is constructed for each dimension, and the criteria for assigning a given rating or score in that dimension are elaborated. In dimension IV, two subscales are defined, whereas all other dimensions contain only one scale.

Groups with whom this instrument has been used: Adults

Norms: N/A

Format: A document that is divided into three sections.

Administration time: 15 to 30 minutes

Scoring time: 20 minutes

Computer scoring? No

Administrator training and qualifications: N/A

Fee for use: No

Available from: American Association of Community Psychiatrists
www.wpic.pitt.edu/aacp/find.html

Eating Attitudes Test (EAT-26)

The following screening questionnaire is designed to help you determine if your eating behaviors and attitudes warrant further evaluation. The questionnaire is **not intended to provide a diagnosis.** Rather, it identifies the presence of symptoms that are consistent with a possible eating disorder.

Answer these as honestly as you can, and then score questions using the instructions at the end.

Please mark a check to the right of each of the following statements:	Always	Usually	Often	Some-times	Rarely	Never	Score
1. Am terrified about being overweight.	☐	☐	☐	☐	☐	☐	☐
2. Avoid eating when I am hungry.	☐	☐	☐	☐	☐	☐	☐
3. Find myself preoccupied with food.	☐	☐	☐	☐	☐	☐	☐
4. Have gone on eating binges where I feel that I may not be able to stop.	☐	☐	☐	☐	☐	☐	☐
5 Cut my food into small pieces.	☐	☐	☐	☐	☐	☐	☐
6. Aware of the calorie content of foods that I eat.	☐	☐	☐	☐	☐	☐	☐
7. Particularly avoid food with a high carbohydrate content (i.e. bread, rice, potatoes, etc.)	☐	☐	☐	☐	☐	☐	☐
8. Feel that others would prefer If I ate more.	☐	☐	☐	☐	☐	☐	☐
9. Vomit after I have eaten.	☐	☐	☐	☐	☐	☐	☐
10. Feel extremely guilty after eating.	☐	☐	☐	☐	☐	☐	☐
11. Am preoccupied with a desire to be thinner.	☐	☐	☐	☐	☐	☐	☐
12. Think about burning up calories when I exercise.	☐	☐	☐	☐	☐	☐	☐
13. Other people think that I am too thin.	☐	☐	☐	☐	☐	☐	☐
14. Am preoccupied with the thought of having fat on my body.	☐	☐	☐	☐	☐	☐	☐
15. Take longer than others to eat my meals.	☐	☐	☐	☐	☐	☐	☐
16. Avoid foods with sugar in them.	☐	☐	☐	☐	☐	☐	☐
17. Eat diet foods	☐	☐	☐	☐	☐	☐	☐
18. Feel that food controls my life.	☐	☐	☐	☐	☐	☐	☐
19. Display self-control around food.	☐	☐	☐	☐	☐	☐	☐
20. Feel that others pressure me to eat.	☐	☐	☐	☐	☐	☐	☐
21. Give too much time and thought to food.	☐	☐	☐	☐	☐	☐	☐
22. Feel uncomfortable after eating sweets.	☐	☐	☐	☐	☐	☐	☐
23. Engage in dieting behavior.	☐	☐	☐	☐	☐	☐	☐
24. Like my stomach to be empty.	☐	☐	☐	☐	☐	☐	☐
25. Have the impulse to vomit after meals.	☐	☐	☐	☐	☐	☐	☐
26. Enjoy trying new rich foods.	☐	☐	☐	☐	☐	☐	☐
						Total Score =	

Eating Attitudes Test (EAT-26) (continued)

A) Have you gone on eating binges where you feel that you may not be able to stop? __ No   Yes __   How many times in the last 6 months? _____

B) Have you ever made yourself sick (vomited) to control your weight or shape? __ No   Yes __   How many times in the last 6 months? _____

C) Have you ever used laxatives, diet pills or diuretics (water pills) to control your weight or shape? __ No   Yes __   How many times in the last 6 months? _____

D) Have you ever been treated for an eating disorder?   __ No   Yes __   When? _____

EAT-26' David M. Garner (1982) Note: The EAT-26 has been made available with permission of the authors.

Step 1: EAT-26 ITEM SCORING			
Score each item as indicated below and put score in box to the right of each item			
Items # 1-25:		Item # 26 only:	
Always	= 3	=	0
Usually	= 2	=	0
Often	= 1	=	0
Sometimes	= 0	=	1

Step 2: Total EAT-26 Score	
	Total =
Add item scores together for a Total EAT-26 score:	

Step 3: Behavioral Questions	
	Total =
Did you score Yes on Questions A, B, C or D?	

Step 4: Underweight
Determine if you are significantly underweight according to the table to the right

Step 5: Referral	No	Yes
If your EAT-26 score is **20 or more**		
or if you answered **YES** to any questions A-D		
or if your **weight** is below the number on the weight chart to the right		
Please discuss your results with your physician or therapist		

Significantly Underweight According to Height (Body Mass Index of 18)*			
Height (inches)	Weight (pounds)	Height (inches)	Weight (pounds)
58	86	68	118
58	88	68	120
59	89	69	121
59	90	69	124
60	91	70	125
60	93	70	127
61	95	71	128
61	96	71	131
62	99	72	132
62	100	72	134
63	101	73	135
63	103	73	138
64	105	74	140
64	106	74	141
65	108	75	144
65	109	75	146
66	112	76	147
66	113	76	149
67	114	77	152
67	117	77	154

*Note: The table on the previous page indicates the body weights for heights considered to be "significantly underweight" according to a Body Mass Index (BMI) of 18. BMI is a simple method of evaluating body weight taking height into consideration. It applies to both men and women. There is some controversy regarding whether or not BMI is the best method of determining relative body weight and it is important to recognize that it is possible for someone to be quite malnourished even though they are above the weight listed in the table. In order to determine if you are "significantly underweight", locate your height (without shoes) on the table and see if the corresponding body weight (in light indoor clothing) is below that listed. If so, you are considered "significantly underweight" and should speak to your physician or therapist about your weight. To Calculate Body Mass Index (BMI) exactly; Weight (pounds) Divided by Height in Inches; Divide this again by Height in Inches and Multiply by 703

$$BMI = (lbs) \div (inches) \div (inches) \times 703$$

Spiritual Well-Being Scale (SWBS)

Purpose: A general indicator of well-being that may be used for the assessment of both individual and group spiritual well-being. It provides an overall measure of the perception of spiritual quality of life, as well as subscale scores for Religious and Existential Well-Being. The Religious Well-Being subscale provides a self-assessment of one's relationship with God, while the Existential Well-Being Subscale gives a self-assessment of one's sense of life purpose and life satisfaction.

Clinical utility: The SWBS is composed of 20 items, 10 of which assess religious well-being specifically, and 10 of which assess existential well-being.

Groups with whom this instrument has been used: Adults and children

Norms: Yes

Format: The SWBS is a paper-pencil instrument currently available in English and Spanish.

Administration time: 10-15 minutes

Scoring time: Information not available

Computer scoring? Information not available

Administrator training and qualifications: Information not available

Fee for use: Yes

Available from:

Life Advance, Inc.
81 Front Street
Nyak, NY 10960
Lifeadvance.com

Drinker Inventory of Consequences (DrInC-2L)

Instructions: Here are a number of events that drinkers sometimes experience. Read each one carefully, and circle the number that indicates whether this has <u>EVER</u> happened to you (0 = No, 1 = Yes). If an item does not apply to you, circle zero (0).

Has this EVER happened to you?	No	Yes
1. I have had a hangover or felt bad after drinking.	0	1
2. I have felt bad about myself because of my drinking.	0	1
3. I have missed days of work or school because of my drinking.	0	1
4. My family or friends have worried or complained about my drinking.	0	1
5. I have enjoyed the taste of beer, wine, or liquor.	0	1
6. The quality of my work has suffered because of my drinking.	0	1
7. My ability to be a good parent has been harmed by my drinking.	0	1
8. After drinking, I have had trouble with sleeping, staying asleep, or nightmares.	0	1
9. I have driven a motor vehicle after having three or more drinks.	0	1
10. My drinking has caused me to use other drugs more.	0	1
11. I have been sick and vomited after drinking.	0	1
12. I have been unhappy because of my drinking.	0	1
13. Because of my drinking, I have not eaten properly.	0	1
14. I have failed to do what is expected of me because of my drinking.	0	1
15. Drinking has helped me to relax.	0	1
16. I have felt guilty or ashamed because of my drinking.	0	1
Has this EVER happened to you?	No	Yes
17. While drinking I have said or done embarrassing things.	0	1

	No	Yes
18. When drinking, my personality has changed for the worse.	0	1
19. I have taken foolish risks when I have been drinking.	0	1
20. I have gotten into trouble because of drinking.	0	1
21. While drinking or using drugs, I have said harsh or cruel things to someone.	0	1
22. When drinking, I have done impulsive things that I regretted later.	0	1
23. I have gotten into a physical fight while drinking.	0	1
24. My physical health has been harmed by my drinking.	0	1
25. Drinking has helped me to have a more positive outlook on life.	0	1
26. I have had money problems because of my drinking.	0	1
27. My marriage or love relationship has been harmed by my drinking.	0	1
28. I have smoked tobacco more when I am drinking.	0	1
29. My physical appearance has been harmed by my drinking.	0	1
30. My family has been hurt by my drinking.	0	1
31. A friendship or close relationship has been damaged by my drinking.	0	1
32. I have been overweight because of my drinking.	0	1
33. My sex life has suffered because of my drinking.	0	1
34. I have lost interest in activities and hobbies because of my drinking.	0	1
35. When drinking, my social life has been more enjoyable.	0	1
36. My spiritual or moral life has been harmed by my drinking.	0	1
37. Because of my drinking, I have not had the kind of life that I want.	0	1
Has this EVER happened to you?	No	Yes
38. My drinking has gotten in the way of my growth as a person.	0	1
39. My drinking has damaged my social life, popularity, or reputation.	0	1
40. I have spent too much or lost a lot of money because of my drinking.	0	1

41. I have been arrested for driving under the influence of alcohol.	0	1
42. I have had trouble with the law (other than driving while intoxicated) because of my drinking.	0	1
43. I have lost a marriage or a close love relationship because of my drinking.	0	1
44. I have been suspended/fired from or left a job or school because of my drinking.	0	1
45. I drank alcohol normally, without any problems.	0	1
46. I have lost a friend because of my drinking.	0	1
47. I have had an accident while drinking or intoxicated.	0	1
48. While drinking or intoxicated, I have been physically hurt, injured, or burned.	0	1
49. While drinking or intoxicated, I have injured someone else.	0	1
50. I have broken things while drinking or intoxicated.	0	1

DrInC Scoring Sheet

Physical	Inter-personal	Intra-personal	Impulse Control	Social Responsibility	Control Scale*
1 _____					
		2 _____		3 _____	
	4 _____				5 _____
				6 _____	
	7 _____				
8 _____			9 _____		
			10 _____		
11 _____		12 _____			
13 _____				14 _____	15 _____
		16 _____			
	17 _____	18 _____	19 _____	20 _____	
	21 _____		22 _____		
			23 _____		
24 _____					25 _____
				26 _____	
	27 _____		28 _____		
29 _____	30 _____				
	31 _____		32 _____		
33 _____		34 _____			35 _____
		36 _____			
		37 _____			
		38 _____			
	39 _____			40 _____	
			41 _____		
			42 _____		
	43 _____			44 _____	45 _____
	46 _____		47 _____		
48 _____			49 _____		
			50 _____		
_____ +	_____ +	_____ +	_____ +	_____ =	_____ _____
Physical	Inter-personal	Intra-personal	Impulse Control	Social Responsibility	Total DrInC Score	Control Scale*

INSTRUCTIONS: For each item, copy the circled number from the answer sheet next to the item number above. Then sum each column to calculate scale totals. Sum these totals to calculate the total DrInC score.

* Zero scores on Control Scale items may indicate careless or dishonest responding. On version 2R (Recent Drinking), totals of 5 or less are suspect.

DrInC Profile Sheet

Profile form for WOMEN

LIFETIME (Ever) Consequences (2L)

DECILE SCORES	Total Score	Physical	Inter- personal	Intra- personal	Impulse Control	Social Responsibility
10	42–45				11–12	
9 Very high	39–41		10		10	7
8	37–38	8			9	
7 High	35–36		9		8	6
6	32–34	7	8	8	7	
5 Medium	29–31		7		6	5
4	26–28	6	5–6	7	5	4
3 Low	24–25	5	4		4	3
2	19–23	4		6	3	2
1 Very low	0–18	0–3	0–3	0–5	0–2	0–1

RAW SCORES:

INSTRUCTIONS: Transfer the total scale scores from the DrInC Scoring Form to the raw score line at the bottom of the Profile Sheet. Then for each scale, CIRCLE the same value above it to determine the decile range.

These interpretive ranges are based on a sample of 342 adult women presenting for treatment. Individual scores are therefore ranked as low, medium, or high *relative to women already presenting for treatment*. The normative data are from Project MATCH, a multisite clinical sample. For details of study design see:

Project MATCH Research Group. Rationale and methods for a multisite clinical trial matching patients to alcoholism treatment. *Alcoholism: Clinical and Experimental Research* 17:1130–1145, 1993.

Appendix D: Allen Barriers to Treatment Instrument

DRAFT FORMAT – FEBRUARY 28, 2006

Form Approved
OMB No. 0930-0269
Expiration Date 09-30-2007

DATE: |__|__| |__|__| |2|0|__|__|
  AB_MO   AB_DY   AB_YR

MOTHER'S ID# |__|__|__|__|__|__|__|__|__|__|__|__|__|__|__|
                        AB_MOM

EVALUATION PHASE: Intake |__|1   6-months |__|4   12-months |__|5   Discharge |__|6
AB_INTERVIEW_TYPE

PERSON COMPLETING |_____| GRANT# **TI** |__|__|__|__|__|
                      AB_INTERVIEWER   AB_SITE

ALLEN BARRIERS TO TREATMENT INSTRUMENT

Listed below are reasons that sometimes keep people from getting help. Based on what you are experiencing, have experienced, or have heard about, how much do each of the following treatment program characteristics keep you from getting treatment for alcohol or other drug problems?

Check <u>one box</u> for each statement.

This keeps me from getting help...	A lot	An average amount	A little	Not at all
AB_LACK_OF_INFORMATION 1. Lack of information about and not knowing the location of treatment programs	☐4	☐3	☐2	☐1
AB_WAIT_OPENING_PROG_FULL 2. Having to wait for an opening because the program is full	☐4	☐3	☐2	☐1
AB_BEHAVIOR_OF_STAFF 3. The behavior of treatment program staff toward patients	☐4	☐3	☐2	☐1
AB_SPEAK_TO_MALE_COUNSELOR 4. The possibility of having to speak of my problem with a male counselor	☐4	☐3	☐2	☐1
AB_FAR_FROM_HOME 5. The far distance of treatment programs from my home	☐4	☐3	☐2	☐1
AB_NO_TRANSPORTATION 6. No available transportation to the treatment program	☐4	☐3	☐2	☐1
AB_SPEAK_WHERE_MEN_PRESENT 7. The possibility of having to speak in a group where men are present	☐4	☐3	☐2	☐1
AB_PROGRAM_INCLUDE_MEN_WOMEN 8. Treatment programs that include men as well as women patients	☐4	☐3	☐2	☐1
AB_NO_HELP_STAY_ADDICTION_FREE 9. No help from treatment programs for staying alcohol and/or drug free afterwards	☐4	☐3	☐2	☐1
AB_NO_ABILITY_TEACHING_ME 10. No confidence in the ability of treatment programs to teach me what I need to know as an alcoholic or drug-abusing woman	☐4	☐3	☐2	☐1

AB_FIRST_OTH
What other things about treatment programs keep you from getting help? (Please answer in three lines or less.)

Based on what you are experiencing or have experienced, how much do each of the following <u>personal beliefs, feelings, or thoughts</u>, keep you from getting treatment for alcohol or other drug problems?

Check <u>one box</u> for each statement.

This keeps me from getting help...	A lot	An average amount	A little	Not at all
AB_FEEL_ASHAMED 11. I feel ashamed when I admit to having this problem	☐4	☐3	☐2	☐1
AB_UNABLE_STAY_FREE_AFTER_TREAT 12. In the past I have been unable to stay alcohol-free and/or drug-free after treatment	☐4	☐3	☐2	☐1
AB_CANNOT_PAY_TREATMENT 13. I cannot pay for treatment of this problem	☐4	☐3	☐2	☐1
AB_NO_INSURANCE 14. I do not have health insurance for this problem	☐4	☐3	☐2	☐1
AB_DONT_TRUST_TO_HELP 15. I do not trust doctors, clinics, or hospitals to help	☐4	☐3	☐2	☐1
AB_DRINK_DRUG_NO_PROBLEM 16. I do not feel that drinking and drug use is a problem for me	☐4	☐3	☐2	☐1
AB_HEALTH_NOT_INTERRUPT_LIFE 17. I do not let health problems interrupt my life	☐4	☐3	☐2	☐1
AB_RELIGIOUS_BELIEFS 18. I have religious beliefs about this problem	☐4	☐3	☐2	☐1
AB_HAVE_RESPONSIBILITIES 19. I have responsibilities at home as a mother, wife, or partner	☐4	☐3	☐2	☐1
AB_TAKE_CARE_OWN_HEALTH 20. I was raised to believe I should take care of my own health problems	☐4	☐3	☐2	☐1

AB_SECOND_OTH

What other personal beliefs, feelings, or thoughts keep you from getting help? (Please answer in three lines or less.)

_____

_____

_____

Based on what you are experiencing or have experienced, how much do each of the following issues keep you from getting treatment for alcohol or other drug problems?

Check <u>one box</u> for each statement.

This keeps me from getting help...	A lot	An average amount	A little	Not at all
AB_NO_ENCOURAGEMENT_GET_HELP 21. No encouragement from family and friends to get help for the problem	☐4	☐3	☐2	☐1
AB_NOT_ACCEPTED_ALC_DRUG_FREE 22. Not being accepted by my friends if I am alcohol-free and/or drug free	☐4	☐3	☐2	☐1
AB_NOBODY_CARE_FOR_CHILDREN 23. Having no one in my family or community to take care of my children	☐4	☐3	☐2	☐1
AB_NO_PROGRAM_HELP_STAY_FREE 24. Having no meetings or programs in my community to help me stay alcohol-free and/or drug free	☐4	☐3	☐2	☐1
AB_PARTNER_ANGER_BEING_FREE 25. Anger from my boyfriend, husband, or lover for being alcohol-free and/or drug free	☐4	☐3	☐2	☐1
AB_FEAR_TAKE_CHILDREN_AWAY 26. The fear that my admission of this problem could be used by someone to take my children away	☐4	☐3	☐2	☐1
AB_NO_TIME_OFF_FROM_WORK 27. Not being able to get time off from work	☐4	☐3	☐2	☐1
AB_EVERYONE_EXPECTED_PARTY 28. Living in a community where everyone is expected to party using alcohol and drugs	☐4	☐3	☐2	☐1
AB_PROTECTED_FROM_BAD_RESULTS 29. Being protected from the bad results of my alcohol and/or drug problem by friends, family or coworkers	☐4	☐3	☐2	☐1
AB_ALC_DRUGS_FOR_STRESS 30. Needing alcohol and/or drugs to deal with the stress of daily life in my community	☐4	☐3	☐2	☐1

AB_THIRD_OTH

What other issues keep you from getting help? (Please answer in three lines or less.)

_____

_____

_____

Appendix E: DSM-IV-TR Criteria for Posttraumatic Stress Disorder

A. The person has been exposed to a traumatic event in which both of the following were present:

  (1) The person experienced, witnessed, or was confronted with an event or events that involved actual or threatened death or serious injury, or a threat to the physical integrity of self or others.

  (2) The person's response involved intense fear, helplessness, or horror. Note: In children, this may be expressed instead by disorganized or agitated behavior.

B. The traumatic event is persistently reexperienced in one (or more) of the following ways:

  (3) Recurrent and intrusive distressing recollections of the event, including images, thoughts, or perceptions. Note: In young children, repetitive play may occur in which themes or aspects of the trauma are expressed.

  (4) Recurrent distressing dreams of the event. Note: In children, there may be frightening dreams without recognizable content.

  (5) Acting or feeling as if the traumatic event were recurring (includes a sense of reliving the experience; illusions, hallucinations, and dissociative flashback episodes, including those that occur on awakening or when intoxicated). Note: In young children, trauma-specific reenactment may occur.

  (6) Intense psychological distress at exposure to internal or external cues that symbolize or resemble an aspect of the traumatic event.

  (7) Physiological reactivity on exposure to internal or external cues that symbolize or resemble an aspect of the traumatic event.

C. Persistent avoidance of stimuli associated with the trauma and numbing of general responsiveness (not present before the trauma), as indicated by three (or more) of the following:

(8) Efforts to avoid thoughts, feelings, or conversations associated with the trauma

(9) Efforts to avoid activities, places, or people that arouse recollections of the trauma

(10) Inability to recall an important aspect of the trauma

(11) Markedly diminished interest or participation in significant activities

(12) Feeling of detachment or estrangement from others

(13) Restricted range of affect (e.g., unable to have loving feelings)

(14) Sense of a foreshortened future (e.g., does not expect to have a career, marriage, children, or a normal lifespan)

D. Persistent symptoms of increased arousal (not present before the trauma), as indicated by two (or more) of the following:

(1) Difficulty falling or staying asleep

((2) Irritability or outbursts of anger

(3) Difficulty concentrating

(4) Hypervigilance

(5) Exaggerated startle response

E. Duration of the disturbance (symptoms in Criteria B, C, and D) is more than 1 month.

F. The disturbance causes clinically significant distress or impairment in social, occupational, or other important areas of functioning.

Specify if:

Acute: if duration of symptoms is less than 3 months

Chronic: if duration of symptoms is 3 months or more

Specify if:

With Delayed Onset: if onset of symptoms is at least 6 months after the stressor.

Appendix F: Integration Self-Assessment for Providers

The Women Embracing Life and Living (WELL) Toolkit is designed to help organizations develop plans to improve the quality of care offered to women with co-occurring substance abuse and mental health difficulties and histories of experiencing violence. The toolkit includes

- Instructions for using the WELL Toolkit
- Principles for the Trauma-Informed Treatment of Women with Co-occurring Mental Health and Substance Abuse Disorders (WELL Project 1999)
- Self-Assessment for Providers
- Organizational Self-Assessment
- WELL Planning Tool
- Example of the use of the WELL Planning Tool

The assessment instruments can be used to take an initial measure of an organization's strengths and weaknesses, and to track progress in moving in the desired direction. Organizations that provide direct services to families should use the Self-Assessment for Providers, while State agencies and funding or regulatory agencies should use the Organizational/Agency Self-Assessment. The information from the Self-Assessment can be used in conjunction with the Planning Tool to develop concrete plans to strengthen quality of service in particular areas.

There are many ways of using the Self-Assessment for Providers, depending on the priorities of the organization. The general approach is to

1. Look at one subscale at a time.
2. List the items on which you are not satisfied with your scores.
3. Prioritize them in terms of importance to your agency.
4. Choose a certain target number of items.
5. Develop remedies, steps, and timelines for those items.

An organization can prioritize the subscales and work on only one at a time, or can select items from a number of subscales and then prioritize the items, without reference to subscale. It is a good idea to re-administer the assessment tool on a yearly basis in order to track progress. This assessment should be done for each program administered by your organization. Following is the Self-Assessment for Providers.

Items to be scored on the following Likert Scale:

1. Rarely   2. Occasionally   3. Sometimes
4. Often   5. Consistently

Integration—General

1. ___ Staff is knowledgeable about the way trauma, substance abuse, and mental illness interact.
2. ___ Consumers are provided with psycho-education about the ways in which trauma, substance abuse, and mental illness interact.
3. ___ Service plans address substance abuse, mental illness, and trauma when appropriate.
4. ___ Case management is available which integrates substance abuse, mental health, and violence/trauma services.
5. ___ Multidisciplinary teams can be consulted to address service plan difficulties.
6. ___ Policies and procedures encourage direct care providers to have regular contact (with consent of the consumer) with other service providers who serve the same client.
6. ___ Aftercare plans address substance abuse, mental illness, and trauma.
7. ___ The program appropriately supports direct care staff in participating in supervision and obtaining training.

___Total

Trauma Integrated Into Other Services

7. ___ Staff is knowledgeable about symptoms of trauma.
8. ___ Staff is knowledgeable about domestic violence.
9. ___ Staff is knowledgeable about the risk for retraumatization of victims of violence by staff and peers.
10. ___ Staff is knowledgeable about vicarious traumatization and self-care.
11. ___ Staff is knowledgeable of nonviolent de-escalation techniques.
12. ___ Consumers are assessed regarding their history of experiencing violence.
13. ___ Consumers are assessed regarding their current safety from perpetrators.
14. ___ Consumers are assessed regarding the safety of their current living situation.
15. ___ Psychoeducation is provided for consumers about domestic violence.
16. ___ Psychoeducation is provided for consumers about the symptoms of trauma.
17. ___ Psychoeducation is provided for consumers regarding skills for dealing with trauma symptoms such as grounding and self-soothing.
18. ___ Consumers have access to services for healing from trauma.
19. ___ Consumers have access to safety planning.
20. ___ Consumers have access to legal services.
21. ___ Crisis Prevention Plans are developed in which consumers and providers agree regarding what to do if the behavior of the consumer begins to escalate.
22. ___ Advanced Directives are developed regarding what consumers would like providers to do in the event of a crisis (i.e., who should be notified, where she might be transferred if necessary).
23. ___ Physical restraints are used only as an extreme exception and last resort in accordance with the recommendations of the report of the Massachusetts Department of Mental Health task force on the restraint and seclusion of persons who have been physically or sexually abused.

24. ___ Consumers are instructed in procedures for maintaining each other's confidentiality in order to maintain safety.

25. ___ Procedures are in place to protect both staff and clients if a perpetrator attempts to enter.

26. ___ A "quick response" agreement is in place with local law enforcement should a perpetrator attempt to enter the program.

27. ___ Procedures are in place (which protect the confidentiality of current consumers) for screening new admissions to determine whether they are victimizers of current consumers.

28. ___ A policy is in place to deny admission to the victimizers of a current consumer and refer elsewhere (including certified batterers intervention).

29. ___ Procedures are in place to assist a consumer in accessing a corresponding level of care in another community if it is not safe for her to use the services in her local area.

30. ___ Consumers are helped to grieve the loss of family when it is necessary in order to maintain safety.

31. ___ There is no *arbitrary* exclusion based on domestic violence.

32. ___ Linkages exist with domestic violence providers for referral purposes.

33. ___ Linkages exist with domestic violence providers for consultation purposes.

___Total

Substance Abuse Treatment Integrated Into Other Services

34. ___ Staff has basic knowledge about substance abuse.

35. ___ Psychoeducation is provided for consumers about substance abuse.

36. ___ Consumers are assessed for substance abuse.

37. ___ Linkages exist with substance abuse providers for referral purposes.

38. ___ Linkages exist with methadone providers for referral purposes.

39. ___ Linkages exist with substance abuse providers for consultation purposes.

40. ___ Consumers can participate in the program if they are on methadone.

41. ___ There is no *arbitrary* exclusion based on substance abuse. ___Total

Mental Health Integrated Into Other Services

42. ___ Staff has basic knowledge about mental disorders.

43. ___ Consumers are assessed for mental health problems.

44. ___ Linkages exist with mental health providers for referral purposes.

45. ___ Linkages exist with mental health providers for consultation purposes.

46. ___ Staff has basic knowledge about common side effects of psychotropic medications.

47. ___ Psychoeducation is provided for consumers regarding mental disorders.

48. ___ Policies are in place and provided for consumers regarding what to do if a consumer decompensates psychiatrically.

49. ___ Referrals are made for psychotropic medication evaluation and monitoring.

50. ___ Consumers can participate in the program if they are taking psychotropic medication.

51. ___ There is no arbitrary exclusion based on mental health diagnosis or symptoms.

___Total

Empowerment

52. ___ Staff is knowledgeable about informed consent and confidentiality.

53. ___ Staff is knowledgeable about stigmas.

54. ___ Staff has received training in empowerment-based treatment.

55. ___ Intake assessments include the strengths of consumers.

56. ___ Consumers are given choices regarding which services they access.

57. ___ Consumers may change individual providers of services if they are not satisfied.

58.___ Service plans are individualized.

59.___ Advanced Directives are developed in which consumers indicate what they would like providers to do in the event of a crisis (i.e., whom to notify, where she would like to be transferred to).

60.___ The program meets the Federal guidelines for confidentiality that apply to substance abuse.

61.___ The program meets State confidentiality statutes regarding domestic violence and substance abuse counselors.

62.___ Limits on confidentiality, how records are kept, who has access to information, and how information could be used to the consumer's detriment are carefully explained to consumers before information is collected.

63.___ All discussions of consumer information are done in private settings.

64.___ Policies and procedures are in place for collecting information from diverse groups of consumers about quality of services and for incorporating that feedback into service planning.

65.___ Staff and Board members across the hierarchy of positions include significant numbers of diverse consumers.

66.___ There is appropriate support for consumers moving into a professional role, such as peer leadership training, mentoring, and opportunities to function in an advocacy role.

67.___ All consumers have access to peer support.

___Total

Gender Specific

68.___ Staff is knowledgeable about the specific needs of women.

69.___ Gender-specific services are provided.

70.___ Female consumers can work with female providers if that is their preference.

71.___ Female role models in positions of leadership are available.

___Total

Family Focus

72.___ Psychoeducation is provided for consumers on the intergenerational transmission of substance abuse, mental illness, and violence.

73.___ When a consumer requests services, information is collected regarding her children.

74.___ When a consumer requests services, information is collected regarding her children's need for services.

75.___ There is a means in place for screening children of consumers regarding their need for services.

76.___ Linkages are in place for helping a consumer obtain appropriate services for her children.

77.___ Linkages are in place for helping a consumer obtain appropriate services for other family members.

78.___ In a residential program, there is someone who can assist a consumer in arranging for education of children while she is a resident.

79.___ The program provides a level of parenting education that is appropriate to the level of care (a minimal level being assistance and education regarding communication with children about substance abuse, mental illness, and violence).

80.___ Child care is provided or there is someone who can help a consumer arrange child care that may be necessary for a consumer to receive services.

81.___ Education is provided for a consumer's family (as defined by the consumer) or support system (excluding unsafe relationships).

82.___ Providers work with consumers in advance to develop plans for their children that would be followed in the event that the consumer must be transferred to a more acute level of care.

___Total

Cultural Competence

83.___ Staff is knowledgeable about cultural competence.

84.___ Staff is knowledgeable about the cultures represented by the consumers served.

85.___ Information is collected regarding a consumer's primary language at intake.

86.___ Information is collected regarding a consumer's sexual orientation and identity at intake.

87.___ When a consumer requests services, information is collected regarding her cultural/ethnic/racial identity.

88.___ Differences, including those attributable to class, income, culture, race, ethnicity, disability, language, sexual orientation, religion, and age are incorporated into service planning.

89.___ Language in all intake and training materials is gender neutral and nonviolent.

90.___ Services are available in all languages that are the first language of a large number of the population served.

91.___ Professional translators are provided when necessary, rather than using persons with a personal relationship with the consumer.

92.___ Policies and resources are in place for referring to or obtaining services for consumers who speak languages other than those in which the program provides services.

93.___ There are staff members with the same cultural, racial, and ethnic backgrounds as the consumers being served.

94.___ Policies are in place that state that racism, sexism, homophobia, ageism, and other forms of hatred will not be tolerated.

___Total

Holistic

95.___ Information is collected regarding a consumer's current support system at intake.

96.___ Information is collected regarding a consumer's medical status at intake.

97.___ Information is collected regarding a consumer's legal status at intake.

98.___ Information is collected regarding a consumer's housing status at intake.

99.___ Information is collected regarding a consumer's financial status at intake.

100.___ Psychoeducation is provided for consumers regarding sexually transmitted diseases/HIV/AIDS/Hepatitis C.

___Total

Total scores:

# of 1s—Rarely ___

# of 2s—Occasionally ___

# of 3s—Sometimes ___

# of 4s—Often ___

# of 5s—Consistently ___

Source: WELL Project, Institute for Health and Recovery 2002. For more information about the toolkit contact The Institute for Health and Recovery, (617) 661-3991, or http://www.healthrecovery.org.

Appendix G: Resource Panel Members

Note: The information given indicates each participant's affiliation during the time the panel was convened and may no longer reflect the individual's current affiliation.

Ana Anders, LICSW
Senior Advisor
Special Populations Office
National Institute on Drug Abuse
National Institutes of Health
Bethesda, Maryland

Nancy Bateman, LCSW-C, CAC
Senior Staff Associate
Division of Professional Development and Advocacy
National Association of Social Workers
Washington, D.C.

Duchy Brecht-Trachtenberg, LCSW-C

Jutta H. Butler, B.S.N., M.S.
Public Health Advisor
Practice Improvement Branch
Division of Services Improvement
Center for Substance Abuse Treatment
Substance Abuse and Mental Health Services
Administration
Rockville, Maryland

Colevia Carter
Program Officer
Women's Program
District of Columbia Department of Health
Washington, D.C.

Teresa Chapa, Ph.D.
Senior Social Science Analyst
Center for Mental Health Services
Substance Abuse and Mental Health Services
    Administration
Rockville, Maryland

H. Westley Clark, M.D., J.D., M.P.H., CAS,
    FASAM
Director
Center for Substance Abuse Treatment
Substance Abuse and Mental Health Services
    Administration
Rockville, Maryland

Christina Currier
Public Health Analyst
Practice Improvement Branch
Division of Services Improvement
Center for Substance Abuse Treatment
Substance Abuse and Mental Health Services
    Administration
Rockville, Maryland

Dorynne Czechowicz, M.D.
Medical Officer
Treatment Development Branch
Division of Treatment Research and
    Development
National Institute on Drug Abuse
National Institutes of Health
Bethesda, Maryland

Sandra Dodge, CNP
Women's Health Coordinator
Nursing Division
Indian Health Service
Rockville, Maryland

Marlene EchoHawk, Ph.D.
Health Science Administrator
Division of Behavioral Health
Indian Health Service
Rockville, Maryland

Isabel Ellis, M.S.W.
Public Health Analyst
National Institute on Alcohol Abuse and
    Alcoholism
National Institutes of Health
Rockville, Maryland

Krista Evans
Coordinator
Women's Program
Office of Women's Programs
District of Columbia Department of Health
Washington, D.C.

Jennifer Fiedelholtz
Public Health Analyst
Office of Policy and Program Coordination
Substance Abuse and Mental Health Services
    Administration
Rockville, Maryland

Loretta P. Finnegan, M.D.
Medical Advisor for the Director
Office of the Director
Office of Research on Women's Health
National Institutes of Health
Bethesda, Maryland

Bettie Foley, M.S., CMAC
Associate Director
National Association of Addiction Treatment
    Providers
Chicago, Illinois

Jennifer Godfrey
Intern
Maternal and Child Health Bureau
Health Resources and Services Administration
Rockville, Maryland

Kathrine Hollinger, D.V.M., M.P.H.
Health Program Coordinator
Office of Women's Health
Food and Drug Administration
Rockville, Maryland

Sharon L. Holmes
Director
Office of Equal Employment Opportunity
and Civil Rights
Substance Abuse and Mental Health Services
    Administration
Rockville, Maryland

Leah Holmes-Bonilla
National Mental Health Association
Alexandria, Virginia

Arthur MacNeill Horton, Ed.D., ABPN, APP
Office of the Director
Center for Substance Abuse Treatment
Substance Abuse and Mental Health Services
    Administration
Rockville, Maryland

Ellen Hutchins, M.S.W., M.P.H.
Social Work Consultant
Maternal and Child Health Bureau
Health Resources and Services Administration
Rockville, Maryland

Gwendolyn P. Kieta, Ph.D.
Director
Women's Programs Office
American Psychological Association
Washington, D.C.

Lisa King
Women's Health Specialist
Maternal and Child Health Bureau
Health Resources and Services Administration
Rockville, Maryland

Sheila P. Litzky, M.A.
Statewide Coordinator for Women's Services
Alcohol and Drug Abuse Administration
Spring Grove Hospital Center
Catonsville, Maryland

James J. Manlandro, D.O., FAOAAM, FACOFP
Medical Director
Family Addiction Treatment Services, Inc.
Rio Grande, New Jersey

Carmen Martinez
Manager
Office of Equal Employment Opportunity and
    Civil Rights
Substance Abuse and Mental Health Services
    Administration
Rockville, Maryland

Ann Maskell
Office Manager
Family Addiction Treatment Services, Inc.
Dennisville, New Jersey

Alixe McNeill
Assistant Vice President
The National Council on the Aging
Washington, D.C.

Kathleen Mitchell
Program Director
National Organization on Fetal Alcohol
    Syndrome
Washington, D.C.

Susana Perry
Office of State and Community Programs
Administration on Aging
United States Department of Health and Human
    Services
Washington, D.C.

Melissa V. Rael, USPHS
Senior Program Management Officer
Co-occurring and Homeless Branch
Division of State and Community Assistance
Center for Substance Abuse Treatment
Substance Abuse and Mental Health Services
    Administration
Rockville, Maryland

Rosa M. Reyes
Intern
Center for Substance Abuse Treatment
Substance Abuse and Mental Health Services
    Administration
Rockville, Maryland

Gwen Rubinstein, M.P.H.
Director of Policy Research
Legal Action Center
Washington, D.C.

Hector Sanchez, M.S.W.
Team Leader
Performance Partnership Grant Branch
Division of State and Community Assistance
Center for Substance Abuse Treatment
Substance Abuse and Mental Health Services
    Administration
Rockville, Maryland

Steven J. Shapiro, M.C.J.
Public Health Advisor
Division of Practice and Systems Development
Center for Substance Abuse Treatment
Substance Abuse and Mental Health Services
    Administration
Rockville, Maryland

June Susan Sivilli
Senior Policy Analyst
Office of National Drug Control Policy
Executive Office of the President
Washington, D.C.

Lany Sivongsay
Intern
Office of Policy Coordination and Planning
Center for Substance Abuse Treatment
Substance Abuse and Mental Health Services
    Administration
Rockville, Maryland

Arlene Stanton, Ph.D., NCC
Social Science Analyst
Office of Evaluation, Scientific Analysis and
    Synthesis
Data Infrastructure Branch
Center for Substance Abuse Treatment
Substance Abuse and Mental Health Services
    Administration
Rockville, Maryland

Richard T. Suchinsky, M.D.
Associate Chief for Addictive Disorders and
    Psychiatric Rehabilitation
Mental Health and Behavioral Sciences Services
Department of Veterans Affairs
Washington, D.C.

Appendix H: Cultural Competency and Diversity Network Participants

Note: The information given indicates each participant's affiliation during the time the network was convened and may no longer reflect the individual's current affiliation.

Jacqueline P. Butler, M.S.W., CCDC, LISW
Professor of Clinical Psychiatry
College of Medicine
Substance Abuse Division
University of Cincinnati
Cincinnati, Ohio
African American Workgroup

Deion Cash
Executive Director
Community Treatment & Correction
Center, Inc.
Canton, Ohio
African American Workgroup

Carol S. D'Agostino, C.S.W., CASAC
Director
Geriatric Addictions Program
LIFESPAN of Greater Rochester, Inc.
Rochester, New York
Aging Workgroup

Marty Estrada
Regional Administrator
Correctional Treatment
Florida Addictions and Correctional
Treatment Services, Inc.
Tallahassee, Florida
Hispanic/Latino Workgroup

Nancy Ferreyra
Executive Director
Pacific Research and Training Alliance
Berkeley, California
Disabilities Workgroup

Tonda L. Hughes, Ph.D., R.N.
Associate Professor
College of Nursing
University of Illinois at Chicago
Chicago, Illinois
LGBT Workgroup

Ting-Fun May Lai, M.S.W., CASAC
Director
Asian American Recovery Services, Inc.
New York, New York
Disabilities/Asian Workgroup

Lorene Lake, M.A., Ed.
Executive Director
Chrysalis House, Inc.
Crownsville, Maryland
African American Workgroup

Rachelle A. Martin
Provider Relations Manager
Alcohol, Drug and Mental Health
Board of Franklin County
Columbus, Ohio
African American Workgroup

Alixe McNeill
Assistant Vice President
The National Council on the Aging
Washington, D.C.
Aging Workgroup

Valerie Robinson, M.S., LPC
Director of Training
Danya Institute, Inc.
Central East Addictions Technology Transfer
    Center
Silver Spring, Maryland
African American Workgroup

Hector Sanchez, M.S.W.
Team Leader
Performance Partnership Grant Branch
Division of State and Community Assistance
Center for Substance Abuse Treatment
Substance Abuse and Mental Health Services
    Administration
Rockville, Maryland
Hispanic/Latino Workgroup

Richard T. Suchinsky, M.D.
Associate Chief for Addictive Disorders and
    Psychiatric Rehabilitation
Mental Health and Behavioral Sciences Services
Department of Veterans Affairs
Washington, D.C.
Disabilities Workgroup

Appendix I:
Field Reviewers

Note: The information given indicates each participant's affiliation during the time the review was conducted and may no longer reflect the individual's current affiliation.

Sharon K. Amatetti, M.P.H.
Sr. Public Health Analyst
Office of Program Analysis and Coordination
Center for Substance Abuse Treatment
Substance Abuse and Mental Health Services Administration
Rockville, Maryland

Duiona R. Baker, M.P.H.
Associate Administrator for Women's Services
Substance Abuse and Mental Health Services Administration
Rockville, Maryland

Peggy Bean
Analyst
Perinatal Substance Abuse
California Department of Alcohol and Drug Programs
Sacramento, California

Faye Belgrave, Ph.D.
Professor of Psychology
Department of Psychology
Virginia Commonwealth University
Richmond, Virginia

Mary R. Boyd, Ph.D., R.N.
Associate Professor
College of Nursing
University of South Carolina
Columbia, South Carolina

Suzette E. Brann, J.D., M.B.A.
President
Unlimited Horizons, LLC
Port Tobacco, Maryland

Catherine J. Brow
Specialized Female Services Coordinator
Commission on Alcohol and Drug Abuse
Austin, Texas

Jutta H. Butler, B.S.N., M.S.
Public Health Advisor
Practice Improvement Branch
Division of Services Improvement
Center for Substance Abuse Treatment
Substance Abuse and Mental Health Services
    Administration
Rockville, Maryland

Donna L. Caldwell, Ph.D.
Director of Evaluation and Research
National Perinatal Information Center
Providence, Rhode Island

Sherry Dyche Ceperich
Assistant Professor
Division of Addiction Psychiatry
Virginia Commonwealth University
Richmond, Virginia

Redonna K. Chandler, Ph.D.
Health Scientist Administrator
Services Research Branch
Division of Epidemiology, Services, and
    Prevention Research
National Institute on Drug Abuse
Bethesda, Maryland

Charlotte Chapman, M.S., LPC, CAC
Training Director
Division of Addiction Psychiatry
Mid-Atlantic Addiction Technology Transfer
    Center
Virginia Commonwealth University
Richmond, Virginia

Kaye Chavis
Treatment Consultant
Public Health Programs Director
Bureau of Alcohol and Drug Abuse Services
Tennessee Department of Health
Nashville, Tennessee

Stephanie S. Covington, Ph.D., LCSW
Co-Director
Center for Gender and Justice
Institute for Relational Development
La Jolla, California

Margaret A. Cramer, Ph.D.
Clinical Psychologist/Instructor
Harvard Medical School
Boston, Massachusetts

A. Rebecca Crowell, LCDC, LPC
Executive Director
Nexus Recovery Center
Dallas, Texas

Carol S. D'Agostino, C.S.W., CASAC
Director
Geriatric Addictions Program
LIFESPAN of Greater Rochester, Inc.
Rochester, New York

Sharon DeEsch, M.A., MAC, LCDC
Genesis Counseling Associates, P.C.
Dallas, Texas

Herman Diesenhaus
Social Science Analyst
Center for Substance Abuse Treatment
Substance Abuse and Mental Health Services
    Administration
Rockville, Maryland

Marlene EchoHawk, Ph.D.
Health Science Administrator
Division of Behavioral Health
Indian Health Service
Rockville, Maryland

Darcy Edwards, Ph.D., M.S.W., CADC I
Alcohol and Drug/HIV Services Manager
Counseling and Treatment Services
Oregon Department of Corrections
Salem, Oregon

Saul Feldman, Ph.D.
Chairman & C.E.O.
United Behavioral Health
San Francisco, California

Nancy Ferreyra
Executive Director
Pacific Research and Training Alliance
Berkeley, California

Norma B. Finkelstein, Ph.D., M.S.W.
Executive Director
Institute for Health & Recovery
Cambridge, Massachusetts

Jo Ann Ford, M.A.
Assistant Director
Substance Abuse Resources and Disability
Issues School of Medicine
Wright State University
Dayton, Ohio

Joanne Gampel
Social Science Analyst
Center for Substance Abuse Treatment
Substance Abuse and Mental Health Services
    Administration
Rockville, Maryland

Mary M. Gillespie, Psy.D., CASAC
Psychologist
Hudson Valley Community College
Private Practice
Saratoga Springs, New York

Jennifer Glover, M.S., LPC
Programs Field Representative
Oklahoma Department of Mental Health and
    Substance Abuse Services
Oklahoma City, Oklahoma

Valerie A. Gruber, Ph.D., M.P.H.
Assistant Clinical Professor
University of California
Senior Psychologist Division of Substance Abuse
    and Addiction Medicine
San Francisco General Hospital
San Francisco, California

Joanne M. Hall, Ph.D., R.N.
Associate Professor
College of Nursing
University of Tennessee
Knoxville, Tennessee

Deborah Hollis, M.A.
Director
Division of Substance Abuse Quality and
    Planning
Michigan Department of Community Health
Lansing, Michigan

Kathryn S. Icenhower, Ph.D., LCSW
Executive Director
SHIELDS for Families Project, Inc.
Los Angeles, California

Lauren Jansson, M.D.
Director of Pediatrics
Center for Addiction and Pregnancy
Johns Hopkins Bayview Medical Center
Baltimore, Maryland

Hendree E. Jones, Ph.D.
Assistant Professor
CAP Research Director
Department of Psychiatry and Behavioral
    Sciences
Johns Hopkins University Center
Baltimore, Maryland

Karol A. Kaltenbach, Ph.D.
Clinical Associate Professor of Pediatrics,
    Psychiatry and Human Behavior
Director, Maternal Addiction Treatment
    Education and Research
Department of Pediatrics
Jefferson Medical College
Thomas Jefferson University
Philadelphia, Pennsylvania

George Kanuck, D.N.Sc.
Public Health Analyst
Center for Substance Abuse Treatment
Substance Abuse and Mental Health Services
    Administration
Rockville, Maryland

Cheryl Ann Kennedy, M.S.W.
Assistant Director
Institute for Health & Recovery
Cambridge, Massachusetts

Nancy Kennedy, Dr.P.H.
Scientific Advisor to the Director
Center for Substance Abuse Prevention
Substance Abuse and Mental Health Services
    Administration
Rockville, Maryland

Mary V. Ker, Ph.D.
Executive Director
Optimal Research and Evaluation
Tucson, Arizona

Michael Warren Kirby, Jr., Ph.D., M.A.,
CAC III
Chief Executive Officer
Arapahoe House, Inc.
Thornton, Colorado

Danica Kalling Knight, Ph.D.
Research Scientist
Institute of Behavioral Research
Texas Christian University
Fort Worth, Texas

Hillary Kunins, M.D., M.P.H.
Medical Director, HUB II Clinic Program
    Coordinator
Division of Substance Abuse
Albert Einstein College of Medicine
Bronx, New York

Carol L. Kuprevich, M.A.
Training Education Administrator
Division of Alcoholism, Drug Abuse and Mental
    Health
Delaware Health and Social Services
New Castle, Delaware

Martha Kurgans, M.A.
Women's Services Program Specialist
Virginia Department of Mental Health,
Mental Retardation and Substance Abuse
    Services
Richmond, Virginia

Linda Christina Latta, Ph.D.
Women's Treatment Coordinator
Chemical Dependency Bureau
Montana State Department of Public Health
    and Human Services
Helena, Montana

Kayla Mary Leopold, LCSW
Site Manager
New Directions Family Treatment Center
CODA, Inc.
Portland, Oregon

Helen J. Levine, Ph.D.
Senior Research Scientist
JSI Research and Training
Boston, Massachusetts

Kimberly A. Lucas
Treatment Specialist
Women's Treatment Coordinator
Delaware Division of Substance Abuse and
    Mental Health
New Castle, Delaware

Ruby J. Martinez, Ph.D., R.N., CS
Assistant Professor
School of Nursing
University of Colorado
Denver, Colorado

Kathleen B. Masis, M.D.
Medical Officer for Behavioral Health
Billings Area Indian Health Service
Billings, Montana

Lisa A. Melchior, Ph.D.
Vice President
The Measurement Group, LLC
Culver City, California

Juana Mora, Ph.D.
Professor
Northridge Chicano/a Studies Department
California State University
Northridge, California

Ruby Neville
Public Health Advisor
Center for Substance Abuse Treatment
Substance Abuse and Mental Health Services
    Administration
Rockville, Maryland

Joanne Nicholson, Ph.D.
Associate Professor
Psychiatry and Family Medicine
University of Massachusetts Medical School
Worcester, Massachusetts

Nancy Nikkinnen, M.D.
Medical Director
Children and Parents Program
Penn-Silver Health Center
Prince George's County Health Department
Forestville, Maryland

William (Bill) Francis Northey, Jr., Ph.D.
Research Specialist
American Association for Marriage and Family
    Therapy
Alexandria, Virginia

Gwen M. Olitsky, M.S.
Founder and C.E.O.
The Self-Help Institute for Training and
    Therapy
Lansdale, Pennsylvania

Dorothy Payne, M.B.A.
AOD Program Consultant
Alcohol and Drug Abuse Prevention
Arkansas Department of Health
Freeway Medical Center
Little Rock, Arkansas

Thomas A. Peltz, LMHC, CAS, M.Ed.
Therapist
Private Practice
Beverly Farms, Massachusetts

David J. Powell, Ph.D.
President
International Center for Health Concerns, Inc.
East Granby, Connecticut

Beverly A. Pringle, Ph.D.
Health Scientist Administrator
National Institute on Drug Abuse
Bethesda, Maryland

Melissa Rael, CAPT., USPHS
Senior Program Management Officer
Center for Substance Abuse Treatment
Substance Abuse and Mental Health Services
    Administration
Rockville, Maryland

Barbara E. Ramlow
Acting Director
Institute on Women and Substance Abuse
University of Kentucky
Lexington, Kentucky

José Rivera, J.D.
President
Rivera, Sierra and Company, Inc.
Brooklyn, New York

Valerie Robinson, M.S., LPC
Director of Training
Danya Institute, Inc.
Silver Spring, Maryland

Maurilia Rodriguez, Ph.D., R.N., CDE
Diabetes Consultant
Houston, Texas

Laurie Roehrich, Ph.D.
Associate Professor
Department of Psychology
Indiana University of Pennsylvania
Indiana, Pennsylvania

James Rowan, M.A., CAC III
Program Manager
Case Management and Offender Services
Arapahoe House, Inc.
Thornton, Colorado

Paula G. Ruane
Marketing Director
Gaudenzia, Inc.
Harrisburg, Pennsylvania

Judith Rubin
Instructor
School of Social Work
San Francisco State University
San Francisco, California

Suzanne A. Rymer
Director
Health and Social Work Services
Mature Services, Inc.
Akron, Ohio

JoAnn Y. Sacks, Ph.D.
Principal Investigator
National Development and Research
Institutes, Inc.
New York, New York

Andrea Savage, Ph.D.
Associate Professor
School of Social Work
Hunter College
New York, New York

Karen Saylors, Ph.D.
Director of Research and Evaluation
Family and Child Guidance Clinic
Native American Health Center
Oakland, California

Sheryl A. Schrepf, M.S.W.
Consultant
Nebraska Coalition for Women's Treatment
Lincoln, Nebraska

Meri Shadley, Ph.D., M.F.T., LADC
Associate Professor
Center for the Application of Substance Abuse
    Technologies
College of Education
University of Nevada, Reno
Reno, Nevada

David E. Smith, M.D.
Founder and President
Haight Ashbury Free Clinics, Inc.
San Francisco, California

Diane Batt Smith, LADC
Substance Abuse Program Coordinator
Division of Alcohol and Drug Abuse
Vermont Department of Health
Burlington, Vermont

Virginia Steadman
Director of Women's Issues
Alcohol and Substance Abuse Services
Mississippi Department of Mental Health
Jackson, Mississippi

Marceil Ten Eyck, MC
Psychotherapist/Consultant
Kirkland, Washington

Elaine Tophia, M.S.W.
Executive Director
National Opioid Treatment Clinician
    Association
Decatur, Georgia

Karen Urbany
Public Health Advisor
Center for Substance Abuse Treatment
Substance Abuse and Mental Health Services
    Administration
Rockville, Maryland

Nancy R. VanDeMark, M.S.W.
Director
Research and Program Evaluation
Arapahoe House, Inc.
Thornton, Colorado

Beverly Vayhinger, Ph.D.
Program Director
Children and Parents Program
Prince George's County Health Department
Forestville, Maryland

Suzanne L. Wenzel, Ph.D.
Senior Behavioral Scientist
RAND
Santa Monica, California

Sharon Wilsnack, Ph.D.
Professor
School of Medicine & Health Sciences
Department of Neuroscience
University of North Dakota
Grand Forks, North Dakota

Helen Wolstenholme, M.S.W., LCSW, CCAS
Women's Treatment Coordinator
Substance Abuse Services Section
North Carolina Division of Mental
Health/Developmental Disabilities/Substance
    Abuse Services
Raleigh, North Carolina

Carolyn A. Work, M.A.
Training Director
Institute for Research, Education and Training
    in Addictions
Pittsburgh, Pennsylvania

Loretta Young Silvia, M.Ed., Ph.D.
Associate Professor of Psychiatry
Department of Psychiatry and Behavioral
    Medicine
Wake Forest University School of Medicine
Winston-Salem, North Carolina

Nancy Young, Ph.D.
Director
Children and Family Futures
Irvine, California

Shaila Yeh, M.S.W.
Senior Associate
Children and Family Futures
Irvine, California

Joan E. Zweben, Ph.D.
Executive Director
The 14th Street Clinic and Medical Group
East Bay Community Recovery Project
University of California
Berkeley, California

Janet K. Zwick
Director
Division of Health Promotion, Prevention and
    Addictive Behaviors
Iowa Department of Public Health
Des Moines, Iowa

Appendix J: Acknowledgments

Numerous people contributed to the development of this TIP, including the TIP Consensus Panel (see p. xi), the KAP Expert Panel (see p. xv), the Federal Resource Panel, (see appendix G), the KAP Cultural Competency and Diversity Network (see appendix H), and TIP Field Reviewers (see appendix I).

In addition, Rose M. Urban, M.S.W., J.D., LCSW, LCAS, served as the CDM KAP Executive Deputy Project Director. Roberta Hochberg served as the CDM KAP Managing Project Co-Director. Claudia A. Blackburn, M.S., Psy.D., served as the CDM KAP Expert Content Director. Other CDM KAP personnel included Susan Kimner, Deputy Project Director/ Editorial Director; Jessica L. Culotta, Managing Editor; Amy Conklin, Editor; Janet Humphrey, M.A., former Editor; Virgie D. Paul, M.L.S., Librarian; Lee Ann Knapp, Quality Assurance Editor.

JBS KAP personnel included Barbara Fink, R.N., M.P.H., KAP Managing Project Co-Director; Dennis Burke, M.S., M.A., former Product Development Manager; Wendy Caron, Senior QA Editor; Leah Bogden, Junior Editor; and Frances Nebesky, Senior QA Editor.

Sandra Clunies, M.S., I.C.A.D.C., served as Content Advisor. Catalina Bartlett, M.A., Randi Henderson, B.A., Susan Hills, Ph.D., Helen Oliff, and Mary Lou Rife, Ph.D., were writers.

Index

Caucasian population
    acculturation effect on substance use
        disorders, 24
    misuse of OTC cough and cold medications
        and, 48
    primary substance of abuse on admission
        to treatment, 32
CBT. *See* Cognitive-behavioral therapy
"Celebrating Families"™, 153
Center for Epidemiologic Study Depression
    Scale
    description and uses, 67
Center for Substance Abuse Treatment. *See also*
    specific publications
    comprehensive model of care, 4, 15
Congress's funding of, 273
        Residential Women and Children/
            Pregnant and Postpartum Women
            programs, 100, 273, 281
Centers for Disease Control and Prevention
    HIV association with injecting drugs, 52
    life expectancy for women, 14
Cervical cancer
    alcohol use and abuse and, 42
    substance use disorders and, 7
Chan, C.S.
    Asian/Pacific American lesbian and
        bisexual women, 126
Chang, G.
    T-ACE compared with MAST and AUDIT,
        64
*The Change Book: A Blueprint of Technology
    Transfer,* 194
Chasnoff, I.J.
    5Ps screening for pregnant women, 65
Chen, H.
    cirrhosis mortality, 54
Child care. *See also* Children
    as an obstacle to treatment, 86
    detoxification issues, 97
    immediate and short-term services, 291
    issue overview, 10–11, 13
    onsite, 141, 288, 290
    outpatient treatment and, 98
    residential treatment programs and,
        100–101
    therapeutic, 288
    women in the criminal justice system and,
        134

Child custody. *See also* Children
    African Americans and, 110
    issue overview, 10
    loss of custody as a treatment obstacle, 85,
        87, 88
    mothers in treatment who wish to
        relinquish care, 154
    parent-child visiting and, 153–154
    regaining custody, 153
    women in the criminal justice system and,
        134
Child protective services
    co-occurrence of a substance use disorder
        and involvement in the child welfare
        system, 87
    reunification of mothers and children
        after treatment, 101
    treatment referral and, 31
    treatment retention and referral to or
        involvement with, 139
Child welfare system
    confidentiality issues, 87, 88
    linking women with, 289–290
    prevalence of co-occurring disorders
        among women in, 158
Children. *See also* Adolescents; Age factors;
    Child care; Child custody; Child welfare
    system; *Comprehensive Substance Abuse
    Treatment Model for Women and Their
    Children*; Services for children of women in
    substance abuse treatment
    accompanying their mothers in residential
        treatment settings, 86, 100–101, 141
    information about mothers' substance use
        disorders, 152–153
    physical and sexual abuse by parents, 156
Children with special needs
    accompanying mothers in residential
        treatment, 154
    assessment of, 154
Cigarette smoking. *See* Tobacco use
Cirrhosis
    African Americans and, 111
    alcohol use and, 40, 41
    hepatitis C virus and, 54
    substance use disorders and, 7
CIWA-Ar. *See* Clinical Institute Withdrawal
    Assessment

Cultural competence
    Hispanic/Latina clients and, 107
    Improving Cultural Competence in Substance Abuse Treatment, 32
    treatment of Native Americans and, 122–123
    of treatment programs, 86
Cultural Competency and Diversity Network participants, 323–324
Culture. *See also* Psychosocial and cultural history; Racial/ethnic factors; Sociocultural context
    acculturation effect on substance use disorders, 24, 26
    cultural relevance and, 58
    negative attitudes toward substance abuse as an obstacle to treatment, 85–86
    physiological effects of substance abuse and, 38–39
    screening and assessment and, 58–60

D
Danger Assessment
    description and uses, 71
DATOS. *See* Drug Abuse Treatment Outcome Study
Day, N.
    birth outcomes and marijuana use, 52
Decategorization
    definition, 293
Demographics
    African Americans, 109
    Asian/Pacific Americans, 115
    Hispanic/Latina population, 104
    lesbian and bisexual women, 123–124
    Native Americans, 119
    older women, 127
    Rural American women, 130–131
    sociodemographics of treatment retention, 138
Demonstration Grant Program for Residential Women and their Children
    Lessons Learned: Residential Substance Abuse Treatment for Women and Their Children, 108
Depression. *See also* Postpartum depression
    co-occurring substance use, 23–24, 173–174

description, 173
factors increasing a women's chance of depression prior to deliver of a baby, 158, 160
hepatitis C virus treatment and, 54
older women and, 127
physical or sexual abuse survivors and, 22
racial/ethnic factors, 21, 173
screening instruments, 67–68
sexual orientation and, 21
substance abuse treatment and, 174
Detoxification, ASAM Levels I-IV
    description, 96, 285
    length of, 97
    pregnancy and, 97–98, 151
    trauma victims and, 97
    treatment after, 97
    women with dependent children and, 97
Detoxification and Substance Abuse Treatment (TIP 45), 78, 96, 98
Developmental characteristics of women
    life-course issues, 13
    physiological effects of substance abuse and, 39–40
Developmental services for children, 288
Diabetes
    alcohol consumption and, 40
Diagnostic and Statistical manual of Mental Disorders, Fourth Edition, Text Revision
    postpartum depression criteria, 159
    posttraumatic stress disorder symptoms and criteria, 70, 161, 311–312
    substance abuse definition and treatment, 16, 275
    Texas Christian University Drug Screen II and, 62
    trauma criteria, 154
Dialectical behavior therapy
    eating disorders, 176
Discrimination
    substance use disorder risk factor, 24
Disordered eating
    definition, 175
Divorce
    risk factor for substance use disorders, xviii, 19–20
Domestic violence. *See also* Interpersonal violence; Trauma
    substance use disorders and, 23

Drabble, L.
        sexual orientation and substance use, 21
DrinC. *See* Drinker Inventory of Consequences
Drinker Inventory of Consequences
        description and uses, 79
        text of, 302–306
Drug Abuse Treatment Outcome Study
        age factors in treatment retention, 138
Drug use monitoring
        range of concerns, 287
DSM-IV-TR. *See Diagnostic and Statistical manual of Mental Disorders, Fourth Edition, Text Revision*

E

Early and Periodic Screening, Diagnostic, and Treatment
        description, 294
Early intervention, ASAM Level 0.5
        approaches for, 96
        motivational interviewing, 96
        during pregnancy, 96
        services included, 95
        treatment goals, 95–96
EAT-26. *See* Eating Attitudes Test-26
Eating Attitudes Test-26
        description and uses, 73
        text of, 299–301
Eating disorders. *See also specific disorders*
        biopsychosocial context, 176
        co-occurring substance use, 23–24, 175–176
        compulsive eating, 72–73
        definitions (figure), 175
        difficulty of detecting, 174–175
        misuse of over-the-counter drugs and, 47
        mortality rates, 72
        nutritional counseling and, 177
        percent of women in substance abuse treatment with, 72
        personality disorders and, 176
        prevalence of, 174
        screening for, 72–73
        treatment for substance use disorders and, 176–177
Economic issues
        overview, 2
Ecstasy. *See* Methylenedioxy-methamphetamine
Education. *See also* Training
        discrimination and opportunities for, 24

in parenting and child development, 289
        remediation and support for women in treatment, 289
        services for children, 291
        substance abuse education, 285–286, 288
        trauma-informed treatment approach and, 166
        treatment retention and level of, 138
        vocational and academic, 292
Elderly persons. *See also* Older women
        physiological effects of substance abuse and, 40
        substance dependence issues, 14
        women as caregivers for, 14
Eliason, M.
        definitions of "lesbian," "gay," and "bisexual," 124
Employment. *See also* Unemployment
        complexity of women's work lives, 13
        discrimination and, 24
        readiness services, 289
        support services, 292
Endometrial cancer
        alcohol use and, 42
Enhancing Motivation for Change in Substance Abuse Treatment (TIP 35), 96, 143
EPSDT. *See* Early and Periodic Screening, Diagnostic, and Treatment
Ethnic factors. *See* Racial/ethnic factors
Evans, S.M.
        cocaine effects on menstruation, 46
Executive Orders
        establishment of tribal colleges for Native Americans, 123
Eyler, F.D.
        prenatal cocaine exposure effects, 49

F

Faith-based initiatives. *See also* Religious and spiritual practices
        for early intervention, 96
Faith-based organizations. *See also* Religious and spiritual practices
        support for women, 292
Fals-Stewart, W.
        couples therapy and treatment outcomes, 138

Hispanic/Latina population and, 105
Native Americans and, 120
Methylenedioxy-methamphetamine
gender differences in metabolism and
effects of, 46–47
Mexican Americans
acculturation effect on substance use
disorders, 24
alcohol use by women, 105
MHSF-III. *See* Mental health Screening Form-
III
MI. *See* Motivational interviewing
Michigan Alcohol Screening Test
compared with T-ACE, 64
compared with TWEAK, 63
Miles, D.R.
pregnancy and co-occurring disorders,
139
Miller, D.
*The Addiction and Trauma Recovery
Integration Model*, 171
Trauma Reenactment Model, 171
Miller, Jean Baker
Toward a New Psychology of Women, 144
M.I.N.I. *See* Mini-International
Neuropsychiatric Interview
Mini-International Neuropsychiatric Interview
description and uses, 67
Mood disorders. *See also* Depression; *specific
disorders*
postpartum depression and, 158
Moos, B.S.
benefits of Alcoholics Anonymous for
women, 186
Moos, R.H.
benefits of Alcoholics Anonymous for
women, 186
Mora, J.
alcohol use by Mexican American women,
105
key questions for clinicians with Hispanic/
Latina clients, 107
Morgenstern, J.
case management study, 92
Motivational interviewing
pregnancy and, 96
Multidimensional Measure of Religiousness/
Spirituality
description and uses, 79–80

N

Najavits, L.M.
posttraumatic stress disorder in women
with substance use disorders, 163–164
Seeking Safety, 145, 147, 164, 171–172
Woman's Addiction Workbook, 145, 147
Nanehahal, K.
alcohol use and stroke, 41
Narcotics Anonymous
description, 291
NAS. *See* Neonatal abstinence syndrome
National Association for Children of Alcoholics
"Celebrating Families"™, 153
National Center for Health Statistics, National
Health Interview
tobacco use prevalence, 28
National Center on Addiction and Substance
Abuse
initiation of substance use among women,
27
National Comorbidity Study
co-occurring substance use and mental
disorders, 23
National Epidemiologic Survey on Alcohol and
Related Conditions
inverse relationship between rates of
alcohol dependence and age, 127–128
National Institutes of Health
racial and ethnic disparities in health, 103
National Medical Expenditures Survey
prescription drug use among women, 26
National Survey on Drug Use and Health
cost of treatment, 11
description, 26
illicit drug use by women, 26
misuse of OTC cough and cold
medications, 47–48
percent of females with substance
dependence or abuse, 1
percentages of reasons for not receiving
substance use treatment in the past
year among women aged 18-49 who
needed treatment and who perceived a
need for it: 2004-2006 (figure), 85
substance abuse among Native Americans,
119, 120
National Survey on Drug Use and Health 2003
age factors in substance use disorders, 30
prescription drug use among women, 26

Office of the Surgeon General. *See also* Surgeon General
    effect of mothers' smoking cessation on their children, 28
Office on Women's health
    educational materials on eating disorders, 177
Older women. *See also* Age factors; Elderly persons
    clinical treatment issues, 130
    demographics, 127
    resiliency factors, 130
    risk factors for alcohol dependence and prescription drug abuse, 127
    in Rural America, 130
    signs of alcohol-dependence and/or drug abuse, 128
    substance use among, 127–128, 130
    timing of onset of alcohol dependence, 127
Opioids
    African Americans and, 110
    Asian/Pacific Americans and, 117
    birth outcomes and, 50–51
    gender differences in metabolism and effects of, 47
    withdrawal from, 66, 98
Opportunistic diseases
    substance use disorders and, 7
Organization of the TIP, 15
Organizational change
    administrative strategies for, 193–196
Osteoporosis
    alcohol use and, 42, 45
    substance use disorders and, 7, 14
    tobacco use and, 42, 45
OTC drugs. *See* Over-the-counter drugs
Outpatient treatment, ASAM Level I. *See also* Intensive outpatient treatment, ASAM Level II
    appropriate use of, 98
    child care and, 98
Outreach
    effectiveness of, 88
    major components, 88, 283
    PROTOTYPES Outreach Program (figure), 91
    trauma-informed treatment approach and, 166

Over-the-counter drugs
    admission of women for treatment of abuse of, 32–33
    gender differences in metabolism and effects of, 47–48
Overexercising
    definition, 175

P

Page, R.M.
    negative self-image, 21
Panic disorders
    co-occurring substance use, 23–24
Paranjape, A.
    questions to use in screening for interpersonal violence, 71
Parenting
    children who are not in a mother's care, 153–154
    children with special needs, 154
    desire of women to be caring and competent parents, 151
    education in parenting and child development, 289
    inadequate role models and, 151
    issue overview, 10–11, 13
    recovery and, 151–152
    women with histories of trauma and, 153
Parenting programs
    onsite child care and child specialists, 152
    topics for parenting skills and relationship building, 152
    women's coping skills and, 152
Partial fetal alcohol syndrome
    description, 49
Partners. *See also* Marital status
    curricula for relationships in recovery, 145–146
    dynamic of one partner being the supplier and the other using the drug, 20, 27
    effect of partner substance abuse, 20
    ending significant relationships, 145
    entering or staying in treatment and, 20
    intimate partner violence screening tool (figure), 72
    involving male partners in women's treatment, 20, 145–147
    safety issues for clients, 145
    support from, 10, 21

R

Racial/ethnic factors. *See also* Culture;
    Substance abuse among specific population
    groups and settings; *specific races and
    ethnicity*
        depression, 21, 173
        health disparities, 103
        misuse of OTC cough and cold
            medications, 48
        percentage of admissions to substance
            abuse treatment programs by racial/
            ethnic group in 2006 (figure), 33
        physiological effects of substance abuse,
            38–39
        primary substance of abuse among women
            admitted for substance abuse treatment
            by racial/ethnic group by percentage
            (figure), 34
        reluctance to seek treatment, 86
        screening and assessment, 58–60
        treatment admissions characteristics of
            racial/ethnic groups, 31–32, 33
Reader guidelines, 15
Recovery management
        continuing care, 181–182
        executive summary, xxii–xxiii
        overview, 181
Recreational services for children, 290–291
Refinancing
        definition, 293–294
Relapse
        client characteristics and, 183–184
        during the continuing care period, 181–
            182
        heroin use and, 98
        postpartum relapse prevention, 184–186
        posttraumatic stress disorder and, 164
        women-specific predictors of relapse and
            reactions to relapse (figure), 184
Relational Systems Change Model, 144, 194
Relationships. *See also* Partners; *specific
    relationships*
        curricula for relationships in recovery,
            145–146
        disconnections, 143
        exploring the history and influence of
            relationships: sociogram, 148–149
        importance of in women's lives, 138, 143
        relational model approach to therapy,
            144, 194

skills related to improving the quality of,
            143–144
Religious and spiritual practices. *See also* Faith-
    based initiatives
        African Americans and, 111
        assessment and, 79–80
        Hispanic/Latina population and, 109
        Multidimensional Measure of
            Religiousness/Spirituality, 79–80
        as protective factors, 21
Religious Practice and Beliefs measurement, 79
    Spiritual Well-Being Scale, 80
Religious Practice and Beliefs measurement
        description and uses, 79
Reproductive issues. *See also* Pregnancy
        alcohol consumption, 40, 41–42
        substance use disorders, 7–8
Research. *See also specific studies and study
    authors*
        benefits of consumer input, 187–188
        issue overview, 2
Residential and inpatient treatment
        appropriate uses for, 99
        child care and, 86, 141, 287
        children accompanying their mothers in,
            86, 100–101, 141
        components, 99–100
        creating a healing environment, 188
        effectiveness of, 99
        length of stay, 99, 100
        settings for, 99
Residential Women and Children/Pregnant and
    Postpartum Women programs
        funding for, 273
        importance of, 281
        outcomes, 100
Resource Panel members, 319–322
The Revised Conflict Tactics Scale
        description and uses, 71
Risk factors
        childhood sexual and physical abuse,
            156–157
        co-occurring disorders, 23–24
        continuing care period and, 182
        discrimination, 24
        familial substance abuse, 18–19
        family of origin characteristics, xviii, 19
        genetic, 19
        hepatitis C virus, 53–54
        marital status, 19–20

depression, 67–68

General Health Questionnaire, 67

general screening instruments, 67

Level of Care Utilization System for
Psychiatric and Addiction Services, 68

Mental Health Screening Form-III, 67

Mini-International Neuropsychiatric
Interview, 67

posttraumatic stress disorder, 68–70

trauma, 68–70

Screening for substance abuse

AUDIT, 62

CAGE, 62–63, 74

CAGE-AID, 63

comfort level of the counselor or
healthcare professional, 61–62

general alcohol and drug screening, 62–63

goal of, 61

instrument selection, 61

TCUDS II, 62

Screening instruments for pregnant women

5Ps, 65

T-ACE, 64–65

TWEAK, 63–64

Sedative-hypnotics

older women and, 128

withdrawal from, 66, 97, 98

Seeking Safety (Najavits), 145, 147, 164, 171–172

Seizures

alcohol withdrawal and, 97

Selective serotonin reuptake inhibitors

depression treatment, 174

eating disorder treatment, 176

Self-harm

screening instruments, 68

Sellers, E.M.

hormonal changes and alcohol
consumption, 42

Service delivery issues

treatment retention and, 141

Services for children of women in substance
abuse treatment

clinical support services, 290–291

description, 279

whole-family perspective for, 281

Services Grant Program for Residential
Treatment for Pregnant and Postpartum
Women

*Lessons Learned: Residential Substance
Abuse Treatment for Women and Their
Children*, 108

Sexual abuse. *See also* Trauma

African Americans and, 110

history of as a risk factor for substance
use disorders, 156–157

impact of trauma and prenatal care, 102

lesbian and bisexual women and, 22, 156

Native Americans and, 120

by parents, 156

questions regarding (figure), 71

screening for, 70–71

sexuality and, 150

socioeconomic factors, 70

survivor self-medication for depression or
anxiety, 22

Sexual dysfunction

substance abuse treatment and, 150

Sexual orientation. *See also* Lesbian and
bisexual women

demographics, 123–124

physiological effects of substance abuse
and, 39

risk factor for substance use disorders,
20, 21–22

screening and assessment and, 60

substance abuse and healthy development
of, 147

as a treatment obstacle, 86

Sexuality

fear of sex while abstinent, 147, 150

sexual and interpersonal violence, 150

sexual concerns during early recovery,
147, 150

sexual dysfunction, 150

sexual identity, 147

sexually transmitted diseases, 150

treatment for substance abuse and
changes in, 147

Sexually transmitted diseases. *See also* HIV/
AIDS; *specific diseases*

clinical issues, 150

increased risk for among women who
abuse substances, 150

substance abuse and, 80–81

Short Acculturation Scale for Latinos

description, 59

Simmel, C.
    partner's influence on a woman's
        recovery, 145
Simoni, J.M.
    "Triangle of Risk" for HIV/AIDS, 122
Singer, L.T.
    prenatal cocaine exposure effects, 50
Smith, A.M.
    birth outcomes and marijuana use, 52
Social characteristics of women
    accessing treatment for substance abuse,
        12
    caregiver role, 11
    client-counselor expectations, 12
    family/partner support, 10
    help-seeking behavior, 11
    interpersonal stressful life events and, 12
    pregnancy, parenting, and child care,
        10–11
    social relationships and family history,
        9–13
    stigma as a barrier to treatment, 12–13, 85
Sociocultural context. *See also* Culture
    Bronfenbrenner's ecological model, 2–4
    CSAT's comprehensive model of care, 4
    identity and gender expectations, 13
    treatment obstacles, 85–86
    a woman's life in context (figure), 3
Socioeconomic status
    African Americans, 109
    Hispanic/Latina population, 104, 105
    interpersonal violence and, 70
    Native Americans, 119
    physiological effects of substance abuse
        and, 39
    risk factor for substance use disorders, 26
    Rural American women, 130, 131
    screening and assessment and, 60
    sexual abuse and, 70
Spiritual practices. *See* Faith-based initiatives;
    Religious and spiritual practices
Spiritual Well-Being Scale
    description and uses, 80, 301
SSRIs. *See* Selective serotonin reuptake
    inhibitors
Staffing issues
    clinical supervision, 190, 192–193
    male staff members, 188–189
    organizational change, 193–196

    training, 189–190
    women-centered staff, 188
StaT
    description and uses, 71
    intimate partner violence screening tool
        (figure), 72
States
    concentrations of Asian/Pacific
        Americans, 115
    concentrations of Hispanic/Latina women,
        104
    concentrations of Native Americans, 119
    guidance to states: treatment standards
        for women with substance use
        disorders, 196
    mandated reporting of child abuse or
        neglect, 88
    Medicaid programs, 294
    services needed in women's substance
        abuse treatment (figure), 93–95
    state standard examples of gender-specific
        treatment (figure), 195–196
STDs. *See* Sexually transmitted diseases
Stevens, S.J.
    socioeconomic status of urban Native
        American women, 120
Stigma
    as an obstacle to treatment, 12–13, 85
Strategies for treatment engagement
    case management, 91–92
    integration and centralization of services,
        87–88
    outreach services, 88
    pretreatment intervention groups, 91
Stroke
    alcohol use and, 41
Structural obstacles to treatment
    child care issues, 86
    cultural competence of programs, 86
    program structure, 87
    transportation issues, 87
    women with disabilities, 87
Structured Behavioral Outpatient Rural
    Therapy
    description, 133
Substance abuse
    definition, 16
*Substance Abuse: Administrative Issues in
    Outpatient Treatment* (TIP 46), 98

therapist characteristics and, 139, 140, 141–142

treatment environment and, 139–140

type of treatment services and, 140–141

Treloar, C.

partner relationship effect on substance use, 27

Tuberculosis

illicit drug use and, 52

TWEAK

compared with CAGE, 63

compared with Michigan Alcohol Screening Test, 63

compared with the T-ACE, 63–64

description and uses, 63

TWEAK Questionnaire: Women (figure), 64

12-Step programs

effectiveness of, 186

relapse prevention and, 186

treatment outcomes, 182

U

Ulcers

alcohol use and, 41

Underhill, B.

sexual orientation and substance use, 21

Unemployment. *See also* Employment

Native Americans and, 119

risk factor for substance use disorders, 26

Unified fiscal planning

description, 293–294

U.S. Department of Agriculture

light, moderate, and heavy drinking definitions, 41

U.S. Department of Health and Human Services

light, moderate, and heavy drinking definitions, 41

Office on Women's health, 177

U.S. Department of Justice

estimate of the percent of females in the criminal justice system who are dependent on or abusing drugs, 134

U.S. Preventive Services Task Force

questions to use in screening for depression, 67

V

Vannicelli, M.

cultural competence of treatment programs, 86

Violence. *See* Domestic violence; Interpersonal violence

Viral Hepatitis and Substance Use Disorders, 55

Volk, R.J.

screening by healthcare providers, 74

W

WCDVS. *See* Women, Co-Occurring Disorders and Violence Study

Web sites

Level of Care Utilization System for Psychiatric and Addiction Services, 68

Mini-International Neuropsychiatric Interview, 67

National Center for PTSD, 70

Office on Women's health, 177

SAMHSA's Women, Co-Occurring Disorders and Violence Study, 170

Texas Christian University Drug Screen II, 62

Weiderpass, E.

cancer and alcohol use, 42

Weir, B.W.

socioeconomic status effect on screening, 60

Widowed women

alcohol use and, 128

physical and mental health issues, 14

Williams Lake Band, Canada

alcohol- and drug-free community example, 123

Wilsnack, S.C.

sexual orientation and substance use, 21

Withdrawal. *See* Screening for acute safety risk related to serious intoxication or withdrawal; *specific drugs*

Woman's Addiction Workbook (Najavits), 145, 147

Women, Co-Occurring Disorders and Violence Study

description, 71, 152, 170

including consumers in all aspects of the study design, 187

Women Embracing Life and Living (WELL)
Project
    description, 165
    Self-Assessment for Providers, 313–317
    Toolkit, 313
Women for Sobriety
    description, 186
Women of color
    definition, 16
    sexual orientation and, 126
    treatment retention and, 138
Women-Specific Health Assessment
    description and uses, 81
Women with disabilities. *See also* Cognitive
    impairment; Learning Disabilities
    co-occurring mental disorders and, 134
    factors increasing the likelihood of
      substance abuse and dependence, 134
    interpersonal violence screening and, 72
    obstacles to treatment, 87
    substance use among, 133–134
    trauma history and, 134
Women's Addiction Workbook, 79
Women's Recovery Group
    manual-based relapse prevention (figure),
      185
    relapse prevention and, 183–184, 185

Women's treatment issues and needs. *See also*
    Pregnancy
    co-occurring disorders, 157–177
    influence of family, 143–145
    parenting, 151–154
    partner relationships, 145–147
    relational model approach, 144
    relationships and the need for connection,
      143
    sexuality, 147, 150
    tobacco use, 177–179
    trauma history, 154–157
World Health Organization
    alcohol as a risk factor of diseases, 40
Wraparound services
    definition, 293
WRG. *See* Women's Recovery Group

Y

Young, N.K.
    co-occurrence of a substance use disorder
      and involvement in the child welfare
      system, 87
Youth Risk Behavior Survey 2007
    prevalence of alcohol and other drug use
      among adolescent Hispanic/Latina
      females, 105

Z

Zlotnick, C.
    family therapy and treatment outcomes,
      138

SAMHSA TIPs and Publications Based on TIPs

What Is a TIP?

Treatment Improvement Protocols (TIPs) are the products of a systematic and innovative process that brings together clinicians, researchers, program managers, policymakers, and other Federal and non-Federal experts to reach consensus on state-of-the-art treatment practices. TIPs are developed under the Substance Abuse and Mental Health Services Administration's (SAMHSA's) Knowledge Application Program (KAP) to improve the treatment capabilities of the Nation's alcohol and drug abuse treatment service system.

What Is a Quick Guide?

A Quick Guide clearly and concisely presents the primary information from a TIP in a pocket-sized booklet. Each Quick Guide is divided into sections to help readers quickly locate relevant material. Some contain glossaries of terms or lists of resources. Page numbers from the original TIP are referenced so providers can refer back to the source document for more information.

What Are KAP Keys?

Also based on TIPs, KAP Keys are handy, durable tools. Keys may include assessment or screening in-struments, checklists, and summaries of treatment phases. Printed on coated paper, each KAP Keys set is fastened together with a key ring and can be kept within a treatment provider's reach and consulted fre-quently. The Keys allow you, the busy clinician or program administrator, to locate information easily and to use this information to enhance treatment services.

Ordering Information

Publications may be ordered or downloaded for free at http://store.samhsa.gov. To order over the phone, please call 1-877-SAMHSA-7 (1-877-726-4727) (English and Español).

TIP 1 State Methadone Treatment Guidelines—Replaced by TIP 43

TIP 2 Pregnant, Substance-Using Women—Replaced by TIP 51

TIP 3 Screening and Assessment of Alcohol- and Other Drug-Abusing Adolescents—Replaced by TIP 31

TIP 4 Guidelines for the Treatment of Alcohol- and Other Drug-Abusing Adolescents—Replaced by TIP 32

TIP 5 Improving Treatment for Drug-Exposed Infants

TIP 6 Screening for Infectious Diseases Among Substance Abusers—Archived

TIP 7 Screening and Assessment for Alcohol and Other Drug Abuse Among Adults in the Criminal Justice System—Replaced by TIP 44

TIP 8 Intensive Outpatient Treatment for Alcohol and Other Drug Abuse—Replaced by TIPs 46 and 47

TIP 9 Assessment and Treatment of Patients With Coexisting Mental Illness and Alcohol and Other Drug Abuse—Replaced by TIP 42

TIP 10 Assessment and Treatment of Cocaine- Abusing Methadone-Maintained Patients—Replaced by TIP 43

TIP 11 Simple Screening Instruments for Outreach for Alcohol and Other Drug Abuse and Infectious Diseases—Replaced by TIP 53

TIP 12 Combining Substance Abuse Treatment With Intermediate Sanctions for Adults in the Criminal Justice System—Replaced by TIP 44

TIP 13 Role and Current Status of Patient Placement Criteria in the Treatment of Substance Use Disorders

Quick Guide for Clinicians

Quick Guide for Administrators

KAP Keys for Clinicians

TIP 14 Developing State Outcomes Monitoring Systems for Alcohol and Other Drug Abuse Treatment

TIP 15 Treatment for HIV-Infected Alcohol and Other Drug Abusers—Replaced by TIP 37

TIP 16 Alcohol and Other Drug Screening of Hospitalized Trauma Patients

Quick Guide for Clinicians

KAP Keys for Clinicians

TIP 17 Planning for Alcohol and Other Drug Abuse Treatment for Adults in the Criminal Justice System—Replaced by TIP 44

TIP 18 The Tuberculosis Epidemic: Legal and Ethical Issues for Alcohol and Other Drug Abuse Treatment Providers—Archived

TIP 19 Detoxification From Alcohol and Other Drugs— Replaced by TIP 45

TIP 20 Matching Treatment to Patient Needs in Opioid Substitution Therapy—Replaced by TIP 43

TIP 21 Combining Alcohol and Other Drug Abuse Treatment With Diversion for Juveniles in the Justice System

Quick Guide for Clinicians and Administrators